V. M. Der Kaloustian A. K. Kurban

Genetic Diseases of the Skin

With a Foreword by F. Clarke Fraser

With 441 Figures

Springer-Verlag
Berlin Heidelberg New York 1979

Vazken M. Der Kaloustian, M. D., Associate Professor of Pediatrics, American University of Beirut and American University Hospital, Beirut, Lebanon

Amal K. Kurban, M. D., Professor and Head, Division of Dermatology, American University of Beirut and American University Hospital, Beirut, Lebanon

ISBN 3-540-09151-3 Springer-Verlag Berlin Heidelberg New York
ISBN 0-387-09151-3 Springer-Verlag New York Heidelberg Berlin

Library of Congress Cataloging in Publication Data. Der Kaloustian, Vazken, M., 1937. Genetic Diseases of the Skin. Bibliography: P. Includes index. 1. Skin — Diseases — Genetic aspects. I. Kurban, Amal, K., 1928, joint author. II. Title. [DNLM: 1. Skin diseases — Familial and genetic] RL72.D46   616.5'042   78-25740

Reproduction of the figures: Brend'amour Simhart & Co., Munich

Typesetting, printing, and bookbinding by Universitätsdruckerei Brühl, Lahn-Gießen.

2121/3130-543210

*To Lebanon, our country, land of
bountiful giving, torn and devastated
during the writing of this book*

Foreword

The two organs of the body most accessible to examination are the eye and the skin and its appendages. That is why, it is said, ophthalmological genetics is in such flourishing good health. Dermatological genetics does not seem to have benefited so much from the skin being on the outside, and there are but few dermatological counterparts to the volumes of Sorsby, Waardenburg, Franceschetti and François, among others. But thanks to the growing interest in medical genetics, and the modern sophisticated techniques of molecular, biochemical, and ultrastructural examination, dermatology is beginning to catch up, as the appearance of this volume testifies.

Because of the growing body of knowledge and the heightened awareness of genetics by both patients and physicians, dermatologists not only will be asked more often about the inheritance of skin conditions they diagnose but increasingly will have the opportunity to diagnose a variety of inborn errors and syndromes by their dermatologic manifestations. On the other hand, syndromologists, clinical geneticists, and physicians are continually seeing patients with diagnostic clues in the skin that they must be able to appreciate. For both groups this book will be a new and valuable source of help.

Spring 1979
        F. CLARKE FRASER, Ph.D., M.D.
        Molson Professor of Human Genetics
        Departments of Biology and Paediatrics
        McGill University
        Montreal, Quebec, Canada

Preface

The past two decades have witnessed dramatic and fundamental progress in the biologic sciences in general and human genetics in particular. The rapidly developing field of molecular biology has shed light on our understanding of such basic concepts as the nature of the gene, the structure of the DNA molecule, and the mechanisms of protein synthesis. Methods have been devised for the study and mapping of human chromosomes. The knowledge of enzymatic deficiencies and lysosomal pathology has elucidated the pathogenesis of many inherited diseases and helped our understanding of normal biologic mechanisms. The new methods of fibroblast culture have enabled human geneticists to avoid the drawback of the long generation time of the species. The techniques of heterozygote detection and amniocentesis have opened new horizons in medical genetics and particularly genetic counseling. Finally, certain therapeutic measures for genetic diseases have been attempted and have already given rewarding results.

Within this general context, the genetic aspects of dermatologic diseases have also received significant attention. The two fields of genetics and dermatology have been complementary in their accomplishments in basic biologic research. Certain dermatologic diseases have helped in elucidating genetic facts and mechanisms (e.g., Anderson-Fabry disease and X-linkage of α-galactosidase with "lyonization" of its locus). Similarly, genetics has helped us in our understanding of the pathogenesis and pathophysiology of certain dermatologic diseases (e.g., defective DNA repair replication in xeroderma pigmentosum). The easy accessibility of the skin makes it, among the human tissues, the system par excellence for observation, study, and experimentation. Even minor skin lesions may be important in detecting various biologic processes and in initiating the understanding of basic mechanisms.

Cockayne's *Inherited Abnormalities of the Skin*, published in 1933 [1], was the first attempt to bring together in one volume information on inherited disorders of the skin scattered throughout the world literature. Since then, three other books have become milestones in this endeavor: *L'Hérédité en Médecine* by A. Touraine, published in 1955 [2], *Clinical Genodermatology* by Butterworth and Strean, published in 1962 [3], and *Vererbung von Hautkrankheiten* by Gottron and Schnyder (Handbuch der Haut- und Geschlechtskrankheiten. J. Jadassohn, Vol. 7), published in 1966 [4]. Finally, Volume VII, Part XII of *The Clinical Delineation of Birth Defects*, published in 1971 [5], deals with diseases of the skin, hair, and nails and has been a welcome addition, with its up-to-date information and excellent photographs.

Our present effort is a continuation of the work of these predecessors. We have attempted to present, in a concise, extensively illustrated manner, current information on disorders that are of definite or probable hereditary or genetic origin affecting the skin and its appendages. This book is not intended to be an exhaustive review of each entity or to include all the controversial theories and postulates in which today's literature abounds. We try to give factual information on diseases and traits with cutaneous manifestations, underlining their systemic associations and pathophysiologic mechanisms.

The book is aimed at serving not only dermatologists and medical geneticists, but also pediatricians, internists, and all those interested in birth defects and developmental anomalies. Our general plan for each disease includes information on clinical presentation, pathology and pathophysiology, inheritance, and treatment. However, for various reasons this format was not always suitable. In the case of certain well-known diseases such as psoriasis, stress was put on the hereditary aspects rather than on a detailed description of the clinical manifestations. Likewise, groups of diseases (e.g., the immune deficiency disorders) have been presented in table form for easy comparison and assimilation of information. In addition, we were forced, because of space limitation, to omit material that might otherwise have been included. For this and other omissions, we beg the reader's indulgence. However, we have covered, in relative detail, recent advances in some very rare diseases such as xeroderma pigmentosum and progeria that provide basic information relating to fundamental biologic and medical problems like aging and cancer.

The classification of the diseases presented some difficulties. Since the basic pathogenetic mechanism and pathophysiology are not known in the majority of the disorders, we had to classify them according to the presenting signs. As a syndrome may have several presenting signs, it may be discussed under different headings. We have tried to avoid this by presenting the disorder according to its most striking sign and using cross-references. Where the pathogenetic mechanisms are known (e.g. metabolic disorders, immune deficiency diseases, chromosomopathies), the disorders are classified accordingly. The investigators' names have been mentioned in the text when they were the first to report a certain disease; the others are referred to by reference number only. Whenever eponyms are used, the possessive form is avoided (e.g., Down syndrome, Gaucher disease).

To facilitate the use of the book we have included the following features: a detailed table of contents preceding each chapter, an appendix listing for the various disorders their differential diagnoses based on dermatologic signs, a short list of references following each entry, a glossary, and a subject index. An introduction to human genetics is presented for a basic understanding of concepts and terminology. Unfortunately, we could not discuss principles of population genetics because of lack of space. For these, and other information on genetics, the reader is referred to *Principles of Human Genetics* by Stern [6], *Genetics in Medicine* by Thompson and Thompson [7], and *Medical Genetics: Principles and Practice* by Nora and Fraser [8].

We are indebted to McKusick's fourth edition of *Mendelian Inheritance in Man*, published in 1975 [9], as a guide to the various disorders considered to be inherited. We have added a few conditions that have appeared subsequently in the 1978 edition [10]. Other main references that we have used are *Lysosomes and Storage Diseases* edited by Hers and Van Hoof [11], *Mental Retardation* by Holmes and colleagues [12], *Recognizable Patterns of Human Malformation* by Smith [13], *The Metabolic Basis of Inherited Disease*, edited by Stanbury, Wyngaarden, and Fredrickson [14], and *Human Cytogenetics* by Hamerton [15], as well as various medical journals and yearbooks.

Although we have tried hard to make this book as useful and as accurate as possible, we are certain that errors and deficiencies have escaped our attention. We would greatly appreciate suggestions or criticism from our readers aimed at the improvement of our presentation.

Beirut, Lebanon V. M. DER KALOUSTIAN
Spring 1979 A. K. KURBAN

References

1. Cockayne, E.A.: Inherited abnormalities of the skin and its appendages. London: Oxford University Press 1933
2. Touraine, A.: L'hérédité en médecine. Paris: Masson 1955
3. Butterworth, T., Strean, L.P.: Clinical genodermatology. Baltimore: Williams & Wilkins Co. 1962
4. Gottron, H.A., Schnyder, U.W.: Vererbung von Hautkrankheiten. In: Handbuch der Haut- und Geschlechtskrankheiten. J. Jadassohn. Erg.-Werk, Bd. 7. Berlin, Heidelberg, New York: Springer 1966
5. Bergsma, D. (ed.): The clinical delineation of birth defects. Part XII: Skin, hair and nails. Vol. VII, No. 8. Baltimore: Williams & Wilkins Co. 1971
6. Stern, C.: Principles of human genetics, 3rd ed. San Francisco: Freeman 1973
7. Thompson, J.S., Thompson, M.W.: Genetics in medicine, 2nd ed. Philadelphia: Saunders, W.B. Co. 1973
8. Nora, J.J., Fraser, F.C.: Medical genetics: principles and practice. Philadelphia: Lea & Febiger 1974
9. McKusick, V.A.: Mendelian inheritance in man, 4th ed. Baltimore: Johns Hopkins University Press 1975
10. McKusick, V.A.: Mendelian inhertiance in man. 5th ed. Baltimore: Johns Hopkins University Press 1978
11. Hers, H.G., Van Hoof, F. (eds.): Lysosomes and storage diseases. New York: Academic Press 1973
12. Holmes, L.B., Moser, H.W., Halldórsson, S., Mack, C., Pant, S.S., Matzilevich, B.: Mental retardation. New York: Macmillan Co. 1972
13. Smith, D.W.: Recognizable patterns of human malformation, 2nd ed. Philadelphia: Saunders, W.B. Co. 1976
14. Stanbury, J.B., Wyngaarden, J.B., Fredrickson, D.S. (eds.): The metabolic basis of inherited disease, 4th ed. New York: McGraw-Hill Book Co. 1978
15. Hamerton, J.L.: Human cytogenetics. Vols. I and II. New York: Academic Press 1971

Special Acknowledgments

We are indebted to many whose help made this book possible. In particular, we wish to express our thanks to Mrs. Phyllis Bergman and Mrs. Helena Kurban for competent and patient editorial assistance; Drs. Ronald Bergman and Adel Afifi for encouragement and advice; Drs. John Malak, Khalil A. Feisal, Samir Deeb, and Shukrallah Zaynoun for reading parts of the manuscript; Dr. Marilyn Preus for her help in the chapters on chromosomal anomalies and dermatoglyphics; Dr. E. Reece for her advice on the chapter on immunologic disorders; Miss Mona Barakat for assistance in accumulating the clinical material; Mrs. Margaret Abbott for sorting out valuable photographs; Mrs. C. Suer and Miss Ani Kehkejian for typing the whole manuscript under difficult circumstances and sometimes even under heavy shelling during the Lebanese civil war; Mrs. M. Forster for additional secretarial assistance; and Mr. Antranig Chelebian for the diagrams. We wish to thank also the staff members of the Saab Memorial Medical Library (American University of Beirut) for their help.

The kind support of Drs. Victor A. McKusick and F. Clarke Fraser is greatly appreciated.

We are grateful to the many colleagues from all over the world who contributed pictures of their patients.

Part of this work was supported by a grant from the Lebanese National Council for Scientific Research.

Finally, we wish to acknowledge the patient cooperation of the staff of Springer-Verlag.

Contents

Chapter 1   Introduction to Human Genetics

Contents

Molecular Genetics

Molecular genetics has made giant strides during the past three decades. DNA (deoxyribonucleic acid) was synthesized in vitro, its intimate structure was elucidated, the genetic control of enzyme and virus synthesis was discovered, and the genetic code was deciphered.

Structure of DNA

Genetic information is coded in DNA. DNA is a macromolecule with three types of components: a sugar (deoxyribose), a phosphate, and a base. There are four types of bases in DNA. Two are purines [adenine (A) and guanine (G)] and two are pyrimidines [thymine (T) and cytosine (C)]. The structure of the DNA molecule represents a "double helix" (Fig. 1.1). The backbones of the helices are formed by the alternating ribose and phosphate molecules from which the bases project. The bases of the helices pair by hydrogen bonds: A pairs with T, and G with C. DNA serves two main functions: self-replication and coding for proteins.

DNA Repair

With the help of the enzyme DNA *polymerase*, self-replication occurs with great accuracy. Although the DNA molecule is subject to injurious environmental factors such as radiation, it has very effective processes of repair. Ultraviolet (UV) irradiation produces bonds between neighboring thymines on the same DNA strand and creates dimers. The formation of the dimers is considered an "injury" and an abnormal situation. The repair of the damage involves four steps [1], each requiring the action of a specific enzyme (Fig. 1.2): an endonuclease, an exonuclease, a polymerase, and a ligase. Certain dermatologic diseases have a deficiency in one of the enzymes involved in DNA repair. For example, in xeroderma pigmentosum the cells are unable to perform adequately the first step in repair

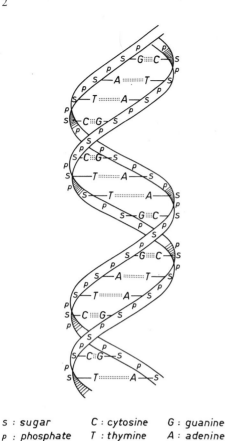

s : sugar   C : cytosine   G : guanine
p : phosphate T : thymine   A : adenine

Fig. 1.1. The double helix. (For description, see text)

1. Under the effect of ultraviolet light a thymine dimer is formed.

2. An endonuclease breaks the helix near the dimer.

3. The region of the thymine dimer is excised by an exonuclease.

4. Synthesis of a new strand occurs with the help of DNA polymerase.

5. The two ends of the strand are joined by the polynucleotide ligase.

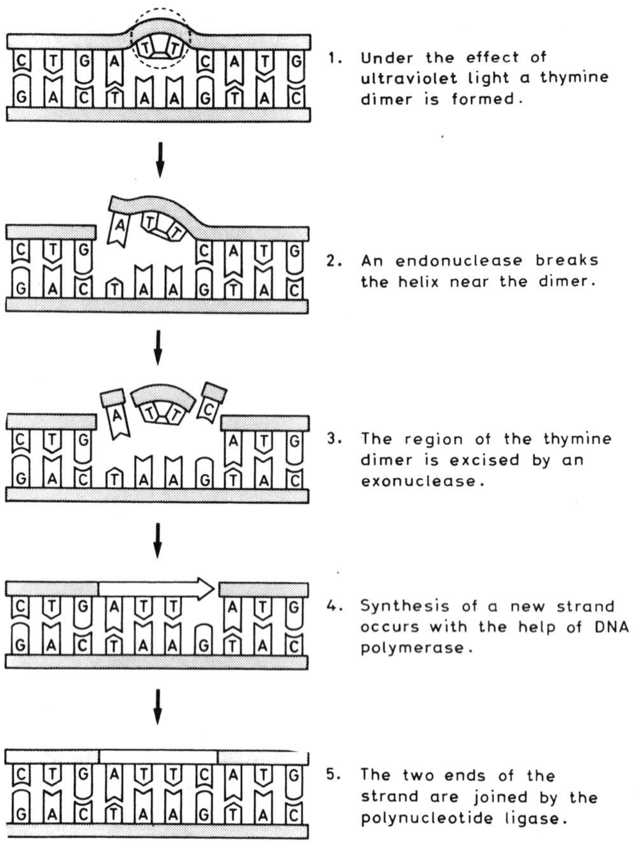

Fig. 1.2. DNA repair. For description, see text. (Adapted from Watson, J.D.: Molecular biology of the gene, 2nd ed., p. 294. New York: Benjamin, W.A. Inc. 1970, with permission)

of damage to DNA (see also p. 151). In certain other dermatologic diseases deficiency in repair mechanisms is also implicated. These deficiencies may elucidate degenerative processes or shed light on the pathophysiology of malignant transformation.

RNA and Protein Synthesis

Expression of genetic information into proteins involves the transcription (nucleic acid→nucleic acid) of the genetic message from DNA to RNA and the translation (nucleic acid→protein) from RNA to protein (Fig. 1.3).
On a single DNA helix each sequence of three bases (triplet) codes for a specific amino acid, although the amino acid in question may be coded by different triplets. The sequence of triplets on the DNA helix determines the sequence of amino acids in a polypeptide chain. A *gene* represents a segment of DNA molecule coding for a single polypeptide.

RNA is a nucleic acid similar in its structure to DNA but different in two respects: (a) the sugar is ribose instead of deoxyribose and (b) the fourth base is uracil instead of thymine. There are three main types of RNA: messenger (mRNA), transfer (tRNA), and ribosomal (rRNA). mRNA is a nucleic acid molecule transcribed by the enzyme RNA polymerase using one of the DNA strands as a template. mRNA carries the genetic message from the nucleus to the cytoplasm where protein synthesis occurs.
In the cytoplasm, mRNA binds to the ribosomes which are structures composed of ribosomal RNA (rRNA) and proteins. Subsequently, amino acids are transferred to the site of protein synthesis by means of a special type of RNA, called transfer RNA (tRNA). Each amino acid is transferred by its own specific tRNA (covalently linked by a specific enzyme). The various tRNA-amino acid molecules are bound to triplet *codons* on mRNA. The binding is guided by virtue of the complementary base sequence between the mRNA codons and anticodons

Fig. 1.3. An interpretation of protein biosynthesis. For description, see text. (Adapted from Thompson and Thompson: Genetics in medicine, 2nd ed., p. 43. Philadelphia: Saunders, W.B. Co. 1973, with permission)

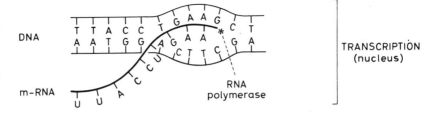

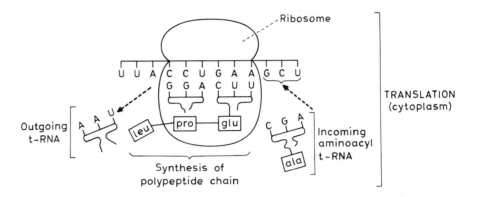

on tRNA molecules (Fig. 1.3). At any one time only two aminoacyl-tRNAs bind to the ribosome-mRNA complex. Peptide bond formation occurs between two amino acids linked to the two adjacent tRNAs on the ribosome. Thus, the sequences of bases in DNA dictate the sequences of amino acids in polypeptides. These, in turn, determine the phenotype of the individual and the characteristics of the species.

Mutation

The term mutation is generally used for changes either in the chromosomal structure detectable cytologically or in the DNA at the level of a base pair. The latter type of change is called a *point* mutation and is responsible for specific alterations in protein molecules [2].

Mutations may be due to chemical mutagens, physical agents (e.g., X-rays, UV light), or viruses. They may also be associated with advanced paternal age as, for example, in achondroplasia, Apert syndrome, and fibrodysplasia ossificans. Point mutations change a base in the triplet, thus coding for a different amino acid. This changes the structure of the polypeptide chain, producing a variant protein. Protein variants (structural proteins or enzymes) that arise from mutations may still function normally or produce an abnormality in the physiology of the organism. Point mutations may also involve the insertion or loss of a single base in the DNA.

This results in a "frame-shift" and the synthesis of a new amino acid sequence beyond the mutation, producing a nonfunctional protein.

Biochemical Genetics

Protein Variants

The significance of protein variants was recognized and appreciated by Sir Archibald Garrod at the turn of the century [3]. They characterize the individuality of each being and also introduce into populations the polymorphisms which may be important in the processes of adaptation and evolution of the species [4]. On the other hand, particular variants, or combinations of variants, may be pathologic or represent different degrees of susceptibility or resistance to certain diseases. For example, hemoglobin S (HbS) differs from hemoglobin A (HbA) in a mutation in the chain of the globin molecule. This mutation results in the change of one amino acid (glutamic acid to valine). The change is due to a single base substitution (thymine to adenine) in DNA. Even though the mutation leading to HbS is pathogenic, there are more than 400 different types of hemoglobin, most of them due to point mutations, which do not necessarily lead to pathology [5].

The heterogeneity of proteins is expressed qualitatively and quantitatively. The variants are identified by electrophoresis, immunologic and enzymatic methods, heat stability, and response to inhibitors.

Inherited Metabolic Disorders

Certain mutations may produce changes in *structural* proteins and result in disorders such as Marfan syndrome or Clouston type of ectodermal dysplasia (see p. 113). Others produce disturbances in circulating *transport* proteins such as hemoglobin, lipoproteins, and other plasma proteins. A number of diseases are due to defects in membrane transport, involving carrier substances that behave in a way similar to enzymes. Finally, mutations produce changes in *enzymes* resulting in important metabolic derangements. From his observations on alkaptonuria, albinism, cystinuria, and pentosuria, Sir Archibald Garrod had already developed in 1908 the concept that certain diseases are due to a defect in the activity of specific enzymes [6, 7]. By 1978, 160 inherited enzymatic deficiencies had been discovered [8]. These may be harmless (e.g., pentosuria with a deficiency of xylitol dehydrogenase) or result in clinical disorders. The clinical manifestations of the enzymatic deficiency may be due to accumulation of a precursor prior to the enzymatic block (phenylketonuria, lysosomal storage diseases) or deficiency of the reaction product (albinism).

Lysosomal Diseases

An important group of enzymatic deficiencies comprises the lysosomal diseases. Many of these have been clinically known since the turn of the century (Gaucher, Tay-Sachs, Fabry, Niemann-Pick, Hunter, and Hurler diseases). However, their pathophysiology has been elucidated only recently.

The biochemical concept of lysosomes as membrane-bound particles containing acid hydrolases emerged around 1955 [9, 10]. About 10 years later, the lysosomal localization of the enzyme deficiency in Pompe disease established the concept of "inborn lysosomal disease" [11, 12]. This concept focused attention on two easily detectable characteristics, one morphologic and the other biochemical: (a) abnormal deposits within the lysosomes and (b) severe deficiency in a single enzyme which normally digests the stored substance [13]. The lysosomal diseases that interest the dermatologist are mainly fucosidosis, Fabry disease, Gaucher disease, Niemann-Pick disease, aspartylglycosaminuria, Farber disease, and the mucopolysaccharidoses.

Inheritance in Man

In man, inheritance of traits may be monogenic, multigenic, or may be the result of the transmission of an abnormal chromosome (e.g., a deletion or a translocation).

Single Gene Inheritance

Single gene inheritance can be autosomal dominant, autosomal recessive, X-linked dominant, or X-linked recessive. The pattern of inheritance of a certain trait may be apparent from pedigree studies. These are very important, since they represent one of the first steps in the thorough study of inherited diseases. They should be included in all case histories in which a familial disease is suspected. They are a must in all pediatric records. The symbols commonly used are standard and generally accepted (Fig. 1.4).

The distinction between "dominant" and "recessive" genes is not absolute. By definition, a "recessive" gene has no detectable expression in a heterozygote under the conditions of study and analysis. Diseases involving enzymes with decreased activity behave as recessives because in the heterozygous situation the amount of normal enzyme produced by the allele allows a normal metabolic function. In heterozygotes in which the abnormal gene codes for a structural protein, the mutant allele acts as a dominant, since all cells that have the mutant produce the structurally abnormal protein. As a result of changes in the physical properties of the protein, heterozygotes may show phenotypic abnormalities even though only about half of the protein is of the mutant type. Thus, amino acid substitutions are expected in the collagen or elastic fiber proteins of the dominantly inherited forms of the Ehlers-Danlos syndrome and in the keratin in the case of a dominant abnormality of the hair such as monilethrix. In the Clouston variety of ectodermal dysplasia the gene involved is the structural gene for a matrix polypeptide [14]. Similarly, since the trait of the Marfan syndrome behaves as a dominant, most probably the pathogenesis of the syndrome is not due to an enzymatic deficiency. On the other hand, in over 160 of the 521 certain recessives an enzyme deficiency has been demonstrated [8].

Single gene defects are transmitted according to Mendel's laws [15]. The following are the characteristics of *autosomal dominant* inheritance (Fig. 1.5):

Fig. 1.4. Symbols commonly used in recording pedigrees

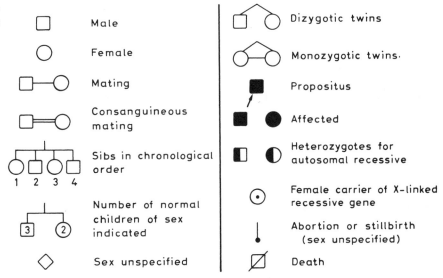

PROTOTYPE OF PEDIGREE

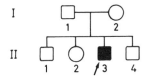

Generations are numbered with roman numerals and range from the earliest at the top of the pedigree to the most recent at the bottom

1. The trait appears in every generation. There is no "skipping" except when the "penetrance" is reduced (see below).

2. An affected person heterozygous for the trait transmits it to half of his or her children.

3. At least one of the parents of an affected person is also affected except when the penetrance is reduced (see below).

4. Males and females can have and transmit the trait equally.

By 1978, 736 "proved" dominant traits had been identified [8]; 182 of these have dermatologic manifestations. Acanthosis nigricans, keratosis follicularis, and erythrokeratodermia variabilis are examples of dominant inheritance.

Two traits are said to be *codominant* when their genes are allelic and are both expressed in a heterozygote. For example, in blood group AB both the gene for A and that for B are expressed.

The following are the characteristics of *autosomal recessive* inheritance (Fig. 1.6):

1. When the parents are heterozygous and phenotypically normal the trait appears only in the children homozygous for the mutant gene.

2. On the average one-fourth of the children of heterozygous parents are affected.

3. Males and females have an equal risk of being affected.

By 1978, 521 "proved" recessive traits had been identified [8]; 160 of these have dermatologic manifestations. Acrodermatitis enteropathica, epidermolysis bullosa dystrophica, Hartnup disease, and Letterer-Siwe disease are examples of recessive inheritance.

In the case of consanguineous marriages, the risk of a carrier of a rare recessive trait marrying another carrier is much higher. Thus, children of consanguineous marriages run an increased risk of suffering from autosomal recessively inherited diseases. This risk may be increased by 100-fold, but in absolute terms it is still small, being of the order of 1 % [16]. This is the biologic basis of the prohibition of cousin marriage in many societies.

X-linked recessive inheritance (Fig. 1.7) has the following characteristics:

1. The trait is much more common in males than females. All males carrying the X-linked gene express the trait. Females are affected when they are

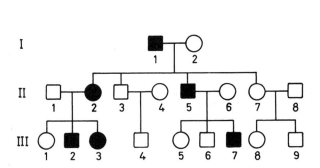

Fig. 1.5. Stereotype pedigree of autosomal dominant inheritance

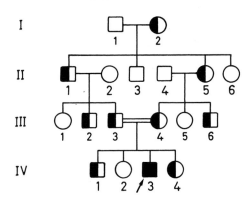

Fig. 1.6. Stereotype pedigree of autosomal recessive inheritance

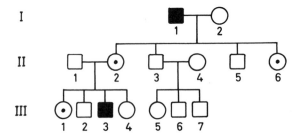

Fig. 1.7. Stereotype pedigree of X-linked recessive inheritance

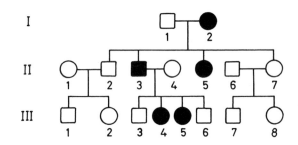

Fig. 1.8. Stereotype pedigree of X-linked dominant inheritance

homozygous and in certain heterozygous cases (see The Lyon Hypothesis, p. 9).

2. An affected man passes his X-linked gene to half of his daughters who become carriers. He does not transmit it to any of his sons.

3. A carrier woman passes her X-linked gene to half of her sons who manifest the trait and to half of her daughters who become carriers.

Fabry disease (diffuse angiokeratoma) and dyskeratosis congenita are examples of X-linked recessive traits.

X-linked dominant inheritance (Fig. 1.8) has the following characteristics:

1. Affected men transmit the trait to all their daughters and to none of their sons.

2. Heterozygous women are affected. They transmit the trait to half of their sons and half of their daughters.

Keratosis follicularis spinulosa cum ophiasi is an example of X-linked dominant inheritance. Certain diseases can also be inherited as X-linked dominant with lethality in the hemizygous male. Dermatologic diseases with the latter form of inheritance are focal dermal hypoplasia (FDH) and, probably, type I orofaciodigital (OFD) syndrome. By 1978, 107 "proved" X-linked traits had been identified [8], 29 of which have dermatologic manifestations.

Y-linked genes occur only in males. They are transmitted to all the sons and none of the daughters. The only genes definitely known to be on the Y chromosomes are those coding for testis-determining factors. They are located on the short arm of the chromosome [8]. It has been suggested that one or more genes concerned with stature are on the Y chromosome [8]. Although Y-linkage may not be completely excluded, "hairy ears" seem more likely to be inherited as autosomal dominant with a strong male influence [8].

Typical pedigree patterns can be altered by certain mechanisms such as reduced penetrance, variable expressivity, pleiotropism, genetic heterogeneity, variability of the age of onset, sex limitation, interaction of two or more gene pairs, and environmental factors.

Certain traits may be modified by other genes and by environmental influences to such an extent that they may not be recognizable even though the gene causing the trait is present. In these cases this gene or trait is said to be *nonpenetrant*. Thus, certain autosomal dominant traits with reduced penetrance may "skip" a generation (see above).

Expressivity is the variation of degree of expression that a trait may have. In clinical medicine, a certain gene with variable expressivity may produce mild, moderate, or severe disease. A *forme fruste* is an extremely mild and clinically insignificant expression of an abnormality. Variable expressivity and formes frustes are noted especially in autosomal dominant inheritance.

Pleiotropism is the production of multiple phenotypic effects by a mutant gene or gene pair. For example, the primary defect in phenylketonuria is the specific enzyme deficiency. Secondary effects are severe mental retardation, excretion of phenylketones in the urine, and dilution of pigmentation. Pleiotropism is especially important to dermatology because many systemic genetic disorders have cutaneous features [17]. Thus, keeping in mind the possibility of pleiotropism, one should avoid the mistake of considering two aspects of the same genetic disease as two different closely linked diseases that segregate together.

Genetic heterogeneity of a disease may also give confusing pedigrees. Thus, inherited congenital deafness may be the result of two autosomal recessive traits at two different gene loci. Two deaf individuals, each homozygous for a recessive trait at a different locus, will have normal children, because their offspring will be heterozygous for each of the loci (see below, p. 12).

Other situations that may give confusing pedigrees are *sex-limited traits* (e.g., male-limited autosomal dominant precocious puberty, X-linked testicular feminization syndrome) and *sex-influenced traits* (e.g., autosomal dominant hemochromatosis, which is more common in males).

Genetic diseases that are not congenital and have a relatively late age of onset may also be confusing in pedigrees (e.g., intermittent porphyria, in which the onset is not until early adulthood).

Isoalleles are multiple wild-type alleles that appear to have identical phenotypic effects, except when observed in heterozygous combinations with a mutant allele. Such a mutant allele is responsible for the nail-patella syndrome (see p. 197). In this autosomal dominant disorder, the grade of severity shows a much higher correlation between affected sibs than between offspring and affected parent [18].

Polygenic Inheritance

Polygenic inheritance (also called *quantitative*) is difficult to analyze genetically. Representative examples in man are the total fingerprint ridge count (TRC), stature, and skin color [19]. In this type of inheritance the variability with respect to a given

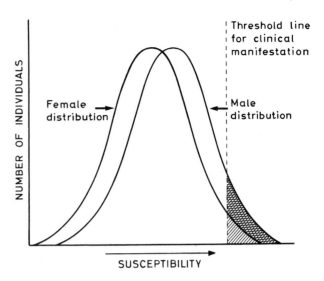

Fig. 1.9. Quasi-continuous variation in polygenic inheritance. For description, see text

trait follows a normal distribution curve. However, even though the distribution is continuous, a threshold effect for certain phenotypic manifestations may make it appear discontinuous [20]. Thus, diseases with a polygenic inheritance represent the area beyond a specific threshold in the normal continuous phenotypic curve resulting from the effect of multiple genes (Fig. 1.9).

Inheritance through Anomalous Chromosomes

A phenotype that is due to an abnormality of chromosome structure (deletion, translocation, or inversion) or number follows a pattern of inheritance similar to that of autosomal dominant genes. However, some minute familial chromosomal rearrangements are beyond our present means of detection [21].

Twins in Medical Genetics

Twins have a special place in medical genetics because they help to determine whether a disease is the result of genetic or environmental factors. Thus, diseases caused wholly or partly by genetic factors have a higher concordance rate in monozygotic (identical) than in dizygotic (fraternal) twins [22].

The Human Chromosomes

Classification and Techniques

Studies on the human chromosome complement began with Flemming's work in 1882 [23]. However, it was not until 1956 that the correct normal human chromosomal number of 46 was established by Tjio and Levan [24]. Later, the rapid increase in our knowledge of human chromosomes necessitated the establishment of a standard international system of nomenclature ("The Denver Classification") [25].

Of the 46 chromosomes in human cells, 44 are autosomes and 2 are sex chromosomes. The autosomes constitute 22 homologous pairs. The sex chromosomes are two Xs in normal females and an X and a Y in normal males (Fig. 1.10). Each pair of autosomes is serially numbered from 1 to 22 in descending order of length and grouped according to the position of the centromere. The chromosomes are described as metacentric, submetacentric, or acrocentric, depending on whether the centromere is at the center of the chromosome, near the center, or near the end, respectively. The acrocentric chromosomes (except the Y) possess small terminal projections known as satellite bodies. The autosomes are divided into seven recognizable groups, identified by the letters A through G, each group consisting of chromosomes of similar morphology and distinct from the other groups.

In 1966 [26], a set of symbols designating certain normal or unusual chromosome features was proposed and generally accepted (see Table 1.1). From 1970 on, to facilitate a more accurate examination of human chromosomes, several "banding" techniques were developed: Q banding, quinacrine fluorescence [27]; C banding, centromeric banding [28]; R banding, reverse banding [29]; and G banding, Giemsa banding [30]. Q and G banding patterns are essentially the same. R banding patterns are the reverse of those of G banding. C banding demonstrates mainly the centromeric area.

These techniques allow identification of each human chromosome individually, since each chromosome has a particular and specific banding pattern. The Giemsa or G banding technique is the one generally adopted because it is inexpensive, provides accurate information to distinguish individual chromosomes and particular areas of each chromosome, and facilitates the identification of specific chromosomal aberrations. All four banding methods (Q, C, R, and G) are helpful under different circumstances and complementary in the information they provide (Fig. 1.10).

Table 1.1. Symbols used for the designation of karyotypes

p	Short arm of chromosome
q	Long arm of chromosome
r	Ring chromosome
t	Translocation
i	Isochromosome
/	Diagonal line indicating mosaicism
+	Extra chromosome or part of chromosome
−	Missing chromosome or part of chromosome
45, X	X0 Turner karyotype
47, XX, 21+	Karyotype of female with trisomy Down syndrome
45, X/46, XX/47, XXX	Triple cell line mosaic
46, XY, 5p−	Karyotype of male with Cri du Chat syndrome
46, XY, t(4p−; 15q+)	Karyotype of male with balanced translocation between short arm of chromosome 4 and long arm of chromosome 15
46, XX qi	Karyotype of female with isochromosome of the long arm of an X chromosome

By 1971, when a standardization conference was held in Paris, the development of the banding techniques made it necessary to enlarge the standard system of nomenclature. The detailed system of nomenclature recommended by the Paris conference is still not frequently used in the general medical literature, and thus is not described here.

Human chromosome analysis can be performed by direct techniques or culture techniques. Direct techniques involve the bone marrow, gonadal tissue (for meiotic studies), or other material such as peritoneal and pleural effusions, cerebrospinal fluid (CSF), and cells from various solid tumors. Culture techniques involve mainly the bone marrow, peripheral blood, and skin, and less so the testis, ovary, and most fetal tissues [31].

The peripheral blood is easily accessible and thus represents the most convenient tool for human chromosomal analysis. Lymphocytes grow and divide rapidly in culture but such cultures are short-lived. Since the technique is relatively easy and reliable, it is used for routine karyotyping [32]. Skin cultures, which are also easily accessible, provide long-term multiplication of fibroblasts for many generations. Fibroblast cultures are used for chromosome analysis and for different biochemical and histochemical studies [33, 34]. Freezing of fibroblasts in liquid nitrogen in repositories allows their culture and analysis at a later date [32].

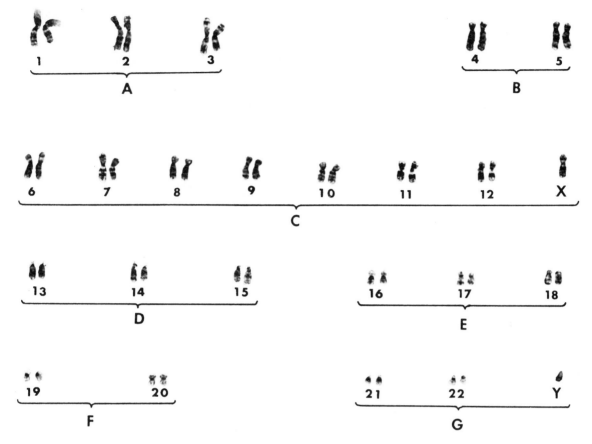

Fig. 1.10. Metaphase chromosomes from a normal male – Giemsa banding. (Courtesy of Dr. D. Kalousek)

The Sex Chromatin Body

During interphase the chromosomes are elongated and cannot be distinguished individually. The nuclear material appears granular. In 1949, Barr and Bertram [35] noted that a previously detected mass of chromatin in the nuclei of some nerve cells was frequently present in cells from females but not males. This body, known as the "sex chromatin" or "Barr body" (Fig. 1.11), can be identified in nerve cells, epithelial cells, and fibroblasts, although buccal smears are routinely used [32].

Sex chromatin is present if there are two or more X chromosomes in the cell. The detection of a Barr body depends on the stage of the cell in the cell cycle and the orientation of the nucleus on the slide. Thus, even normal females reveal Barr bodies in only 50% of their epithelial cells at one time.

The sex chromatin is formed, in a normal female, by the condensation of one X chromosome during interphase. This explanation is supported by cytologic, autoradiographic [36], and clinical observations [37]. The number of sex chromatin bodies is one less than the number of X chromosomes. This finding is very important in detecting abnormalities of X chromosome number by the easy method of buccal smear examination.

With quinacrine fluorescence techniques, the distal part of the long arm of the Y chromosome fluoresces intensively at metaphase. The Y chromosome can also be identified as a fluorescent body at the periphery of the nucleus in cells at interphase (Fig. 1.12). This technique allows the recognition of one or more Y chromosomes and is useful as a diagnostic or investigative technique [38–40]. Identification of the Barr body and a fluorescent Y at interphase is used for sex determination and can be performed on the same specimen.

The Lyon Hypothesis

Males with one X form as much of the product of X-linked structural genes as females with two X chromosomes. For many years, the mechanism of this "dosage compensation" was unknown. The Lyon hypothesis, formulated in 1961 [41, 42], explains dosage compensation in terms of a single

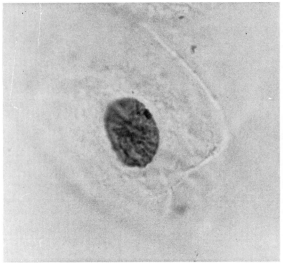

Fig. 1.11. The sex chromatin or Barr body. Note faint contour of cell and dark chromatin body at the nuclear membrane. (Courtesy of Dr. D. Kalousek)

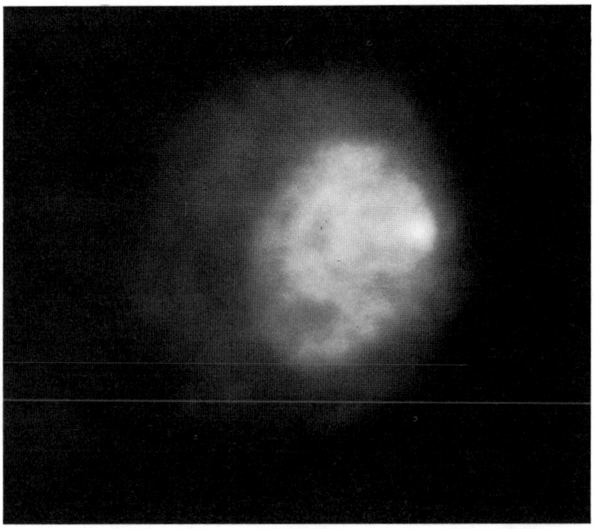

Fig. 1.12. Fluorescent Y chromosome in interphase nucleus. (Courtesy of Dr. G. Khudr)

active X chromosome following the inactivation of the second X chromosome in normal females. It is assumed that the inactive X chromosome forms the sex chromatin body of the interphase nuclei [37].

The Lyon hypothesis further states that the inactivation occurs early in embryonic life, that the original *decision* is *random*, so that in some cells the paternal and in others the maternal X will be inactive, and that once the *decision* is made, the descendants of each X chromosome (active or inactive) will behave like the parent X in clones of cells. Thus, inactivation would be *random* but *fixed*. The mechanism of X inactivation is not clear. Reports on localized derepression of the human inactive X chromosome in mouse-human cell hybrids may help in the future understanding of this mechanism of X inactivation [43].

Females heterozygous for the A and B electrophoretic variants of glucose-6-phosphate dehydrogenase (G6PD) have two populations of cells in skin fibroblast cultures: one with the A type and the other with the B [44]. This is evidence for "lyonization." It also reveals that normal women heterozygous for X-linked genes are "mosaics." Several other loci reveal lyonization: the Hunter syndrome (mucopolysaccharidosis type II) [45]; the X-linked locus for chronic granulomatous disease [46]; hypoxanthine-guanine phosphoribosyltransferase (HGPRT, the deficiency of which causes the Lesch-Nyhan syndrome) [47]; α-galactosidase (the deficiency of which causes Fabry disease) [48]; X-linked hypohidrotic ectodermal dysplasia [49]; phosphorylase kinase [50]; phosphoglycerate ki-

nase (PGK) [51]; and the locus for the dihydrotestosterone receptor [52]. Evidence for inactivation is equivocal for the Xg blood group locus [53–55]. Since "lyonization" is random, females heterozygous for X-linked genes have varying proportions of cells in which a particular allele is active and thus show a considerable phenotype variability [42, 56].

Mitosis and Meiosis

Mitosis and meiosis are the two mechanisms of cell division in man. They consist of several stages: prophase, metaphase, anaphase, and telophase.

In mitotic prophase the chromosomes become distinct, condensed, and divide into two identical chromatids, joined together by the *centromere* or *kinetochore*. At metaphase they are lined up in the middle of the cell at the *metaphyseal plate*. The human karyotypes are analyzed after cell division has been stopped at this stage with colchicine. Mechanisms leading to anomalies of chromosomal number (nondisjunction or anaphase lag) occur during anaphase. In mitosis, each one of the daughter cells is identical with the parent cell and has the same diploid number of chromosomes.

Meiosis is a division specific to gametogenesis and has two important characteristics: a stage for extensive genetic recombination between homologous chromosomes followed by a reductional division whereby the daughter cells have 23 chromosomes each (22 autosomes and 1 sex chromosome).

During meiosis one member of each homologous pair of chromosomes is distributed independently and randomly with regard to the single member of each of the other pairs. This means that there are 2^{23} or 8,388,608 different possible combinations of chromosomes in a gamete derived from a single mother cell. Moreover, portions of the paternal and maternal chromosomes are exchanged during synapsis through "crossing over." It is important to note here that although the X and Y chromosomes pair end to end at meiotic metaphase, recombination does not occur and there is no evidence of exchange of genetic material between the X and Y.

Chromosomal Aberrations

The association of a numerical chromosomal aberration with a syndrome was described for the first time in 1959 [57]. It was demonstrated that children with "mongolism" (Down syndrome) have 47 chromosomes in each somatic cell instead of the normal 46.

The most important mechanism leading to a *numerical aberration* is "*nondisjunction*." This represents failure of paired chromosomes or sister chromatids to disjoin at anaphase either in mitotic division or in the first or second meiotic division. In the case of the Down syndrome the nondisjunction involves chromosome 21, the resulting zygote with 47 chromosomes having 3 chromosome 21s (trisomy 21). Among other syndromes resulting from nondisjunction are the Turner syndrome (X0), the Klinefelter syndrome (XXY), the XXX syndrome, and trisomy 18. When nondisjunction occurs more than once in gametogenesis, the zygote may be XXXY, XXXX, XXYY, XXXXX, or XXXXY. Although X0 is relatively common, Y0 is lethal. Moreover, autosomal monosomy is generally considered as lethal except for some rare cases [58, 59].

If nondisjunction occurs during an early cleavage division of the zygote, the offspring would have two or more lines of cells with different chromosomal numbers. Such individuals are called "mixoploids" or "mosaics."

Anaphase lag is another mechanism leading to numerical aberration of chromosomes. It occurs when one member of a chromosomal pair fails to synapse, does not move correctly on the spindle, and is not included in the respective daughter cell [60].

The different *aberrations of chromosome structure* are deletions, inversions, translocations, isochromosomes, dicentrics, acentrics, and rings.

A *deletion* is the loss of a portion of a chromosome either terminally or interstitially. *Inversions* involve two breaks on the same chromosomal arm with inversion of the segment upon reunion. A pericentric inversion includes the centromere whereas a paracentric inversion does not. *Translocation* involves exchange of chromosome segments between two nonhomologous chromosomes. Robertsonian translocations (centric fusion) are a special type in which the breaks occur at the centromeres and whole chromosome arms are exchanged. An *isochromosome* is an abnormal chromosome with two arms of equal length and bearing the same loci in reverse sequence. It is formed by a transverse division of the centromere rather than by the usual longitudinal division. A *dicentric* chromosome and an *acentric* fragment may be formed by a single crossover in a paracentric inversion. However, they can also arise in other ways. A *ring* chromosome results from a terminal deletion of both arms with rejoining of the ends carrying the centromere.

Chromosomal aberrations are responsible for the production of many dysmorphogenetic syndromes and conditions associated with mental retardation [61]. They are also present in a high percentage of human abortions [62] and are associated with many neoplasias.

Although we know little about the genetic and environmental factors that predispose to chromosomal aberrations, it is suspected that late maternal age [63], genes which increase chromosomal instability in somatic cells [64], radiation [65], chemicals [65], and certain chromosomal abnormalities themselves [66] may be involved in their pathogenesis.

The prevalence of chromosomal abnormalities in live-born infants is about 1 per 200; this may be as frequent as 4% if all fetuses are considered. About half of the live-born affected patients have autosomal anomalies and half have sex chromosomal abnormalities [67].

Assignment of Genes to Human Chromosomes

The assignment of a locus to the X or Y chromosome is relatively simple and can be achieved by studying pedigrees which reveal a specific pattern of inheritance. The assignment of loci to autosomes and their mapping [68] is more complicated and involves the study of traits and linkage groups in families [69], deletion mapping and gene dosage effects [70–72], deductions from the amino acid sequence of proteins [68], in situ DNA–RNA annealing ("hybridization") [73, 74], and study of traits and chromosomes in somatic cell hybrids [75–86].

Linkage

Linkage is the occurrence of two loci on the same chromosome sufficiently close to prevent completely independent assortment. If two loci are on separate nonhomologous chromosomes or on the same chromosome but sufficiently far apart, independent assortment will occur. The distance between two loci determines the amount of crossing over that goes on between them. The measure of crossing over is determined by the proportion of recombinant individuals among the offspring. If 10% of offspring are of the recombinant type, the two loci are said to be 10 *map units* apart. The presence of 50% of offspring of the recombinant type is very suggestive of independent assortment [69].

Examples of linkage groups are AB0 blood groups with the nail-patella syndrome [87, 88] or AB0 blood groups with xeroderma pigmentosum [89].

Genetic Heterogeneity

Genetic heterogeneity [4] refers to the situation in which identical or very similar phenotypes are the result of different genetic defects. A few dermatologic conditions in which heterogeneity has been recognized include albinism, the Ehlers-Danlos syndrome, hyperkeratosis palmaris et plantaris, ichthyosis, intestinal polyposis, and xeroderma pigmentosum.

Genetic heterogeneity of human diseases may be demonstrated by genetic methods, analysis of phenotype, biochemical analysis, physiologic studies, and coculturing experiments [8].

Genetic Methods

Mode of Inheritance. A disease that may follow either one of three modes of inheritance is genetically heterogeneous. Examples are spastic paraplegia, the Charcot-Marie-Tooth peroneal muscular atrophy, and the Ehlers-Danlos syndrome.

Nonallelism of Recessives in Pedigree Studies. For example, parents who are homozygous for two recessive genes causing congenital deafness produce children with normal hearing.

Linkage Relationships. For example, the fact that one form of elliptocytosis is linked to the Rh blood group locus, but at least one other form is not, indicates that genes at more than one locus are responsible for this disease.

Analysis of Phenotype

Two conditions may be phenotypically very similar, but a characteristic clinical finding may distinguish one from the other. For example, the Hurler and the Hunter diseases (mucopolysaccharidoses I and II) are distinguishable by the presence of corneal clouding in the Hurler syndrome.

Biochemical Analysis

The Tay-Sachs and Sandhoff diseases are clinically similar. Genetically, however, they are heterogeneous since patients with Tay-Sachs syndrome lack the electrophoretic variant A of hexosaminidase, whereas patients with Sandhoff syndrome lack both the A and B variants.

Physiologic Studies

The X-linked hemophilias can be distinguished by the mutual cross-correction of the clotting defect. This means that they are due to defects which are results of different mutant genes. Also, there are at least two types of homocystinuria: one responds to vitamin B_6 therapy and one does not.

Studies of Cells in Culture

Coculturing of Cells. A mixed culture of two cell strains with a biochemical anomaly may correct the anomaly and thus reveal heterogeneity. Fibroblasts cultured from the skin of patients with the Hurler and Hunter syndromes reveal accumulation of mucopolysaccharides [45]. It has been shown [90] that the biochemical defect in fibroblasts can be corrected by coculturing cells from patients with these two diseases. In this instance, the correction is mediated through enzymes released into the culture medium.

Cell Hybridization Studies. Somatic cell hybridization may be produced between two animal cell lines, between an animal and a human cell line, and between two human cell lines. It probably occurs as an infrequent spontaneous event in culture. But it can be enhanced by the addition of certain UV-irradiated viruses to the mixed culture of two different cell lines [75]. Under such conditions the cells clump together, the cytoplasms of neighboring cells coalesce, and cells containing varying numbers of nuclei are formed. These polykaryon hybrids are able to synthesize proteins, RNA, and DNA. Nuclei of polykaryon hybrids entering mitosis together usually fuse and form a single large nucleus. The prototype for studies of this kind are experiments performed on cells obtained from patients with the usual type of xeroderma pigmentosum and patients with xeroderma pigmentosum associated with severe mental retardation (de Sanctis-Cacchione syndrome). Both of these cell lines are defective in repair of UV-damaged DNA. In heterokaryotic hybrids of the two cell lines, however, the defect in DNA repair disappears due to complementation [40]. Other complementation studies revealing genetic heterogeneity have also been reported during the past few years [91].

Prevention and Treatment of Genetic Diseases

Prevention

The conception or birth of a child with a genetic disease can be prevented in one of the following ways.

Genetic Counseling. Genetic counseling is the information provided to patients and especially their parents about a specific genetic disease. This information may also be provided to couples who plan to get married and who have a family history of a genetic disease. The information is sought generally to prevent the birth of an affected child. The questions may be centered on specific problems such as late maternal age, parental consanguinity, and multiple abortions.

Important prerequisites for proper genetic counseling include accurate diagnosis and proper knowledge of the disease. An accurate diagnosis is a must, since certain phenotypes may be due to environmental causes, but may mimic specific genetic diseases. These are the "phenocopies." For example, toxoplasmosis may mimic a recessive syndrome of microcephaly and chorioretinopathy [8]. Similarly, in the Creutzfeldt-Jakob disease, the distinction between genetic disease and slow virus infection is not always clear-cut [8]. Counseling necessitates also a thorough knowledge of the pat-

tern of inheritance of diseases determined by a single gene. Some genetic diseases are heterogeneous and may have more than one pattern of inheritance (e.g., the Ehlers-Danlos syndrome). Thus, it is very important to know the exact variety in question for proper counseling. In the case of multigenic conditions, a statistical knowledge of incidence or recurrence rate of the disease is necessary.

Ideally, genetic counseling should be provided by a team comprising physicians trained in genetics, basic scientists, social workers, psychologists, and administrators [92, 93]. This team should be located in a university hospital or medical center. However, it is practically impossible to have this type of facility available wherever and whenever genetic counseling is needed. Thus, if the specialist in a certain field (e.g., dermatology) is reasonably well-versed in the principles of genetics and up to date in his own field of specialty, he may act as counselor even away from a major medical center. Yet, considering the complexity of some genetic problems, he should not hesitate to consult the team of specialists whenever possible.

Artificial Insemination. If both parents are heterozygous for an autosomal recessive gene, artificial insemination can be resorted to using the sperm of a person known not to be heterozygous for the specific gene.

Prenatal Diagnosis. This is possible mainly with the relatively new methods of amniocentesis and fetoscopy [94, 95]. Amniocentesis consists of aspirating a few milliliters of amniotic fluid around the 16th week of pregnancy and performing on its cells and fluid cytogenetic and biochemical tests for the detection of chromosomal anomalies or hereditary metabolic disorders. Fetoscopy involves the introduction of a special fine fiberoptic tube into the amniotic sac to visualize the fetus and detect dysmorphic anomalies. It is just at its beginning and may prove to be a useful procedure in the near future, especially for the diagnosis of the more gross congenital malformations. In the hands of an adequately trained obstetrician, amniocentesis is a reasonably safe procedure for both mother and baby. However, the testing of the amniotic fluid and cells for chromosomal anomalies, and especially for metabolic disorders, needs a highly trained and experienced group of cytologists and biochemists. Such testing should necessarily be performed in a well-equipped medical center. An induced abortion can be resorted to if an affected baby is diagnosed. This, of course, may have many psychological, religious, ethical, and legal implications, which should be carefully assessed before undertaking the procedure of amniocentesis.

Treatment

Patients with genetic diseases require a lot of understanding and moral support because of the generally chronic nature of their condition. Yet, in many cases, they may be greatly helped by specific therapeutic regimens. The degree of improvement varies according to the type of disease and the available therapeutic measure [95].
There are several different approaches to treatment.

Controlling the External Environment. This consists of avoiding trauma in the case of a disease like the Ehlers-Danlos syndrome, heat in anhidrotic ectodermal dysplasia, fractures in Menkes syndrome, cold injury in sickle cell disease, and UV light in xeroderma pigmentosum and albinism.

Dietary Treatment. Exclusion of specific food items or restrictions may prevent untoward effects of a genetic disease (e.g., galactose intake should be restricted in galactosemia; phenylalanine in phenylketonuria) [96].
Supplementation of specific food items or a chemical will improve or cure deficiency states (e.g., administration of arginine in argininosuccinicaciduria; nicotinic acid in Hartnup disease; vitamin B_6 in homocystinuria; zinc sulfate in acrodermatitis enteropathica) [96, 97].

Pharmacologic Approach. Certain drugs help specific genetic diseases while others exacerbate the symptoms and signs of other genetic diseases. Thus, barbiturates should be avoided in patients with acute intermittent porphyria. On the other hand, angioedema due to C_1-esterase deficiency should be treated with kallikrein inhibitors and antifibrinolytic agents. In primary hormone deficiencies (e.g., hypothyroidism) the specific hormone should be administered.

Administration of Gene Products. Replacement of gene products is well-established for the coagulation defects and immunoprotein deficiencies.
A significant amount of research has recently been directed to the treatment of genetic diseases by enzyme replacement [98]. This has been particularly evident in the field of lysosomal storage diseases (e.g., Fabry disease [99], Gaucher disease [100], mucopolysaccharidoses I, II, III, VII [101–103]). This type of treatment consists mainly of the intravenous administration of normal human plasma or leukocyte preparations. Purified enzyme has also

been used in certain instances. Although the preliminary attempts have not been completely successful, the future seems promising.

References

1. Watson, J.D.: Molecular biology of the gene, 2nd ed., pp. 292–295. New York: Benjamin, W.A. Inc. 1970
2. Harris, H.: The principles of human biochemical genetics, 2nd ed., pp. 13–17, 91–125, 277–338. Amsterdam: North Holland Publishing Co. Inc. 1975
3. Childs, B.: Sir Archibald Garrod's conception of chemical individuality: a modern appreciation. New Engl. J. Med. *282*, 71–77 (1970)
4. Childs, B., Der Kaloustian, V.M.: Genetic heterogeneity. New Engl. J. Med. *279*, 1205–1212, 1267–1274 (1968)
5. McKusick, V.A.: Mendelian inheritance in man, 5th ed., pp. 145–200. Baltimore: Johns Hopkins University Press 1978
6. Garrod, A.E.: Inborn errors of metabolism (Croonian lectures). Lancet *1908 II*, 1–7, 73–79, 142–148, 214–220
7. Harris, H. (ed.): Garrod's inborn errors of metabolism (reprinted with a supplement), pp. 5–23. London: Oxford University Press 1963
8. McKusick, V.A.: Mendelian inheritance in man, 5th ed., pp. x–xxiii. Baltimore: Johns Hopkins University Press 1978
9. de Duve, C., Pressman, B.C., Gianetto, R., Wattiaux, R., Appelmans, F.: Tissue fractionation studies. 6. Intracellular distribution patterns of enzymes in rat-liver tissue. Biochem. J. *60*, 604–617 (1955)
10. de Duve, C., Wattiaux, R.: Functions of lysosomes. Ann. Rev. Physiol. *28*, 435–492 (1966)
11. Hers, H.G.: Glucosidase deficiency in generalized glycogen-storage disease (Pompe's disease). Biochem. J. *86*, 11–16 (1963)
12. Hers, H.G.: Inborn lysosomal diseases. Gastroenterology *48*, 625–633 (1965)
13. de Duve, C.: Foreword. In: Lysosomes and storage diseases. Hers, H.G., Van Hoof, F. (eds.), pp. 17–19. New York: Academic Press 1973
14. Gold, R.J.M., Scriver, C.R.: Properties of hair keratin in an autosomal dominant form of ectodermal dysplasia. Amer. J. hum. Genet. *24*, 549–561 (1972)
15. Watson, J.D.: Molecular biology of the gene, 2nd ed., pp. 1–31. New York: Benjamin, W.A. Inc. 1970
16. Nora, J.J., Fraser, F.C.: Medical genetics: principles and practice, p. 92. Philadelphia: Lea & Febiger 1974
17. McKusick, V.A.: Genetics and dermatology or if I were to rewrite Cockayne's inherited abnormalities of the skin. J. invest. Derm. *60*, 343–359 (1973)
18. McKusick, V.A.: Human genetics, 2nd ed., p. 85. Englewood Cliffs: Prentice-Hall, Inc. 1969
19. Stern, C.: Model estimates of the number of gene pairs involved in pigmentation variability of the Negro-American. Hum. Hered. *20*, 165–168 (1970)
20. Carter, C.O.: Genetics of common disorders. Brit. med. Bull. *25*, 52–57 (1969)
21. de Grouchy, J., Aussannaire, M., Brissaud, H.E., Lamy, M.: Aneusomie de recombinaison: three further examples. Amer. J. hum. Genet. *18*, 467–484 (1966)
22. Thompson, J.S., Thompson, M.W.: Genetics in medicine, 2nd ed., pp. 307–318. Philadelphia: Saunders, W.B. Co. 1973
23. Flemming, W.: Beiträge zur Kenntnis der Zelle und ihrer Lebenserscheinungen. III. Arch. mikr. Anat. *20*, 1–86 (1882)

24. Tjio, J.H., Levan, A.: The chromosome number of man. Hereditas *42*, 1–6 (1956)

25. Book, J.A., Chu, E.H.Y., Ford, C.E., Fraccaro, M., Harnden, D.G., Hsu, T.C., Hungerford, D.A., Jacobs, P.A., Lejeune, J., Levan, A., Makino, S., Puck, T.T., Robinson, A., Tjio, J.H., Catcheside, D.G., Muller, H.J., Stern, C.: A proposed standard system of nomenclature of human mitotic chromosomes. Amer. J. hum. Genet. *12*, 384–388 (1960)

26. Chicago Conference: Standardization in human cytogenetics. Birth Defects *2*, 2 (1966)

27. Caspersson, T., Lomakka, G., Zech, L.: The 24 fluorescence patterns of the human metaphase chromosomes – distinguishing characters and variability. Hereditas *67*, 89 (1971)

28. Arrighi, F.E., Hsu, T.C.: Localization of heterochromatin in human chromosomes. Cytogenetics *10*, 81–86 (1971)

29. Dutrillaux, B., Lejeune, J.: Sur une nouvelle technique d'analyse du caryotype humain. C.R. Acad. Sci. [D] (Paris) *272*, 2638–2640 (1971)

30. Sumner, A.T., Evans, H.J., Buckland, R.A.: New technique for distinguishing between human chromosomes. Nature (Lond.) New Biol. *232*, 31–32 (1971)

31. Hamerton, J.L.: Human cytogenetics, Vol. I, pp. 14–25. New York: Academic Press 1971

32. Hamerton, J.L.: Human cytogenetics, Vol. I, pp. 290–309. New York: Academic Press 1971

33. Thompson, J.S., Thompson, M.W.: Genetics in medicine, 2nd ed., pp. 11–12. Philadelphia: Saunders, W.B. Co. 1973

34. Davidson, R.G.: Application of cell culture techniques to human genetics. In: Modern trends in human genetics. 1. Emery, A.E.H. (ed.), pp. 143–180. New York: Appleton-Century-Crofts 1970

35. Barr, M.L., Bertram, E.G.: A morphological distinction between neurones of the male and female, and the behavior of the nucleolar satellite during accelerated nucleoprotein synthesis. Nature (Lond.) *163*, 676–677 (1949)

36. Miller, O.J.: Autoradiography in human cytogenetics. In: Advances in human genetics. Harris, H., Hirschhorn, K. (eds.), Vol. 1, pp. 35–130, New York: Plenum Press 1970

37. Hamerton, J.L.: Human cytogenetics, Vol. I, pp. 131–191. New York: Academic Press 1971

38. Khudr, G., Benirschke, K.: Fluorescence of the Y chromosome: a rapid test to determine fetal sex. Amer. J. Obstet. Gynec. *110*, 1091–1095 (1971)

39. Bell, A.G., Corey, P.N.: A sex chromatin and Y body survey of Toronto newborns. Can. J. Genet. Cytol. *16*, 239–250 (1974)

40. De Weerd-Kastelein, E.A., Keijzer, W., Bootsma, D.: Genetic heterogeneity of xeroderma pigmentosum demonstrated by somatic cell hybridization. Nature (Lond.) New Biol. *238*, 80–83 (1972)

41. Lyon, M.F.: Gene action in the X-chromosome of the mouse (*Mus musculus* L.) Nature (Lond.) *190*, 372–373 (1961)

42. Lyon, M.F.: Sex chromatin and gene action in the mammalian X-chromosome. Amer. J. hum. Genet. *14*, 135–148 (1962)

43. Kahan, B., DeMars, R.: Localized derepression on the human inactive X-chromosome in mouse-human cell hybrids. Proc. nat. Acad. Sci. (Wash.) *72*, 1510–1514 (1975)

44. Davidson, R.G., Nitowsky, H.M., Childs, B.: Demonstration of two populations of cells in the human female heterozygous for glucose-6-phosphate dehydrogenase variants. Proc. nat. Acad. Sci. (Wash.) *50*, 481–485 (1963)

45. Danes, B.S., Bearn, A.G.: Hurler's syndrome. A genetic study in cell culture. J. exp. Med. *123*, 1–16 (1966)

46. Windhorst, D.B., Holmes, B., Good, R.A.: A newly defined X-linked trait in man with demonstration of the Lyon effect in carrier females. Lancet *19671*, 737–739

47. Migeon, B.R., Der Kaloustian, V.M., Nyhan, W.L., Young, W.J., Childs, B.: X-linked hypoxanthine-guanine phosphoribosyl transferase deficiency: heterozygote has two clonal populations. Science *160*, 425–427 (1968)

48. Romeo, G., Migeon, B.R.: Genetic inactivation of the α-galactosidase locus in carriers of Fabry's disease. Science *170*, 180–181 (1970)

49. Passarge, E., Fries, E.: X chromosome inactivation in X-linked hypohidrotic ectodermal dysplasia. Nature (Lond.) New Biol. *245*, 58–59 (1973)

50. Migeon, B.R., Huijing, F.: Glycogen storage disease associated with phosphorylase kinase deficiency: evidence for X inactivation. Amer. J. hum. Genet. *26*, 360–368 (1974)

51. Deys, B.F., Grzeschik, K.H., Grzeschik, A., Jaffe, E.R., Siniscalco, M.: Human phosphoglycerate kinase and inactivation of the X chromosome. Science *175*, 1002–1003 (1972)

52. Meyer, W.J., III, Migeon, B.R., Migeon, C.J.: Locus on human X chromosome for dihydrotestosterone receptor and androgen insensitivity. Proc. nat. Acad. Sci. (Wash.) *72*, 1469–1472 (1975)

53. MacDiarmid, W.D., Lee, G.R., Cartwright, G.E., Wintrobe, M.M.: X-inactivation in an unusual X-linked anemia and the Xg^a blood group. Clin. Res. *15* (Abstr.), 132 (1967)

54. Race, R.R., Sanger, R.: Blood groups in man, 5th ed. Oxford: Blackwell Scientific Publications 1968

55. Fialkow, P.J., Lisker, R., Giblett, E.R., Zavala, C.: Xg locus: failure to detect inactivation in females with chronic myelocytic leukaemia. Nature (Lond.) *226*, 367–368 (1970)

56. Nance, W.E.: Genetic tests with a sex-linked marker: glucose-6-phosphate dehydrogenase. Cold Spr. Harb. Symp. quant. Biol. *29*, 415–425 (1964)

57. Lejeune, J., Gautier, M., Turpin, R.: Etude des chromosomes somatiques de neuf enfants mongoliens. C.R. Acad. Sci. [D] (Paris) *248*, 1721–1722 (1959)

58. Halloran, K.H., Breg, W.R., Mahoney, M.J.: 21 monosomy in a retarded female infant. J. med. Genet. *11*, 386–389 (1974)

59. DeCicco, F., Steele, M.W., Pan, S., Park, S.C.: Monosomy of chromosome no. 22: a case report. J. Pediat. *83*, 836–838 (1973)

60. Hamerton, J.L.: Human cytogenetics, Vol. I, pp. 192–231. New York: Academic Press 1971

61. Holmes, L.B., Moser, H.W., Halldórsson, S., Mack, C., Pant, S.S., Matzilevich, B.: Mental retardation, pp. 145–191. New York: Macmillan Co. 1970

62. Khudr, G.: Cytogenetics of habitual abortion. A review. Obstet. gynec. Surg. *29*, 290–310 (1974)

63. Hamerton, J.L.: Human cytogenetics, Vol. II, pp. 197–200. New York: Academic Press 1971

64. German, J.: Some genes which increase chromosomal instability in somatic cells and predispose to cancer. In: Progress in medical genetics. Steinberg, A.G., Bearn, A.G. (eds.), Vol. VIII, pp. 61–101. New York: Grune & Stratton 1972

65. Bloom, A.D.: Induced chromosomal aberrations in man. In: Advances in human genetics. Harris, H., Hirschhorn, K. (eds.), Vol. 3, pp. 99–172. New York: Plenum Press 1972

66. Hamerton, J.L.: Human cytogenetics. Vol. I, pp. 218–220. New York: Academic Press 1971

67. Polani, P.E.: Autosomal imbalance and its syndromes, excluding Down's. Brit. med. Bull. *25*, 81–93 (1969)

68. McKusick, V.A.: Mendelian inheritance in man, 5th ed., p. lvi. Baltimore: Johns Hopkins University Press 1978

69. McKusick, V.A.: Human genetics, 2nd ed., pp. 66–68. Englewood Cliffs: Prentice-Hall, Inc. 1969

70. McKusick, V.A.: Human genetics, 2nd ed., pp. 32–34. Englewood Cliffs: Prentice-Hall, Inc. 1969

71. Marsh, W.L., Chaganti, R.S.K., Gardner, F.H., Mayer, K., Nowell, P.C., German, J.: Mapping human autosomes: evidence supporting assignment of Rhesus to the short arm of chromosome 1. Science *183*, 966–968 (1974)

72. Ferguson-Smith, M.A., Newman, B.F., Ellis, P.M., Thomson, D.M.G., Riley, I.D.: Assignment by deletion of human red cell acid phosphatase gene locus to the short arm of chromosome 2. Nature (Lond.) *243*, 271–273 (1973)

73. Price, P.M., Conover, J.H., Hirschhorn, K.: Chromosomal localization of human hemoglobin structural genes. Nature (Lond.) *237*, 340–342 (1972)

74. McKusick, V.A.: Mendelian inheritance in man, 5th ed., p. 149. Baltimore: Johns Hopkins University Press 1978

75. Ruddle, F.H.: Linkage analysis using somatic cell hybrids. In: Advances in human genetics. Harris, H., Hirschhorn, K. (eds.), Vol. 3, pp. 173–235. New York: Plenum Press 1972

76. Migeon, B.R., Miller, C.S.: Human-mouse somatic cell hybrids with single human chromosomes (group E): link with thymidine kinase activity. Science *162*, 1005–1006 (1968)

77. Migeon, B.R., Childs, B.: Hybridization of mammalian somatic cells. In: Progress in medical genetics. Steinberg, A.G., Bearn, A.G. (eds.), Vol. VII, pp. 1–28, New York: Grune & Stratton 1970

78. Miller, O.J., Allderdice, P.W., Miller, D.A., Breg, W.R., Migeon, B.R.: Human thymidine kinase gene locus: assignment to chromosome 17 in a hybrid of man and mouse cells. Science *173*, 244–245 (1971)

79. Creagan, R.P., Carritt, B., Chen, S., Kucherlapati, R., McMorris, F.A., Ricciuti, F., Tan, Y.H., Tischfield, J.A., Ruddle, F.R.: Chromosome assignments of genes in man using mouse-human somatic cell hybrids: cytoplasmic isocitrate dehydrogenase (IDH 1) and malate dehydrogenase (MDH 1) to chromosome 2. Amer. J. hum. Genet. *26*, 604–613 (1974)

80. Gilbert, F., Kucherlapati, R., Creagan, R.P., Murnane, M.J., Darlington, G.J., Ruddle, F.H.: Tay-Sach's and Sandhoff's diseases: the assignment of genes for hexosaminidase A and B to individual human chromosomes. Proc. nat. Acad. Sci. (Wash.) *72*, 263–267 (1975)

81. Elsevier, S.M., Kucherlapati, R.S., Nichols, E.A., Creagan, R.P., Giles, R.E., Ruddle, F.H., Willecke, K., McDougall, J.K.: Assignment of the gene for galactokinase to human chromosome 17 and its regional localisation to band q21–22. Nature (Lond.) *251*, 633–636 (1974)

82. Tedesco, T.A., Diamond, R., Orkwiszewski, K.G., Boedecker, H.J., Croce, C.M.: Assignment of the human gene for hexose-1-phosphate uridyltransferase to chromosome 3. Proc. nat. Acad. Sci. (Wash.) *71*, 3483–3486 (1974)

83. Creagan, R., Tischfield, J., Ricciuti, F., Ruddle, F.H.: Chromosome assignments of genes in man using mouse-human somatic cell hybrids: mitochondrial superoxide dismutase (indophenol oxidase-B, tetrameric) to chromosome 6. Humangenetik *20*, 203–209 (1973)

84. Jongsma, A., van Someren, H., Westerveld, A., Hagemeijer, A., Pearson, P.: Localization of genes on human chromosomes by studies of human-Chinese hamster somatic cell hybrids. Assignment of PGM$_3$ to chromosome C6 and regional mapping of the PGD, PGM$_1$, and pep-C genes on chromosome A1. Humangenetik *20*, 195–202 (1973)

85. Tischfield, J.A., Ruddle, F.H.: Assignment of the gene for adenine phosphoribosyltransferase to human chromosome 16 by mouse-human somatic cell hybridization. Proc. nat. Acad. Sci. (Wash.) *71*, 45–49 (1974)

86. Douglas, G.R., McAlpine, P.J., Hamerton, J.L.: Regional localization of loci for human PGM and 6PGD on human chromosome one by use of hybrids of Chinese-hamster-human somatic cells. Proc. nat. Acad. Sci. (Wash.) *70*, 2737–2740 (1973)

87. Renwick, J.H., Lawler, S.D.: Genetical linkage between the ABO and nail-patella loci. Ann. hum. Genet. *19*, 312–331 (1955)

88. Renwick, J.H., Schulze, J.: Male and female recombination fractions for the nail-patella: ABO linkage in man. Ann. hum. Genet. *28*, 379–392 (1965)

89. El-Hefnawi, H., Smith, S.M., Penrose, L.S.: Xeroderma pigmentosum – its inheritance and relationship to the ABO blood-group system. Ann. hum. Genet. *28*, 273–290 (1964–1965)

90. Fratantoni, J.C., Hall, C.W., Neufeld, E.F.: Hurler and Hunter syndromes: mutual correction of the defect in cultured fibroblasts. Science *162*, 570–572 (1968)

91. Galjaard, H., Hoogeveen, A., Keijzer, W., de Wit-Verbeek, H.A., Reuser, A.J.J., Ho, M.W., Robinson, D.: Genetic heterogeneity in GM1-gangliosidosis. Nature (Lond.) *257*, 60–62 (1975)

92. Milunsky, A.: Genetic counseling: principles and practice. In: The prevention of genetic disease and mental retardation. Milunsky, A. (ed.), pp. 64–89. Philadelphia: Saunders, W.B. Co. 1975

93. Epstein, C.J.: Who should do genetic counseling, and under what circumstances? Birth Defects *9*, 39–48 (1973)

94. Milunsky, A., Littlefield, J.W., Kanfer, J.N., Kolodny, E.H., Shih, V.E., Atkins, L.: Prenatal genetic diagnosis. New Engl. J. Med. *283*, 1370–1381, 1441–1447, 1498–1504 (1970)

95. Milunsky, A., Atkins, L.: Prenatal diagnosis of genetic disorders. An analysis of experience with 600 cases. J. Amer. med. Ass. *230*, 232–235 (1974)

96. Hsia, Y.E.: Treatment in genetic diseases. In: The prevention of genetic disease and mental retardation. Milunsky, A. (ed.), pp. 277–305. Philadelphia: Saunders, W.B. Co. 1975

97. Der Kaloustian, V.M., Musallam, S.S., Murib, A., Hammad, W.D., Sanjad, S.A., Idriss, Z.H.: Oral treatment of acrodermatitis enteropathica with zinc sulfate. Amer. J. Dis. Child. *130*, 421–423 (1976)

98. Desnick, R.J., Krivit, W., Fiddler, M.B.: Enzyme therapy in genetic diseases: progress, principles, and prospects. In: The prevention of genetic disease and mental retardation. Milunsky, A. (ed.), pp. 317–342. Philadelphia: Saunders, W.B. Co. 1975

99. Brady, R.O., Tallman, J.F., Johnson, W.G., Gal, A.E., Leahy, W.R., Quirk, J.M., Dekaban, A.S.: Replacement therapy for inherited enzyme deficiency. Use of purified ceramidetrihexosidase in Fabry's disease. New Engl. J. Med. *289*, 9–14 (1973)

100. Brady, R.O., Penchev, P.G., Gal, A.E., Hibbert, S.R., Dekaban, A.S.: Replacement therapy for inherited enzyme deficiency. Use of purified glucocerebrosidase in Gaucher's disease. New Engl. J. Med. *291*, 989–993 (1974)

101. Di Ferrante, N., Nichols, B.L., Donnelly, P.V., Neri, G., Hrgovcic, R., Berglund, R.K.: Induced degradation of glycosaminoglycans in Hurler's and Hunter's syndromes by plasma infusion. Proc. nat. Acad. Sci. (Wash). *68*, 303–307 (1971)

102. Dekaban, A.S., Holden, K.R., Costantopoulos, G.: Effects of fresh plasma or whole blood transfusions on patients with various types of mucopolysaccharidosis. Pediatrics *50*, 688–692 (1972)

103. Knudson, A.G., Jr., Di Ferrante, N., Curtis, J.E.: Effect of leukocyte transfusion in a child with type II mucopolysaccharidosis. Proc. nat. Acad. Sci. (Wash.) *68*, 1738–1741 (1971)

Chapter 2   Abnormalities of Keratinization

Contents

Acrokeratoses

Acrokeratosis Verruciformis

This rare disease was first reported by Hopf in 1931 [1].

Clinical Presentation. The eruption appears at birth, in infancy, or in childhood. The lesions consist of skin-colored verrucous or lichenoid papules, typically affecting the dorsa of the hands and fingers. The dorsa of the feet, the palms and soles, and flexors of the fingers, wrists, and forearms may be involved. Occasionally, other sites may be affected. The palmar and plantar lesions appear as translucent punctae. The nails may be white and thickened (Figs. 2.1–2.4).

Pathology and Pathophysiology. There is hyperkeratosis, hypergranulosis, and acanthosis. There is also papillomatosis, which is frequently associated with circumscribed elevations of the epidermis resembling church spires [2]. The latter feature is quite typical of this condition. There is no vacuolization of epidermal cells. The dermis is unremarkable. The association of acrokeratosis verruciformis and keratosis follicularis is so frequent that the former may be considered a forme fruste of the latter [3]. However, the occurrence of acrokeratosis verruciformis in families with Darier disease [4] may point to a coincidental association.

Inheritance. Autosomal dominant [4].

Treatment. If the lesions are few, superficial destruction with electrodesiccation or liquid nitrogen may be attempted. Otherwise there is no specific treatment.

Van den Bosch Syndrome

Van den Bosch described this syndrome in 1959 [5]. It comprises acrokeratosis verruciformis, anhidrosis, skeletal deformity, mental deficiency, and choroideremia. This syndrome is inherited as X-linked recessive.

References

1. Hopf, G.: Über eine bisher nicht beschriebene disseminierte Keratose (acrokeratosis verruciformis). Derm. Z. *60*, 227–250 (1931)
2. Schneller, W.A.: Acrokeratosis verruciformis of Hopf. Arch. Derm. *106*, 81–83 (1972)
3. Waisman, M.: Verruciform manifestations of keratosis follicularis. Including a reappraisal of hard nevi (Unna). Arch. Derm. *81*, 1–14 (1960)
4. Niedelman, M.L., McKusick, V.A.: Acrokeratosis verruciformis (Hopf). A follow-up study. Arch. Derm. *86*, 779–782 (1962)
5. Van den Bosch, J.: A new syndrome in three generations of a Dutch family. Ophthalmologica (Basel) *137*, 422–423 (1959)

Erythrokeratodermias

Erythrokeratodermia Variabilis (Mendes da Costa Syndrome, Keratosis Rubra Figurata, Erythrokeratodermia Figurata Variabilis)

Since 1925, when Mendes da Costa [1] described this rare disorder, many reports have appeared attesting to its two distinctive components, erythema and hyperkeratosis [2, 3].

Clinical Presentation. The disease starts in infancy. There are hyperkeratotic plaques, which are usually persistent, involving the extremities, buttocks, and face. These plaques have sharp margins and may be circinate, polycyclic, or have other configurations. The erythrodermic patches are also sharply demarcated, confluent, and varying in size, location, and duration. The appearance of these patches may be associated with environmental and emotional influences. The erythemas are transient and may last for hours or days. Occasionally, fixed hyperkeratotic patches are superimposed on the erythematous areas.

There are no associated changes in the hair, nails, or internal organs.

Pathology and Pathophysiology. The involved skin shows orthokeratotic hyperkeratosis, moderate to marked acanthosis and papillomatosis, and a normal granular cell layer. The epidermis has a saw-toothed appearance. The vessels in the papillary dermis are straight, prominent, and surrounded by a modest inflammatory infiltrate [4, 5]. There is an increase in the amounts of hydrolytic enzymes in the epidermis [4, 5]. Ultrastructurally, there are increased numbers of unmyelinated nerves in the papillary dermis and a pronounced reduction of keratinosomes in the epidermis [5]. Autoradiographic studies show normal mitotic indices [6]. All of these findings confirm that erythrokerato-

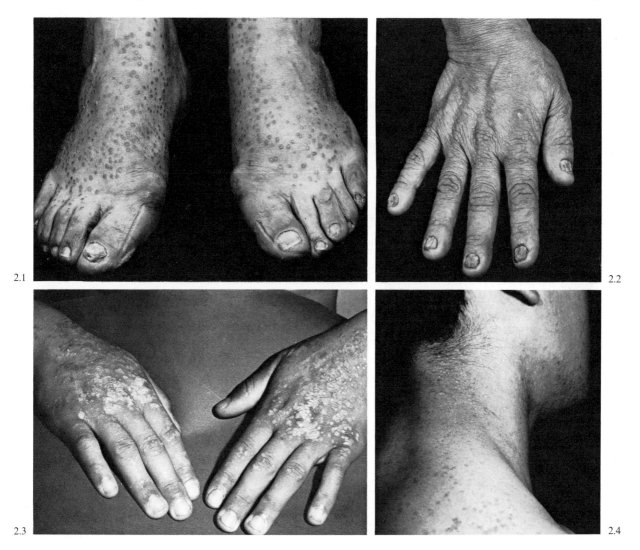

2.1

2.2

2.3

2.4

Figs. 2.1-2.4. Acrokeratosis verruciformis

Fig. 2.1. Skin-colored papules on dorsa of feet. (From McKusick, V.A.: In: The clinical delineation of birth defects. Bergsma, D. (ed.), Vol. VII, No. 8, pt. XII, p. 255. Baltimore: Williams & Wilkins Co. 1971)

Fig. 2.2. Few papules on dorsum of hand. Note thick, whitish nails. (From McKusick, V.A.: In: The clinical delineation of birth defects. Bergsma, D. (ed.), Vol. VII, No. 8, pt. XII, p. 255. Baltimore: Williams & Wilkins Co. 1971)

Fig. 2.3. Numerous papules on the hands

Fig. 2.4. Papules on the neck

dermia variabilis is a disease sui generis and unrelated to ichthyosiform erythrodermia.

Inheritance. Autosomal dominant with variable expressivity [2].

Treatment. Topical steroids may be helpful.

Genodermatose en Cocardes

First described in 1947 by Degos and co-workers [7], this disorder is characterized by asymptomatic, large, circular, erythematous areas with central hyperkeratosis giving the appearance of targets *(en cocarde)*. The lesions disappear spontaneously in a few weeks but recur. Hyperkeratotic lesions on the knees and legs are more persistent. Like erythrokeratodermia variabilis, the lesions of genodermatose en cocardes (GEC) involve the extremities and buttocks and are influenced by heat and cold. The distinctive feature of this disorder is the erythematous rings with central scales [3]. The inheritance follows the autosomal dominant pattern (7). Treatment is symptomatic.

Symmetric Progressive Erythrokeratodermia

The onset is usually in infancy and is characterized by sharply demarcated, erythematous, hyperkeratotic plaques. The sites of involvement are the feet, shins, hands, and fingers (Figs. 2.5 and 2.6). The lesions continue to progress until puberty and may regress later on. Histologically, there is hyperkeratosis, patchy parakeratosis, and marked acanthosis [8,9]. In the involved skin, the rate of cell proliferation is markedly increased because of shortening of the interphase [10]. The inheritance is of the autosomal dominant type. Treatment is symptomatic.

Erythrokeratodermia with Ataxia

In this newly described syndrome, affected individuals develop papulosquamous plaques soon after birth. The usually affected sites are dorsa of hands and feet, wrists, ankles, knees (Figs. 2.7–2.9), and external ears. The plaques have mild variations in intensity and tend to subside in the summer months. After the age of 25 years, the eruption progressively disappears. After the age of 40–45

years, the patients develop neurologic symptoms characterized by abnormal gait, diminution of osteotendinous reflexes with spasticity, occasional muscular pains, and later nystagmus, dysarthria, and severe ataxia [11]. The inheritance is autosomal dominant.

Erythrokeratodermia with Deafness, Physical Retardation, and Neuropathy

In this possibly definite entity, there is a combination of features: skin lesions very suggestive of erythrokeratodermia variabilis, retarded physical growth, bilateral profound perceptive deafness, and bilateral talipes deformity due to a neuropathy. The electromyogram shows no spontaneous activity and the nerve conduction is less than normal. Electron microscopy of the muscle is essentially normal. The inheritance is believed to be autosomal dominant [12].

References

1. Mendes da Costa, S.: Erythrodermia and keratodermia variabilis in mother and daughter. Acta derm.-venereol. (Stockh.) *6*, 255–261 (1925)
2. Brown, J., Kierland, R.R.: Erythrokeratodermia variabilis. Report of three cases and review of the literature. Arch. Derm. *93*, 194–201 (1966)
3. Cram, D.L.: Erythrokeratoderma variabilis and variable circinate erythrokeratodermas. Arch. Derm. *101*, 68–73 (1970)
4. Schellander, F.G., Fritsch, P.O.: Variable erythrokeratoderma. An unusual case. Arch. Derm. *100*, 744–748 (1969)
5. Vandersteen, P.R., Muller, S.A.: Erythrokeratodermia variabilis. An enzyme histochemical and ultrastructural study. Arch. Derm. *103*, 362–370 (1971)
6. Schellander, F.G., Fritsch, P.O.: Variable Erythrokeratodermien. Enzymhistochemische und autoradiographische Untersuchungen an 2 Fällen. Arch. klin. exp. Derm. *235*, 241–251 (1969)
7. Degos, R., Delzant, O., Morival, H.: Erythème desquamatif en plaques, congénital et familial (génodermatose nouvelle?). Bull. Soc. franç. Derm. Syph. *54*, 442 (1947)
8. Orbaneja, J.G., Diez, L.I.: Érythrokératodermie en plaques, symétrique progressive, de croissance excentrique, avec des phases de régression et récidivante par poussées. Ann. Derm. Syph. (Paris) *99*, 21–28 (1972)
9. Touraine, A.: Génodermatoses ichthyosiformes. Proc. 11th Intern. Congr. Dermatol. Acta derm.-venereol. (Stockh.) *3*, 653–658 (1957)
10. Hopsu-Havu, V.K., Tuohimaa, P.: Erythrokeratodermia congenitalis progressiva symmetrica (Gottron). II. An analysis of kinetics of epidermal cell proliferation. Dermatologica (Basel) *142*, 137–144 (1971)
11. Giroux, J.M., Barbeau, A.: Erythrokeratodermia with ataxia. Arch. Derm. *106*, 183–188 (1972)
12. Beare, J.M., Nevin, N.C., Frogatt, P., Kernohan, D.C., Allen, I.V.: Atypical erythrokeratoderma with deafness, physical retardation and peripheral neuropathy. Brit. J. Derm. *87*, 308–314 (1972)

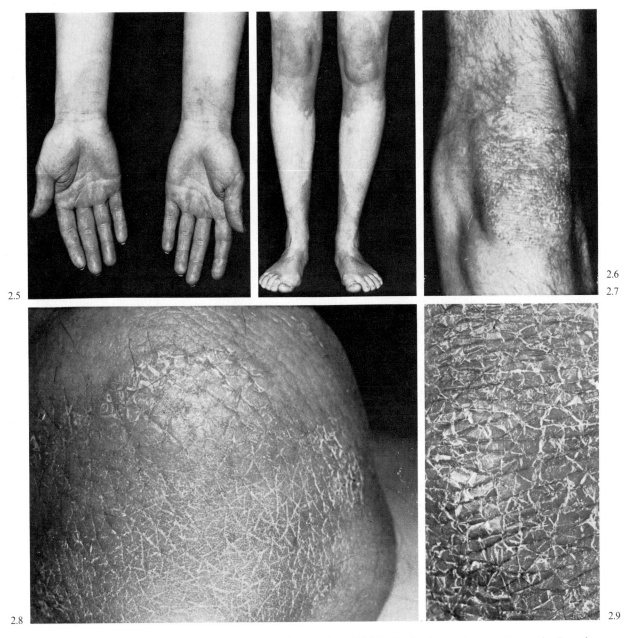

2.5

2.6
2.7

2.8

2.9

Figs. 2.5 and 2.6. Symmetric progressive erythrokeratodermia involving hands, knees, and feet. (Courtesy of Dr.
V. K. Hopsu-Havu)

Figs. 2.7–2.9. Erythrokeratodermia with ataxia. Eruption
on the knee with detail of papulosquamous lesions. (From
Giroux, J. M., Barbeau, A.: Arch. Derm. *106*, 183–188, 1972)

Follicular Keratoses

Keratosis Follicularis
(Darier-White Disease)

Darier [1] and White [2] independently described this uncommon disorder of keratinization in 1889.

Clinical Presentation. The usual age of onset is between 8 and 16 years. The characteristic lesions are initially firm, skin-colored papules which later become greasy, crusted, and yellow or brown. The crusts cover a concavity on the top of the papules. The areas affected are the face, chest, trunk, sacral area, and extremities (Figs. 2.10–2.14). The scalp and flexures, especially the anogenital region, are also frequently involved. Most papules are initially follicular but interfollicular papules are seen as the disease progresses. The papules may remain discrete or coalesce, especially in the flexures, to form fungating, warty, and papillomatous masses which are malodorous and secondarily infected. Over the dorsa of the hands, the papules remain discrete and resemble acrokeratosis verruciformis. On the palms and soles, minute papules or pits may appear. Hemorrhagic macules on the hands and feet may be seen [3]. Occasionally, the lesions are confined to one part of the body in a linear or zosteriform distribution [4, 5], but in such patients there is no family history.

The nails show longitudinal, subungual red or white streaks associated with distal wedge-shaped subungual keratoses [6]. Mucous membrane lesions are uncommon but may be found in many members of some families [7]. The oral lesions appear as pinpointed [7, 8] or flattened papules coalescing to give a pebbly cobblestone appearance [9]. Any part of the oral mucosa can be involved although the lips are usually free. A similar involvement can occur in the hypopharynx and larynx [10], as well as the vulva, esophagus, or rectum [11].

The eruption in Darier disease is aggravated by exposure to sunlight, especially wavelengths of 250–300 nm [12]. Other forms of trauma may also evoke exacerbations. The course of the disease is chronic. Affected individuals are usually of small stature and low intelligence.

A kindred has been recently described in which generalized keratosis follicularis is associated with dwarfism and cerebral atrophy [13]. The inheritance in this kindred is consistent with X-linked recessive pattern.

Pathology and Pathophysiology. The lesions exhibit characteristic changes. There is hyperkeratosis, acanthosis, and papillomatosis. Suprabasal clefts or lacunae are formed by acantholysis. Papillae (villi), lined by a single layer of basal cells, project into these lacunae. In addition, a peculiar form of dyskeratosis results in the formation of *corps ronds* and grains. The *corps ronds*, which consist of large, round basophilic masses surrounded by a clear halo, are found in the upper prickle layer and granular layer. The grains have an elongated, darkly staining nucleus and are found in the keratin layer or as acantholytic cells in the lacunae. In the dermis there is a mild, nonspecific inflammatory infiltrate.

Ultrastructurally, the lacunae and dyskeratoses seem to result from structural defects in the tonofilaments and desmosomes [14] or stretching of the tonofilaments and desmosomes leading to splitting of the latter [15].

Inheritance. Autosomal dominant [7].

Treatment. There is no specific treatment. Vitamin A (100,000–500,000 units daily) may be helpful but the danger of hypervitaminosis A must be remembered. The combination of vitamins A (200,000 units) and E (1,200 units) by mouth may also be helpful [16]. Topical 5-fluorouracil (2%) [17] and tretinoin (0.1%) [18] have been found symptomatically useful.

References

 1. Darier, J.: Psorospermose folliculaire végétante. Ann. Derm. Syph. (Paris) *10*, 597 (1889)
 2. White, J.C.: A case of keratosis (ichthyosis) follicularis. J. cutan. genito-urin. Dis. *7*, 201–209 (1889)
 3. Jones, W.N., Nix, T.E., Jr., Clark, W.H., Jr.: Hemorrhagic Darier's disease. Arch. Derm. *89*, 523–527 (1964)
 4. Kellum, R.E., Haserick, J.R.: Localized linear keratosis follicularis. Response to intralesional vitamin A and simultaneous occurrence of warty dyskeratoma. Arch. Derm. *86*, 450–454 (1962)
 5. Lubritz, R.R., Marascalco, J.: Unilateral Darier's disease. Cutis *9*, 819–821 (1972)
 6. Zaias, N., Ackerman, A.B.: The nail in Darier-White disease. Arch. Derm. *107*, 193–199 (1973)
 7. Getzler, N.A., Flint, A.: Keratosis follicularis. A study of one family. Arch. Derm. *93*, 545–549 (1966)
 8. Gorlin, R.J., Chaudhry, A.P.: The oral manifestations of keratosis follicularis. Oral Surg. *12*, 1468–1470 (1959)
 9. Weathers, D.R., Olansky, S., Sharpe, L.O.: Darier's disease with mucous membrane involvement. A case report. Arch. Derm. *100*, 50–53 (1969)
10. Dellon, A.L., Peck, G.L., Chretien, P.B.: Hypopharyngeal and laryngeal involvement with Darier's disease. Arch. Derm. *111*, 744–746 (1975)
11. Klein, A., Burns, L., Leyden, J.J.: Rectal mucosa involvement in keratosis follicularis. Arch. Derm. *109*, 560–561 (1974)

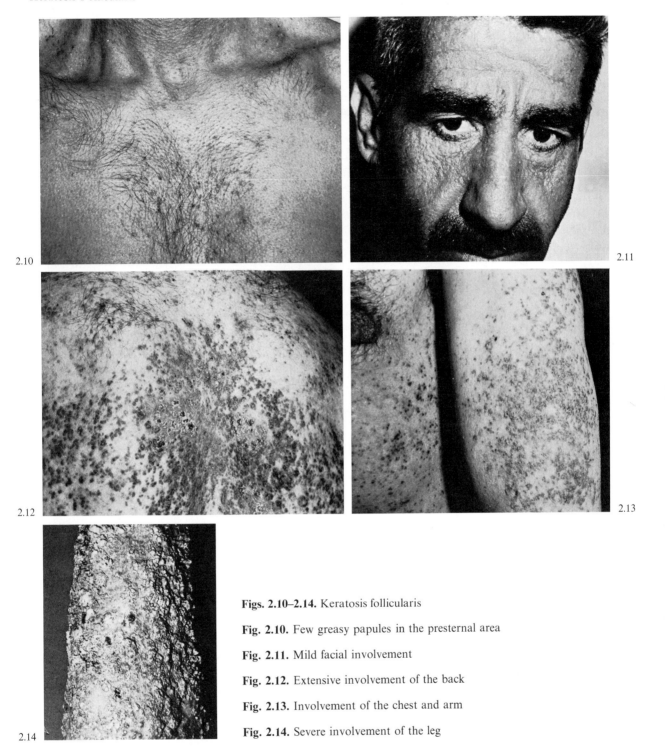

Figs. 2.10–2.14. Keratosis follicularis

Fig. 2.10. Few greasy papules in the presternal area

Fig. 2.11. Mild facial involvement

Fig. 2.12. Extensive involvement of the back

Fig. 2.13. Involvement of the chest and arm

Fig. 2.14. Severe involvement of the leg

12. Heyl, T.: Sunlight and Darier's disease. Brit. J. Derm. *85*, Suppl. 7, 57–59 (1971)
13. Cantu, J.-M., Hernandez, A., Larracilla, J., Trejo, A., Macotela-Ruiz, E.: A new X-linked recessive disorder with dwarfism, cerebral atrophy and generalized keratosis follicularis. J. Pediat. *84*, 564–570 (1974)
14. Caulfield, J.B., Wilgram, G.F.: An electron microscope study of dyskeratosis and acantholysis in Darier's disease. J. invest. Derm. *41*, 57–65 (1963)
15. Mann, P.R., Haye, K.R.: An electron microscope study on the acantholytic and dyskeratotic processes in Darier's disease. Brit. J. Derm. *82*, 561–566 (1970)
16. Ayres, S., Jr., Mihan, R.: Keratosis follicularis (Darier's disease). Response to simultaneous administration of vitamins A and E. Arch. Derm. *106*, 909–910 (1972)
17. Bamshad, J., Hilton, P.E.: Darier's disease: treatment with topical 5-FU. Cutis 8, 555–556 (1971)
18. Goette, D.K.: Zosteriform keratosis follicularis cleared with topically applied vitamin A acid. Arch. Derm. *107*, 113–114 (1973)

Keratosis Pilaris

Keratosis pilaris, in general, is a disorder of keratinization of the hair follicles. The follicular orifices are filled with horny material. The clinical manifestations are follicular papules, which are seen especially over the thighs and arms but may involve other parts of the body (Figs. 2.15 and 2.16). The disorder is present in a large proportion of the normal population but may also be seen in several ichthyotic conditions.

There are, however, several rare disorders that share the presence of lesions of keratosis pilaris but develop in addition early inflammation and later atrophy or scarring. The nomenclature of these disorders is very confusing. One may postulate that the various syndromes represent stages in a single process. It may be worthwhile to recognize three types that differ as to location, presence of papules, and prominence of atrophy.

Ulerythema Ophryogenes (Taenzer) (Keratosis Pilaris Atrophicans Faciei, Keratosis Pilaris Brocq)

Clinical Presentation. From birth or early infancy, erythema with or without follicular papules is present symmetrically on the outer parts of the eyebrows. The lesions extend medially very slowly, resulting in gradual thinning of the eyebrows. The remaining hairs may become atrophic. Occasionally, similar lesions may appear on the cheeks and forehead [1].

Pathology and Pathophysiology. There is hyperkeratosis, atrophy of the epidermis, and follicular plugging. Fibrotic changes appear around the follicles [1].

Inheritance. Autosomal dominant.

Treatment. None is available.

Atrophoderma Vermiculata (Acne Vermoulante, Folliculitis Ulerythematosa Reticulata, Honeycomb Atrophy)

Clinical Presentation. The onset is usually between the ages of 5 and 12 years. There is a symmetric eruption over the cheeks or preauricular areas. The eruption is of pinhead follicular plugs and erythema, leading to reticulate atrophy with pitlike depressions 1 mm deep. The affected cheeks appear waxy (Figs. 2.17 and 2.18). Telangiectasia may be present. Other areas that may be similarly affected are the forehead, upper lip, chin, and ears [2].

Pathology and Pathophysiology. The changes are similar to those of ulerythema ophryogenes.

Inheritance. Not definite. X-linked recessive is possible in certain families.

Treatment. None is available.

Keratosis Pilaris Decalvans (Ichthyosis Follicularis)

Clinical Presentation. Onset is in infancy with the appearance of keratosis pilarislike lesions over the face, scalp, and any or all other hairy areas [3] (Fig. 2.19).

Pathology and Pathophysiology. There is hyperkeratosis of the follicular openings and the intervening skin. The epidermis is flattened. The hair follicles are atrophic and sebaceous glands absent. Sweat glands are normal [3].

Inheritance. Not definite. X-linked recessive is possible in certain families.

Treatment. None is available.

References

1. Davenport, D.D.: Ulerythema ophryogenes. Review and report of a case. Discussion of relationship to certain other skin disorders and association with internal abnormalities. Arch. Derm. *89*, 74–80 (1964)
2. MacKee, G.M., Parounagian, M.B.: Folliculitis ulerythematosa reticulata. J. cut. Dis. *36*, 337 (1918)
3. Zeligman, I., Fleisher, T.L.: Ichthyosis follicularis. Arch. Derm. *80*, 413–420 (1959)

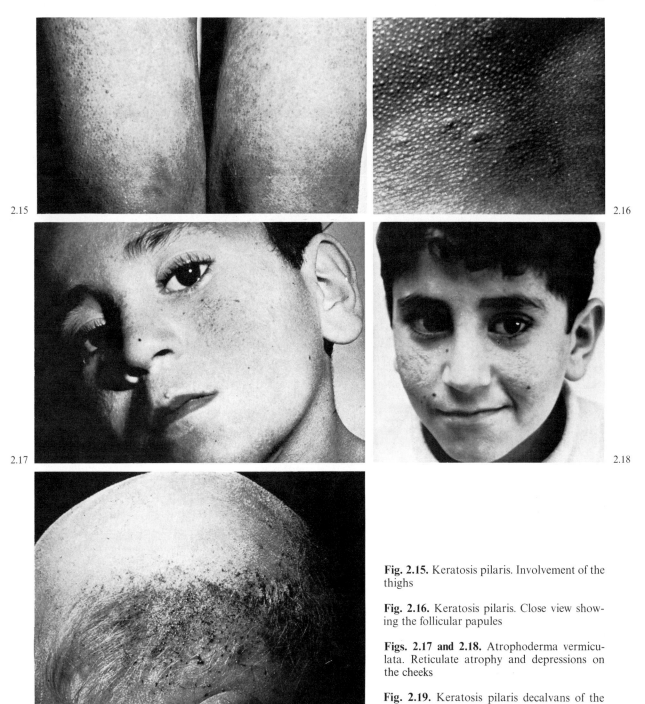

2.15

2.16

2.17

2.18

2.19

Fig. 2.15. Keratosis pilaris. Involvement of the thighs

Fig. 2.16. Keratosis pilaris. Close view showing the follicular papules

Figs. 2.17 and 2.18. Atrophoderma vermiculata. Reticulate atrophy and depressions on the cheeks

Fig. 2.19. Keratosis pilaris decalvans of the scalp

Keratosis Follicularis Spinulosa Decalvans cum Ophiasi

This is an extremely rare condition inherited as an X-linked dominant [1, 2]. Affected individuals have an ophiasic pattern of alopecia in one or more winding streaks on the scalp and sparse facial hair, eyebrows, and eyelashes. The skin of the neck, ears, eyelids, palms, and soles is thickened. Ectropion, photophobia, epiphora, and corneal degeneration (cloudiness and pannus) develop [1]. Affected females show an aborted form of the disease without hair loss or eye changes.

References

1. Jonkers, G.H.: Hyperkeratosis follicularis and corneal degeneration. Ophthalmologica (Basel) *120*, 365–367 (1950)
2. McKusick, V.A.: Mendelian inheritance in man, 5th ed., p. 776. Baltimore: Johns Hopkins University Press 1978

Ichthyosiform Dermatoses

Ichthyosiform dermatoses are inherited disorders of keratinization in which the skin is dry and covered by an accumulation of scales. Cellular kinetic studies and ultrastructural studies of the epidermis in these conditions have helped to formulate a logical and simplified classification of this group of dermatoses [1–3].

Normokinetic ichthyosis
   Ichthyosis vulgaris (autosomal dominant)
   X-linked ichthyosis (X-linked recessive)
Hyperkinetic ichthyosis
   Epidermolytic hyperkeratosis (autosomal dominant)
   Lamellar ichthyosis (autosomal recessive)
     Ichthyosiform erythrodermia
     Harlequin fetus
     Lamellar ichthyosis of the newborn
     Collodion baby
Associated with other defects
   Unilateral Ichthyosiform Erythrodermia with Ipsilateral Malformations
   Ichthyosiform Erythrodermia and Deafness
   Ichthyosis and Cataract
   Ichthyosis with Biliary Atresia
   Ichthyosis with Neutrophil Chemotactic Defect
   Ichthyosis, mental retardation, dwarfism, and renal impairment
   Ichthyosiform dermatosis with systemic lipidosis
   Ichthyosis linearis circumflexa (see p. 34)
   Sjögren-Larsson syndrome (see p. 34)
   Refsum disease (see p. 37)
   Chondrodysplasia punctata (see p. 37)
     Conradi-Hünerman type (autosomal dominant) (see p. 37)
     Severe rhizomelic type (autosomal recessive) (see p. 38)
   Netherton syndrome (see p. 40)

Normokinetic Ichthyosis

Ichthyosis Vulgaris (Ichthyosis Simplex)

Clinical Presentation. This is the mildest and commonest form of ichthyosiform dermatoses. The disorder becomes manifest in childhood between the ages of 1 and 4 years. The scales are fine and flaky but may be larger over the legs. The extensors of the arms and legs are more severely involved while the flexures are usually free (Figs. 2.20–2.22). Follicular hyperkeratosis, especially of the arms and thighs, may be prominent. The face may be involved in childhood but clears later. There is accentuation of the palmar and plantar markings. Manifestations of atopy may be present. The eruption is worse in cold weather and improves in the warmer months. With puberty there is usually improvement.

A bullous variety (ichthyosis, bullous type) has been described in one family [4]. Histologically, it is similar to ichthyosis vulgaris and is probably inherited as autosomal dominant. It is regarded as a separate entity [5].

Pathology and Pathophysiology. Characteristically, there is moderate hyperkeratosis with an attenuated or absent granular cell layer. Occasionally, there may be follicular plugging [6]. Sebaceous glands are small or absent. The dermis shows a sparse lymphohistiocytic perivascular and periappendageal infiltrate [7]. Kinetic studies reveal normal mitotic activity and transit time. Ultrastructurally, the epidermis may be normal or show minimal changes: lack of orientation of the tonofilaments, reduced or abnormal keratohyalin granule synthesis, and increased ribosomal activity. The defect does not seem to be that of overproduction of keratin but rather a possible increased adhesiveness of the scales. Transepidermal water loss is significantly increased [8]. In ichthyosis vulgaris the skin surface pH is higher and the alkali resistance is lower than in healthy skin [9].

Inheritance. Autosomal dominant.

Treatment. The time-honored modalities of treatment are removal of scales (with keratolytic agents and mechanically) and the use of emollients, especially after the skin is moistened. Salicylic acid (6% in propylene glycol, ethanol, and water) was found effective [10]. Similarly, a cream containing 10% urea in an emulsified base controlled the scaliness [11]. More recently, topically applied α-hydroxy acids (lactic and malic acids) were shown to influence the process of keratinization. Such acids, in a 5% concentration in hydrophilic ointment, are effective in ichthyosis vulgaris [12].

Figs. 2.20 and 2.21. Ichthyosis vulgaris. Note fine, flaky scales

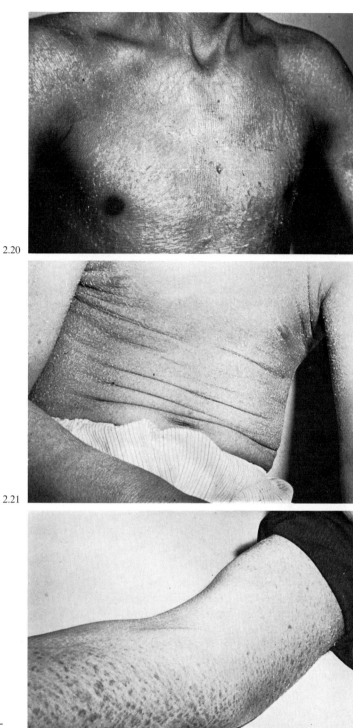

2.20

2.21

Fig. 2.22. Ichthyosis vulgaris. Note involvement of the extensor surfaces and sparing of the flexors

X-Linked Ichthyosis

In essence, the clinical appearance resembles that of ichthyosis vulgaris.

Clinical Presentation. Only males are affected and the onset is in early infancy. The involvement is generalized but is most prominent over the trunk (especially the back), neck, face, and extremities. The flexural surfaces may occasionally be affected, but the palms and soles are free. The scales are brown, thick, and large. In heterozygote females there may be scaliness of the legs (Figs. 2.23–2.25).

Pathology and Pathophysiology. There is compact hyperkeratosis with a nearly normal granular cell layer. There is no follicular plugging [6]. The adnexal structures are within normal limits [7]. The dermis may show a minimal inflammatory infiltrate. Kinetic and ultrastructural studies are similar to those of ichthyosis vulgaris.

Inheritance. X-linked recessive.

Treatment. For general measures see also ichthyosis vulgaris above. Salicylic acid (6% in a mixture of propylene glycol, ethanol, and water [10]) is quite helpful. The topical use of α-hydroxy acids in a hydrophilic base [12] may also be effective. Oral retinoic acid is also helpful [13].

Hyperkinetic Ichthyosis

Epidermolytic Hyperkeratosis (Bullous Ichthyosiform Erythrodermia)

Clinical Presentation. Within the first few weeks of life generalized erythema and scaliness appear. There is shedding of extensive areas of the superficial epidermis leaving moist, raw areas. The erythema gradually subsides. The desquamation, which initially is of fine scales, becomes thick and brown. In the flexures and intertriginous areas the scales assume a verrucous, streaky appearance. From the onset tiny vesicles and larger flaccid bullae appear. The bullae gradually decrease and may cease to appear. However, in about 20% of cases they persist into adult life (Figs. 2.26–2.29).

In some cases, there is a bandlike verrucous lesion (epidermal or linear nevus) that has a histologic picture identical with that of generalized epidermolytic hyperkeratosis [14, 15]. This condition may be considered as a forme fruste of the generalized form. Occasionally the epidermal nevus has

widespread lesions (porcupine man-Lambert family). Associated defects are unusual and life expectancy is normal.

Pathology and Pathophysiology. Characteristically, there is marked compact hyperkeratosis overlying a granular degeneration in the epidermis. In the granular and upper prickle cell layers there are clear spaces around the nuclei, indistinct cellular boundaries, and a thick granular zone with increased, irregular-shaped, basophilic keratohyalinlike and eosinophilic trichohyalinlike bodies [2, 16]. Increased mitotic activity and a rapid cell transit rate have been noted [1]. Ultrastructural studies reveal large areas of perinuclear endoplasmic reticulum filled with ribosomes, mitochondria, and keratinosomes. The tonofilaments are clumped and their association with desmosomes is disturbed. This leads to acantholysis and thus blister formation [17]. However, some investigators believe that these represent a manifestation of staphylococcal impetigo [1]. This may also explain the malodor frequently associated with this condition.

Inheritance. Autosomal dominant.

Treatment. Other than the general use of emollients and keratolytic agents, the use of antibiotics and chemotherapeutic agents to combat the frequent bacterial colonization of the skin is indicated. The use of α-hydroxy acids (especially pyruvic acid) in a hydrophilic ointment is helpful [12]. Topical tretinoin (vitamin A acid) in a concentration of 0.05–0.1% in either alcohol-polyethylene glycol or cream base is effective for symptomatic clearance of the skin [18].

Lamellar Ichthyosis

This is a spectrum of disorders varying in severity but sharing the same mode of inheritance as well as histologic and ultrastructural features.

Ichthyosiform Erythrodermia

This disorder appears at birth, usually with a mild generalized erythema. The skin appears thick and later becomes scaly. The scales are coarse, centrally attached, and more prominent in the flexures (Figs. 2.30 and 2.31). The condition usually lasts throughout life. There is moderate palmoplantar hyperkeratosis. Ectropion is a common finding [19] (Fig. 2.32).

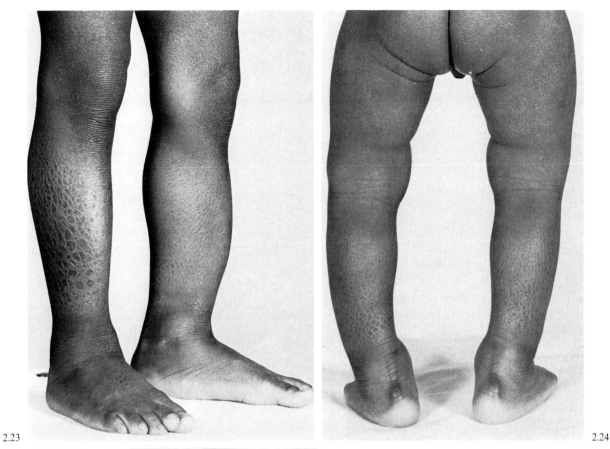

2.23   2.24

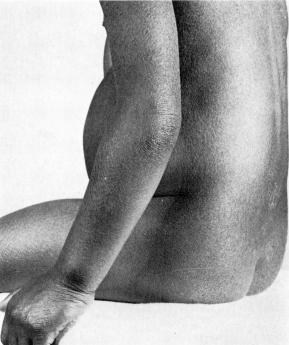

Figs. 2.23–2.25. X-linked ichthyosis. (Courtesy of
Dr. V. A. McKusick. Fig. 25 from Scott, C.I. In: The
clinical delineation of birth defects. Bergsma, D. (ed.),
Vol. VII, No. 8, pt. XII, pp. 243–244. Baltimore:
Williams & Wilkins Co. 1971)

2.25

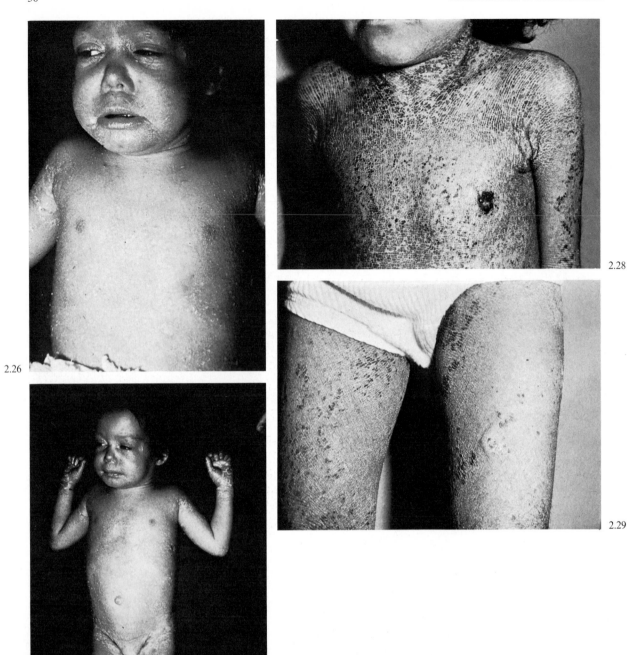

2.26

2.27

2.28

2.29

Figs. 2.26 and 2.27. Epidermolytic hyperkeratosis. Generalized erythema and scaliness with raw areas in axillae and groin

Figs. 2.28 and 2.29. Epidermolytic hyperkeratosis. Thick brown scales. Note bulla on left thigh

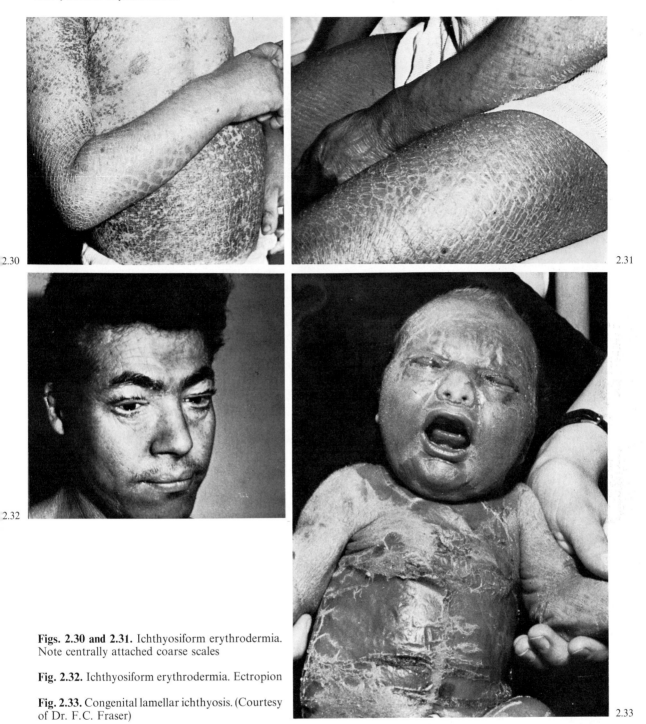

2.30

2.31

2.32

2.33

Figs. 2.30 and 2.31. Ichthyosiform erythrodermia. Note centrally attached coarse scales

Fig. 2.32. Ichthyosiform erythrodermia. Ectropion

Fig. 2.33. Congenital lamellar ichthyosis. (Courtesy of Dr. F.C. Fraser)

Harlequin Fetus (Ichthyosis Fetalis,
Keratome Malignum, Ichthyosis Congenita)

This probably represents a more severe form of
ichthyosiform erythrodermia. The fetus is usually
born prematurely, encased in a thick, horny skin
which appears white initially but within hours
becomes grayish yellow. The thick armorlike skin
splits by deep fissures into polygonal plates. Blood-
stained discharge oozes from the fissures. Vital
respiratory movements are restricted. Secondary
infection and septicemia are frequent complications.
Death is usual in the first few days of life.

Lamellar Ichthyosis of the Newborn

This is the mildest form. The baby is born with a
constricting, parchmentlike collodion membrane
due to the thick stratum corneum (Fig. 2.33). The
membrane usually undergoes peeling within 24 h
and large keratinous sheets are cast off. Recovery is
complete [20].

Collodion Baby

Clinical Presentation. This is not a disease entity but
a condition seen in several ichthyosiform disorders:
epidermolytic hyperkeratosis, ichthyosiform erythrodermia, and X-linked ichthyosis [20]. The infant is
completely enveloped in a thin, dry, shining, brownish yellow layer, perforated with hairs. Shortly after
birth it fissures and peels off leaving a normal-
appearing skin. The skin may persist as normal or
may continue to scale depending on the underlying
ichthyotic disorder.

Pathology and Pathophysiology. In lamellar ichthyosis there is marked hyperkeratosis with a normal or thickened granular cell layer. There may be
acanthosis, follicular plugging, and prominent rete
ridges. The upper dermal vessels are surrounded by
minimal mononuclear infiltrate.
Mitotic activity in the epidermis is increased and cell
transit time is reduced [3]. Ultrastructurally, there is
early development and increased numbers of keratinosomes, and persistence of mitochondria and
nucleated cells high in the granular cell layer [21].
The desmosomes and tonofilaments are normal [1].

Inheritance. Autosomal recessive.

Treatment. In general, emollients and keratolytic
agents are helpful. There is a moderate response to

6 % salicylic acid in propylene glycol under occlusion
[10]. On the other hand, topical tretinoin (vitamin A
acid) [22] and α-hydroxy acids (citric and lactic
acids) [12] have been effective in clearing the skin.
Orally administered 13-*cis* retinoic acid has been
helpful [13].

Associated with Other Defects

Unilateral Ichthyosiform Erythrodermia
with Ipsilateral Malformations

There is a strikingly unilateral distribution of an
erythematous dermatosis associated with hypoplasia or aplasia of bony structures on the same
side. The brain is similarly affected [23]. On the
basis of histologic and kinetic studies it has been
suggested that the dermatosis may be psoriatic
rather than ichthyotic [24]. Inheritance in this
syndrome is autosomal recessive.

Ichthyosiform Erythrodermia and Deafness

In three sibs, ichthyosiform erythrodermia (non-
bullous) associated with deafness has been reported
[25]. Hepatomegaly is present in affected individuals. Inheritance is probably autosomal recessive.

Ichthyosis and Cataract

Cortical cataracts have been described in association
with congenital ichthyosis (lamellar ichthyosis) [26].
Inheritance in this syndrome is autosomal recessive.

Ichthyosis with Biliary Atresia

Two sibs have been described with this combination [27].

Ichthyosis with Neutrophil Chemotactic Defect

In two kindreds affected with "congenital ichthyosis
vulgaris," chemotaxis of leukocytes from the patients (who also had recurrent *Trichophyton rubrum*
infections) and their fathers was defective [28]. This
syndrome is probably inherited as autosomal dominant (see also p. 158).

Ichthyosis and Male Hypogonadism

In one kindred, five males in three generations had congenital ichthyosis and secondary hypogonadism [29]. This syndrome may represent close linkage between hypogonadism and X-linked ichthyosis or more probably a separate mutation that is X-linked recessive [30].

Ichthyosis, Mental Retardation, Dwarfism, and Renal Impairment

Three siblings of unrelated parents exhibited these abnormalities [31]. An autosomal recessive pattern of inheritance is suspected.

Ichthyosiform Dermatosis with Systemic Lipidosis

The skin changes are associated with lipid vacuolation in peripheral blood granulocytes and granulocyte precursors in the marrow and liver [32]. Autosomal recessive inheritance is suggested.

References

1. Frost, P., Van Scott, E.J.: Ichthyosiform dermatoses. Classification based on anatomic and biometric observations. Arch. Derm. 94, 113–126 (1966)
2. Wilgram, G.E., Caulfield, J.B.: An electron microscopic study of epidermolytic hyperkeratosis. Arch. Derm. 94, 127–143 (1966)
3. Frost, P., Weinstein, G.D., Van Scott, E.J.: The ichthyosiform dermatoses. II. Autoradiographic studies of epidermal proliferation. J. invest. Derm. 47, 561–567 (1966)
4. Siemens, H.W.: Dichtung und Wahrheit über die Ichthyosis bullosa mit Bemerkungen zur Systematik der Epidermolysen. Arch. Derm. Syph. (Berl.) 175, 590–608 (1937)
5. Schnyder, U.W.: Inherited ichthyoses. Arch. Derm. 102, 240–252 (1970)
6. Wells, R.S., Kerr, C.B.: The histology of ichthyosis. J. invest. Derm. 46, 530–535 (1966)
7. Feinstein, A., Ackerman, A.B., Ziprkowski, L.: Histology of autosomal dominant ichthyosis vulgaris and X-linked ichthyosis. Arch. Derm. 101, 524–527 (1970)
8. Frost, P., Weinstein, G.D., Bothwell, J.W., Wildnauer, R.: Ichthyosiform dermatoses. III. Studies of transepidermal water loss. Arch. Derm. 98, 230–233 (1968)
9. Tippelt, H.: Zur Hautoberflächen-pH-Messung und Alkali-resistenzprobe bei Hautgesunden und Ichthyosis vulgaris-Kranken. Dermatologica (Basel) 139, 201–210 (1969)
10. Baden, H.P., Alper, J.C.: A keratolytic gel containing salicylic acid in propylene glycol. J. invest. Derm. 61, 330–333 (1973)
11. Pope, F.M., Rees, J.K., Wells, R.S., Lewis, K.G.S.: Outpatient treatment of ichthyosis: a double-blind trial of ointments. Brit. J. Derm. 86, 291–296 (1972)
12. Van Scott, E.J., Yu, R.J.: Control of keratinization with α-hydroxy acids and related compounds. I. Topical treatment of ichthyotic disorders. Arch. Derm. 110, 586–590 (1974)
13. Peck, G.L., Yoder, F.W.: Treatment of lamellar ichthyosis and other keratinizing dermatoses with an oral synthetic retinoid. Lancet 1976 II, 1172–1174

14. Zeligman, I., Pomeranz, J.: Variations of congenital ichthyosiform erythroderma. Report of cases of ichthyosis hystrix and nevus unius lateris. Arch. Derm. 91, 120–125 (1965)
15. Kurban, A.K., Petzoldt, D.: Systematisierter naevus verrucosus mit granulöser Degeneration. Derm. Wschr. 153, 1129–1132 (1967)
16. Ackerman, A.B.: Histopathologic concept of epidermolytic hyperkeratosis. Arch. Derm. 102, 253–259 (1970)
17. Anton-Lamprecht, I., Schnyder, U.W.: Ultrastructure of inborn errors of keratinization. VI. Inherited ichthyoses – a model system for heterogeneities in keratinization disturbances. Arch. Derm. Forsch. 250(3), 207–227 (1974)
18. Schorr, W.F., Papa, C.M.: Epidermolytic hyperkeratosis. Effect of tretinoin therapy on the clinical course and the basic defects in the stratum corneum. Arch. Derm. 107, 556–562 (1973)
19. Sever, R.J., Frost, P., Weinstein, G.: Eye changes in ichthyosis. J. Amer. med. Ass. 206, 2283–2286 (1968)
20. Reed, W.B., Herwick, R.P., Harville, D., Porter, P.S., Conant, M.: Lamellar ichthyosis of the newborn. A distinct clinical entity: its comparison to the other ichthyosiform erythrodermas. Arch. Derm. 105, 394–399 (1972)
21. Vandersteen, P.R., Muller, S.A.: Lamellar ichthyosis. An enzyme histochemical, light, and electron microscopic study. Arch. Derm. 106, 694–701 (1972)
22. Mirrer, E., McGuire, J.: Lamellar ichthyosis – response to retinoic acid (tretinoin). Arch. Derm. 102, 548–551 (1970)
23. Cullen, S.I., Harris, D.E., Carter, C.H., Reed, W.B.: Congenital unilateral ichthyosiform erythroderma. Arch. Derm. 99, 724–729 (1969)
24. Shear, C.S., Nyhan, W.L., Frost, P., Weinstein, G.D.: Syndrome of unilateral ectromelia, psoriasis, and central nervous system anomalies. In: The clinical delineation of birth defects. Bergsma, D. (ed.), Vol. VII, No. 8, pt. XII, pp. 197–293. Baltimore: Williams & Wilkins Co. 1971
25. Desmons, F., Bar, J., Chevillard, Y.: Érythrodermie ichthyosiforme congénitale sèche, surdi-mutité, hépatomégalie, de transmission récessive autosomique. Étude d'une famille. Bull. Soc. franç. Derm. Syph. 78, 585–591 (1971)
26. Pinkerton, O.D.: Cataract associated with congenital ichthyosis. Arch. Ophthal. 60, 393–396 (1958)
27. Gould, A.A.: Ichthyosis in an infant: hemorrhage from umbelicus: death. Amer. J. med. Sci. 27, 356 (1854)
28. Miller, M.E., Norman, M.E., Koblenzer, P.J., Schonauer, T.: A new defect of neutrophil movement. J. lab. clin. Med. 82, 1–8 (1973)
29. Lynch, H.T., Ozer, F., McNutt, C.W., Johnson, J.E., Jampolsky, N.A.: Secondary male hypogonadism and congenital ichthyosis. Association of two rare genetic diseases. Amer. J. hum. Genet. 12, 440–447 (1960)
30. McKusick, V.A.: Mendelian inheritance in man, 5th ed., p. 773. Baltimore: Johns Hopkins University Press 1978
31. Passwell, J.H., Goodman, R.M., Ziprkowski, M., Cohen, B.E.: Congenital ichthyosis, mental retardation, dwarfism and renal impairment: new syndrome. Clin. Genet. 8, 59–65 (1975)
32. Dorfman, M.L., Hershko, C., Eisenberg, S., Sagher, F.: Ichthyosiform dermatosis with systemic lipidosis. Arch. Derm. 110, 261–266 (1974)

Ichthyosis Linearis Circumflexa

Comel was the first to designate this rare disorder in 1949 [1].

Clinical Presentation. Onset is at birth or during the first few months of life [2]. There is initially a diffuse erythema and scaliness. Gradually, the characteristic eruption evolves over the trunk and proximal extremities as polycyclic, migratory, serpiginous erythematous plaques [2, 3]. The periphery shows a distinctive double-edged scale. The face, and occasionally the scalp, may remain erythematous and scaly. There is lichenification of the antecubital and popliteal fossae (Figs. 2.34–2.36).
Hair abnormalities are frequently associated with this disorder. Of 15 patients with trichorrhexis invaginata, 12 had ichthyosis linearis circumflexa [3]. Other reported hair abnormalities are trichorrhexis nodosa, pili torti, and fragile hair. Hyperhidrosis is an inconstant finding [2]. Atopy and aminoaciduria may be present [3].

Pathology and Pathophysiology. There is parakeratosis and acanthosis [2, 3]. The granular cell layer may be accentuated [2]. In the dermis there is a mild perivascular inflammatory infiltrate.
The relationship between ichthyosis linearis circumflexa and Netherton syndrome (see p. 40) is still controversial. It has been proposed that these two entities be considered as one, manifesting as a peculiar defect in keratinization affecting the skin and hair [4]. However, an analysis of findings in patients with structural abnormalities of the hair and ichthyotic skin changes has shown that a variety of combinations exists [3]. It is thus suggested that the two entities remain separate until there is a better understanding of the relationship between ichthyosis linearis circumflexa and other ichthyoses [3].

Inheritance. Probably autosomal recessive.

Treatment. Lubrication of the skin and oral vitamin A (150,000 units daily) result in gradual improvement [2].

References

1. Comel, M.: Ichthyosis linearis circumflexa. Dermatologica (Basel) *98*, 133–136 (1949)
2. Vineyard, W.R., Lumpkin, L.R., Lawler, J.C.: Ichthyosis linearis circumflexa. A variant of congenital ichthyosiform erythroderma. Arch. Derm. *83*, 630–635 (1961)
3. Hurwitz, S., Kirsch, N., McGuire, J.: Reevaluation of ichthyosis and hair shaft abnormalities. Arch. Derm. *103*, 266–271 (1971)
4. Altman, J., Stroud, J.: Netherton's syndrome and ichthyosis linearis circumflexa. Psoriasiform ichthyosis. Arch. Derm. *100*, 550–558 (1969)

Sjögren-Larsson Syndrome

Even though Pardo-Castello and Faz [1] described the association of mental deficiency, ichthyosis, and Little disease in 1932, it was Sjögren and Larsson [2] who, in 1957, delineated this heritable disorder now known by their names.

Clinical Presentation. The skin changes are those of ichthyosiform erythrodermia (lamellar ichthyosis) (Figs. 2.37 and 2.38). These changes are associated with marked mental deficiency and cerebral spastic diplegia (of Little disease type). The spasticity is more marked in the lower extremities with partial contractures (scissor gait). Other features that may be present are dental and osseous dysplasia [3, 4], epilepsy [2, 5], retinal macular degeneration [2, 5, 6], aminoaciduria [3], dysarthria and dysphonia [2, 4], hypertelorism [4], dermatoglyphic abnormalities [4], and exudative enteropathy [7].

Pathology and Pathophysiology. The only documented studies are those of the skin. The changes are characteristic of congenital ichthyosiform erythrodermia.

Inheritance. Autosomal recessive. Formes frustes exist in relatives of patients. In such cases, the only manifestation may be mental retardation with or without spasticity [4].

Treatment. Topical treatment for the skin changes is as described under Lamellar Ichthyosis (see p. 32).

References

1. Pardo-Castello, V., Faz, H.: Ichthyosis-Little's disease. Arch. Derm. Syph. *26*, 915 (1932)
2. Sjögren, T., Larsson, T.: Oligophrenia in combination with congenital ichthyosis and spastic disorders; a clinical and genetic study. Acta psychiat. scand. *32*, Suppl. 113, 1–112 (1957)
3. Williams, R.D.B., Tang, I.L.: Mental defect, quadriplegia and ichthyosis. Report of two cases in one family and a review of the literature. Amer. J. Dis. Child. *100*, 924–929 (1960)
4. Selmanowitz, V.J., Porter, M.J.: Sjögren-Larsson syndrome. Amer. J. Med. *42*, 412–422 (1967)
5. Heijer, A., Reed, W.B.: Sjögren-Larsson syndrome. Congenital ichthyosis, spastic paralysis, and oligophrenia. Arch. Derm. *92*, 545–552 (1965)
6. Gilbert, W.R., Jr., Smith, J.L., Nyhan, W.L.: The Sjögren-Larsson syndrome. Arch. Ophthal. *80*, 308–316 (1968)
7. Hooft, C., Kriekemans, J., van Aker, K., Devos, E., Traen, S., Verdonk, G.: Sjögren-Larsson syndrome with exudative enteropathy. Influence of medium-chain triglycerides on the symptomatology. Helv. paediat. Acta *22*, 447–458 (1967)

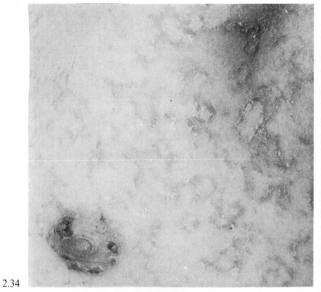

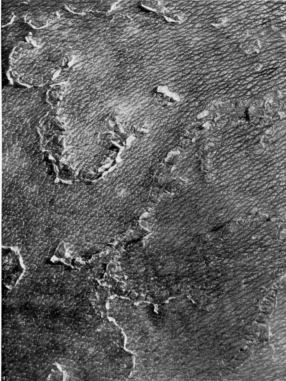

2.34

2.35

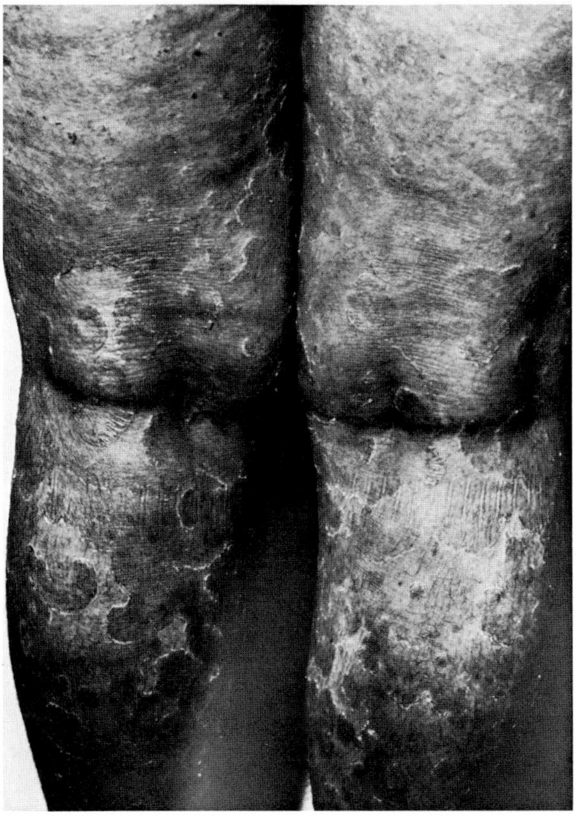

2.36

Figs. 2.34–2.36. Ichthyosis linearis circumflexa

Fig. 2.34. Polycyclic, migratory, serpiginous erythematous eruption. (Courtesy of Dr. W. R. Vineyard)

Fig. 2.35. Note the double-edged scale at the periphery. (From Altman, J., Stroud, J.: Arch. Derm. *100*, 550–558, 1969)

Fig. 2.36. Extensive eruption over the lower extremities. (From Altman, J., Stroud, J.: Arch. Derm. *100*, 550–558, 1969)

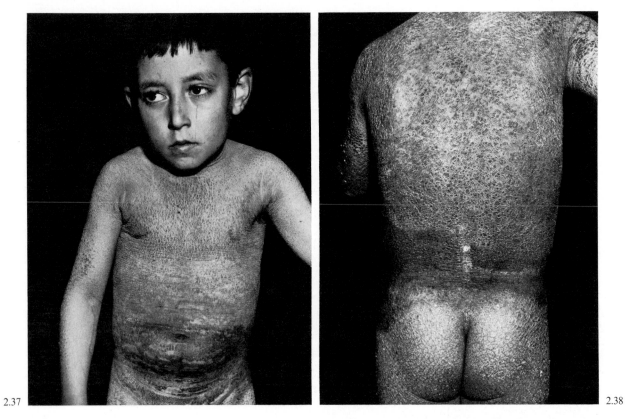

2.37   2.38

Figs. 2.37 and 2.38. Sjögren-Larsson syndrome. Extensive skin involvement. (Courtesy of Dr. A. Sinno)

Refsum Disease
(Heredopathia Atactica Polyneuritiformis)

In 1945 and 1946 Refsum described in a Norwegian community [1] the association of ichthyotic skin changes with retinitis pigmentosa, cerebellar ataxia, and a polyneuritislike condition.

Clinical Presentation. The onset is between the ages of 4 and 7 years and is manifested by anorexia, an unsteady gait, ichthyosis, and progressive neurogenic hearing loss. Funduscopy reveals pigmentary changes in the retina. The patients have night blindness and concentric limitation of the field of vision [1]. There are other cerebellar manifestations as well as a polyneuritislike condition with loss of the deep reflexes, progressive paresis of the limbs distally, and ataxia. There is no mental deficiency. In all patients there is, characteristically, a marked increase in cerebrospinal protein without pleocytosis [1]. Electrocardiographic abnormalities noted in these patients include prolongation of QT and PQ intervals [1].

Pathology and Pathophysiology. The inherited defect is that of storage of the branched-chain fatty acid, phytanic acid (3,7,11,15-tetramethyl-hexadecanoic acid), in the blood and tissues. The defect leading to the storage is in the oxidative pathway for degradation of exogenous phytanic acid and has been characterized as a deficiency in a single enzyme involved in the α-hydroxylation of phytanate, while the enzymes in later steps are present at normal levels [2].
The relationship between phytanate accumulation and the symptoms of Refsum disease is unclear. The displacement of normal structural fatty acids by excess phytanate or a crucial metabolic effect on nervous tissue due to the absence of α-hydroxylating enzyme are postulates to explain the different manifestations. It could still be that the enzymatic biochemical abnormality is not directly responsible for the clinical picture [2].
The diagnosis can be established by detection, in fibroblast culture, of the enzymatic deficiency in phytanate metabolism [2].

Inheritance. Autosomal recessive.

Treatment. The elimination of phytol from the diet leads to clinical improvement [3].

References

1. Refsum, S., Salomonsen, L., Skatvedt, M.: Heredopathia atactica polyneuritiformis in children. J. Pediat. *35*, 335–343 (1949)
2. Herndon, J.H., Jr., Steinberg, D., Uhlendorf, W., Fales, H.M.: Refsum's disease: characterization of the enzyme defect in cell culture. J. clin. Invest. *48*, 1017–1032 (1969)
3. Steinberg, D., Mize, C.E., Herndon, J.H., Jr., Fales, H.M., Engel, W.K., Vroom, F.Q.: Phytanic acid in patients with Refsum's syndrome and response to dietary treatment. Arch. intern. Med. *125*, 75–87 (1970)

Chondrodysplasia Punctata

Conradi-Hünerman Type (Autosomal Dominant)

This rare multisystem disease was first described by Conradi in 1914 [1].

Clinical Presentation. The disorder affects the skeleton, brain, eyes, and skin. The onset is within the first few months of life. The skin changes are found in a high proportion (28%) of affected individuals. The skin is shiny red with rough, dry, whitish adherent scales arranged in a whorl pattern [2]. In most reports the changes are described as resembling ichthyosiform erythrodermia, although occasionally they may resemble pityriasis rubra pilaris [3]. Thickening of the palms and soles may be present. The skin changes, in general, tend to clear spontaneously leaving follicular atrophoderma, especially over the extremities (Fig. 2.39), and cicatricial alopecia (Figs. 2.40 and 2.41). The hair may be coarse, lusterless, sparse, and of irregular diameter. Other skin manifestations are incontinentia pigmentilike pigmentation, seborrheic dermatitis, and dyskeratosis [4].
The affected children are dwarfed, with short limbs, swollen joints, saddle nose, and vertebral abnormalities (Figs. 2.41a and 2.41b). Characteristically, there is stippling of the epiphyses of the bones which develop enchondral ossification. This stippling usually disappears by the age of 3 years. Other skeletal abnormalities are congenital dislocation of the hip, high-arched palate, frontal bossing, craniosynostosis, micro- or macrocephaly, hypertelorism, micrognathia, syndactyly, and clubfoot [4]. Oligophrenia is not infrequent. The ocular manifestations are bilateral cataracts (in 17% of cases) and primary optic atrophy [5]. Other less frequent manifestations are cardiac and gastrointestinal abnormalities [5], involvement of membranous bones [5], aminoaciduria [4], and hypercholesterolemia [5].

Pathology and Pathophysiology. The cutaneous lesions show dyskeratosis. In other tissues, there may be focal mucoid degeneration. In the epiphyseal region, there is disorganization of the cartilage cells and of the process of calcification in areas of enchondral ossification.

Inheritance. Autosomal dominant with variance in expression [6]. Many cases present fresh gene mutations. An X-linked dominant type which is lethal in males has also been described [7]. The features resemble those of the dominant type with the addition of widespread atrophic and pigmented dermal lesions.

Treatment. None is available.

Severe Rhizomelic Type (Autosomal Recessive)

Clinical Presentation. This is a very rare disease. Marked symmetrical shortening of the limbs (rhizomelia) is a significant feature. The changes involve mostly the humeri. Lenticular cataracts are present in 72% of cases. Skin changes (ichthyosiform) occur in 27% of cases. The digits are stubby. There is limitation of movement at the joints with flexion contractures, particularly of the hips, knees, and elbows. Tracheal stenosis may be present. Death from respiratory complications usually takes place during the first year of life [6, 8, 9].

As in the autosomal dominant form, the epiphyses are stippled. However, in this recessive form the spine is only mildly involved and there are areas of calcification outside the margins of the epiphyses, as well as fraying of the metaphyses and coronal cleft in the vertebral bodies [10].

It is worth mentioning that punctate intra- and extracartilaginous calcifications may be found in a variety of hereditary (e.g., Zellweger syndrome) and nonhereditary conditions [2]. A disorder simulating chondrodysplasia punctata is produced by maternal ingestion of anticoagulant (Dicumarol or warfarin) in early pregnancy [11].

References

1. Conradi, E.: Vorzeitiges Auftreten von Knochen und eigenartigen Verkalkungskernen bei Chondrodystrophia fötalis hypoplastica: Histologische und Röntgenuntersuchungen. Jb. Kinderheilk. *80*, 86–97 (1914)
2. Bodian, E.L.: Skin manifestations of Conradi's disease. Chondrodystrophia congenita punctata. Arch. Derm. *94*, 743–748 (1966)
3. Moynahan, E.J.: Genetically determined diseases. In: Recent advances in dermatology. Rook, A. (ed.), No. 3, pp. 323–371. London: Churchill Livingstone 1973
4. Comings, D.E., Papazian, C., Schoene, H.R.: Conradi's disease. Chondrodystrophia calcificans congenita, congenital stippled epiphyses. J. Pediat. *72*, 63–69 (1968)
5. Armaly, M.F.: Ocular involvement in chondrodystrophia calcificans congenita punctata. Arch. Ophthal. *57*, 491–502 (1957)
6. Spranger, J.W., Opitz, J.M., Bidder, U.: Heterogeneity of chondrodysplasia punctata. Humangenetik *20*, 190–212 (1971)
7. Happle, R., Matthiass, H.H., Macher, E.: Sex-linked chondrodysplasia punctata? Clinical Genetics *11*, 73–76 (1977)
8. Fraser, F.C., Scriver, J.B.: A hereditary factor in chondrodystrophia calcificans congenita. New Engl. J. Med. *250*, 272–277 (1954)
9. Beighton, P.: Inherited disorders of the skeleton, pp. 18–21. Edinburgh: Churchill Livingstone 1978
10. Gilbert, E.F., Opitz, J.M., Spranger, J.W., Langer, L.O., Wolgson, J.J., Visekul, C.: Chondrodystrophia punctata-rhizomelic form. Pathologic and radiologic studies of three infants. Eur. J. Pediat. *123*, 89–109 (1976)
11. Pauli, M.P., Madden, J.D., Kranzler, K.J., Culpepper, W., Port, R.: Warfarin therapy initiated during pregnancy and phenotypic chondrodysplasia punctata. J. Pediat. *88*, 506–508 (1976)

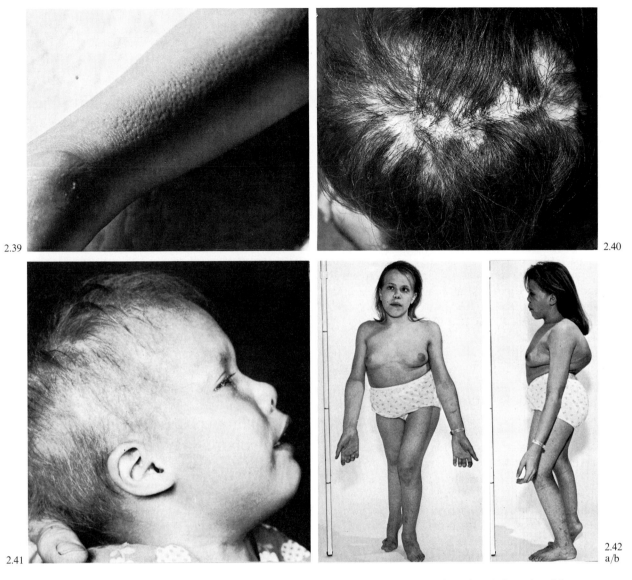

Figs. 2.39–2.42. Chondrodysplasia congenita (Conradi disease)

Fig. 2.39. Follicular atrophoderma. (From Comings, D. E., et al.: J. Pediat. *72*, 63–69, 1968)

Fig. 2.40. Cicatricial alopecia. (From Comings, D.E., et al.: J. Pediat. *72*, 63–69, 1968)

Fig. 2.41. Note sparse, lusterless hair and saddle nose. (Courtesy of Dr. V. A. McKusick, from Scott, C.I.: In: The clinical delineation of birth defects. Bergsma, D. (ed.), Vol. VII, No. 8, pt. XII, p. 309. Baltimore: Williams & Wilkins Co. 1971)

Fig. 2.42a/b. General view of patient. Note short stature, short right femur, kyphoscoliosis, and saddle nose. (From Comings, D.E., et al.: J. Pediat. *72*, 63–69, 1968)

Netherton Syndrome
(Trichorrhexis Invaginata)

In 1958 Netherton [1] described the first case of this syndrome which is characterized by bamboo hair (trichorrhexis invaginata), an ichthyotic skin condition, and, frequently, an atopic diathesis.

Clinical Presentation. The hair is short, dry, and lusterless (Fig. 2.43). The hair abnormality is the most distinctive feature and affects particularly the scalp hair and eyebrows. The "bamboo" defect is seen in all terminal scalp hair. The cup portion of the defect is formed by the proximal portion of the hair shaft and the ball portion by the distal end [2]. The defect is seen in all stages from the abrupt stricture to the fully developed nodes. In addition there may be changes in caliber, as well as transverse linear alterations in the shaft [3]. Vellus hair shows similar but milder defects. The hair abnormality improves with age.

In the majority of patients, the ichthyotic skin changes are those of ichthyosis linearis circumflexa [4] (see p. 34), which is considered a variant of congenital ichthyosiform erythrodermia or lamellar ichthyosis [2, 3] (Figs. 2.44 and 2.45). However, some investigators distinguish a peculiar form of ichthyotic skin changes designated as "psoriasiform ichthyosis" [5], while others associate the distinctive hair abnormalities with a variety of ichthyotic changes [6–8].

Most patients with Netherton syndrome have an atopic diathesis such as urticaria, angioedema, and asthma. Aminoaciduria and hypogammaglobulinemia have been reported in a few patients [2].

Pathology and Pathophysiology. The skin changes are characterized by parakeratosis and acanthosis, with elongated rete ridges and an increased granular cell layer [5]. Plucked hairs may show the bamboo defect (Fig. 2.46), whereas biopsies of the scalp demonstrate the defect at all levels from the surface to the zone of incipient keratinization [2]. It is suggested that a defect in keratinization is responsible for the skin and hair abnormalities.

Inheritance. Autosomal recessive with greater penetrance in females. Occasionally males may be affected [9].

Treatment. The hair changes improve with age. Emollients may be helpful for the skin condition.

References

1. Netherton, E. W.: A unique case of trichorrhexis nodosa – "bamboo hairs". Arch. Derm. *78*, 483–487 (1958)
2. Wilkinson, R.D., Curtis, G.H., Hawk, W.A.: Netherton's disease. Trichorrhexis invaginata (bamboo hair), congenital ichthyosiform erythroderma, and the atopic diathesis. A histopathologic study. Arch. Derm. *89*, 46–54 (1964)
3. Stevanović, D.V.: Multiple defects of the hair shaft in Netherton's disease. Association with ichthyosis linearis circumflexa. Brit. J. Derm. *81*, 851–857 (1969)
4. Price, V.H.: Office diagnosis of structural hair anomalies. Cutis *15*, 231–240 (1975)
5. Altman, J., Stroud, J.: Netherton's syndrome and ichthyosis linearis circumflexa. Psoriasiform ichthyosis. Arch. Derm. *100*, 550–558 (1969)
6. Hurwitz, S., Kirsch, N., McGuire, J.: Reevaluation of ichthyosis and hair shaft abnormalities. Arch. Derm. *103*, 266–271 (1971)
7. Gianotti, F.: La maladie de Netherton. Étude de deux cas et des rapports avec les génodermatoses érythématodesquamatives circinées variables. Ann. Derm. Syph. (Paris) *96*, 147–156 (1969)
8. Degos, R., Larrègue, M.: Maladie de Netherton avec ichtyose vulgaire. Bull. Soc. franç. Derm. Syph. *78*, 636–640 (1971)
9. Julius, C.E., Keeran, M.: Netherton's syndrome in a male. Arch. Derm. *104*, 422–424 (1971)

Palmoplantar Keratodermias
(Palmoplantar Hyperkeratoses)

There are several hereditary disorders of keratinization characterized by diffuse or focal involvement of the palms and soles. These disorders differ in their mode of inheritance, clinical appearance, and other associated abnormalities. Unfortunately the distinctions are not always clear-cut because of overlapping manifestations, interfamily variations, inadequate understanding of etiologic and pathophysiologic factors, and the association of palmoplantar keratodermia with other syndromes. In this presentation the following conditions will be discussed:

Diffuse keratodermia
Keratodermia associated with cancer of the esophagus
Striate keratodermia
Punctate keratodermia
Mutilating keratodermia
Disseminate keratodermia with corneal dystrophy
Progressive keratodermia
Mal de Meleda
Papillon-Lefèvre syndrome
Other keratodermias

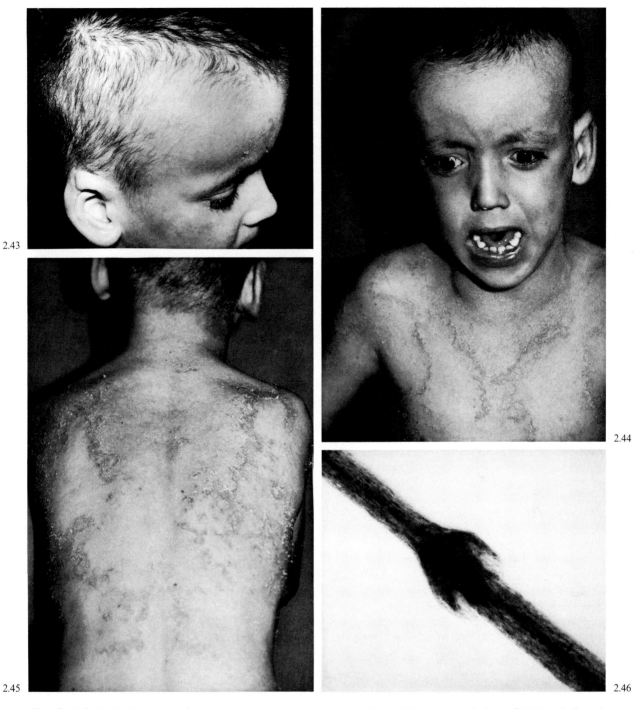

Figs. 2.43–2.46. Netherton syndrome

Figs. 2.44 and 2.45. Note the lesions of ichthyosis linearis circumflexa on the trunk. (Courtesy of Dr. C. E. Julius. Fig. 45 from Julius, C. E., Keeran, M.: Arch. Derm. *104*, 422–424, 1971)

Fig. 2.43. Note sparse hair. (From Julius, C. E., Keeran, M.: Arch. Derm. *104*, 422–424, 1971)

Fig. 2.46. Bamboo hair. (From Julius, C. E., Keeran, M.: Arch. Derm. *104*, 422–424, 1971)

Diffuse Palmoplantar Keratodermia (Tylosis, Keratosis Palmaris et Plantaris, Thost-Unna Syndrome)

This is the commonest form of palmoplantar keratodermia.

Clinical Presentation. In early infancy there may be slight thickening of the palms and soles. However, by the 6th to 12th month, the disorder is well-developed and persists throughout life. There is diffuse, sharply demarcated hyperkeratosis, involving the palmar and plantar surfaces with a narrow erythematous rim. Usually the involvement is bilateral and symmetric. Hyperhidrosis is marked and fissuring may ensue (Figs. 2.47–2.49). Secondary bacterial infection is not uncommon. The nails may be thickened, opaque, or curved, but the hair and teeth are normal. Other associations are rare but may include clinodactyly [1], ainhumlike strictures [2], and clubbed fingers.

Pathology and Pathophysiology. Usually, the histologic picture is nonspecific and consists of marked hyperkeratosis with hypergranulosis and acanthosis [3]. There may be a mild inflammatory infiltrate in the dermis. However, in some families the histologic picture is that of epidermolytic hyperkeratosis (see p. 28) with typical granular degeneration (localized epidermolytic hyperkeratosis) [4, 5]. These findings emphasize the possible heterogeneity of palmoplantar keratodermia.

Inheritance. Autosomal dominant.

Treatment. Traumatic occupations should be avoided. Keratolytic agents, particularly salicylic acid, can be palliative. Recently, topically applied retinoic acid (vitamin A acid), 0.1–0.3% in petrolatum, has given good results [6, 7]. Severe cases can be treated surgically [8–10].

Palmoplantar Keratodermia with Cancer of the Esophagus

Clinical Presentation. Two families have been reported with this condition [11, 12]. The clinical picture is similar to that of diffuse palmoplantar keratodermia except for a delayed onset (between the ages of 5 and 15 years). In such families 70% of the patients with keratodermia develop carcinoma of the esophagus later in life. In the majority of these cases, the carcinoma involves the lower third of the esophagus.

Inheritance. Autosomal dominant.

Keratosis Palmaris et Plantaris Striata (Striate Keratodermia)

Clinical Presentation. Typically, the keratosis is made up of linear confluent streaks. The palms are usually affected and the onset is around puberty. Papillomatous lesions of the buccal mucosa and dotlike opacities in the corneal epithelium have been reported [13].

Inheritance. Autosomal dominant suspected.

Keratosis Punctata Palmaris et Plantaris (Punctate Keratodermia, Keratosis Palmaris et Plantaris Papulosa)

Clinical Presentation. The onset is usually in the second or third decade. The lesions are numerous, yellow-brown, discrete, hard, horny papules [14]. They may be removed, leaving a crater surrounded by a horny wall. The only complaints are related to pain from pressure on the lesions and social embarrassment. Usually there are no associated defects except nail dystrophies [15] manifested by longitudinal fissures, onychomadesis, and onychogryphosis.

A possible variant of this condition is "hereditary papulotranslucent acrokeratoderma" [16], in which asymptomatic, nonscaling, smooth, translucent papules appear on the hands and feet (Fig. 2.50).

Pathology and Pathophysiology. The histologic picture is characterized by marked hyperkeratosis, sharply defined, with depression of the underlying epidermis [14]. There is hypergranulosis. The dermis is unremarkable and free of any inflammatory infiltrate. In some cases a cornoid lamella is seen [17].

Inheritance. Autosomal dominant suspected.

Treatment. There is no specific treatment.

Fig. 2.47. Diffuse palmoplantar keratodermia. Note the involvement of the
mother's palms and the sharp demarca-
tion of the soles of the child

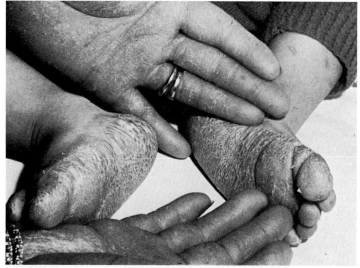

Fig. 2.48. Diffuse palmoplantar keratodermia. Involvement of the palms

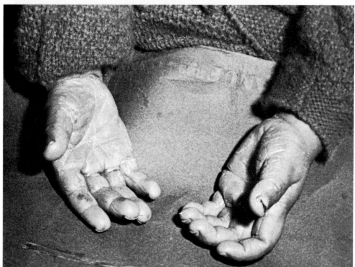

Fig. 2.49. Diffuse palmoplantar keratodermia

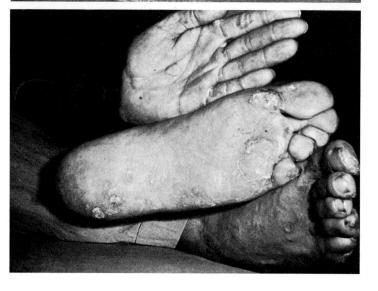

Keratoma Hereditaria Mutilans (Mutilating Keratodermia, Vohwinkel Syndrome, Congenital Deafness with Keratopachydermia and Constrictions of Fingers and Toes)

Clinical Presentation. This rare disorder appears in infancy as diffuse hyperkeratosis of the palms and soles, with a honeycombed surface (Fig. 2.51). Starfish keratoses appear on the dorsa of the hands and feet, linear keratoses on the elbows and knees, and constricting fibrous bands around digits in ainhum fashion. Rare findings are cicatricial alopecia and high-frequency hearing loss [18].

Inheritance. Autosomal dominant.

Disseminate Palmoplantar Keratodermia with Corneal Dystrophy (Richner-Hanhart Syndrome)

Clinical Presentation. This is a very rare disorder characterized by keratodermia of the palms and soles and corneal dystrophy [19]. The keratodermia, which appears between the ages of 12 and 15 years, may have several morphologic appearances: small punctate lesions, slightly elevated circumscribed areas, or coalescence of these areas to form partly diffuse, partly striated keratoses. The eye lesions are superficial corneal opacities in the form of commas and dendritic formations without eyeball irritation. This syndrome is due to a deficiency of hepatic tyrosine aminotransferase. (See Tyrosinemia II, p. 262.)

Inheritance. Autosomal recessive.

Progressive Palmoplantar Keratodermia (Greither Syndrome)

Clinical Presentation. The onset of keratodermia is in infancy. There is progressive thickening of the palms and soles over many years, extending frequently to the sides of the hands and feet. Occasionally, the arms and legs may be involved [20].

Inheritance. Autosomal dominant.

Mal de Meleda (Keratodermia Palmoplantaris Transgrediens)

This rare syndrome gets its name from the Dalmatian island of Meleda (Mljet) where there has been a lot of inbreeding.

Clinical Presentation. During infancy there is palmoplantar erythema followed by hyperkeratosis and thickening. Usually the erythema persists. Gradually, the thickening of the skin extends to the dorsal surfaces of the hands and feet, with the appearance of circumscribed areas on the wrists, forearms, knees, and other sites (Fig. 2.52). Hyperhidrosis, malodor, and eczematization are frequent. Brownish yellow lichenoid plaques may overlie the joints of the hands. Nail abnormalities (koilonychia, subungual keratosis), shortening of the fingers, and persistent perioral erythematous plaques may be found. There are no associated abnormalities of hair, teeth, or eyes, and the intelligence is normal [21].

Inheritance. Autosomal recessive.

Papillon-Lefèvre Syndrome (Palmoplantar Keratodermia with Periodontosis)

This rare syndrome is characterized by palmoplantar keratodermia, premature periodontoclasia, and calcification of the dura [22].

Clinical Presentation. The onset is usually between the 1st and 5th year when erythema and keratodermia appear on the palms and soles and extend to the sides of the hands and feet. There is also extension to the Achilles tendons, external malleoli, tibial tuberosities, dorsa of finger and toe joints, and other sites [22]. Hyperhidrosis and malodor are frequent. The hair may be normal or sparse and some nails may be dystrophic.

The deciduous teeth erupt normally but the gingivae become red, swollen, and boggy. This leads to destruction of the alveolar bone and loss of the deciduous teeth by the age of 4 or 5 years. The process is repeated with the permanent teeth. With loss of all permanent teeth, the gingivae assume their normal appearance. Calcific deposits in the attachment of the tentorium and choroid are frequent [22]. Arachnodactyly and osteolysis of terminal phalanges have been noted in some families [23].

Inheritance. Autosomal recessive.

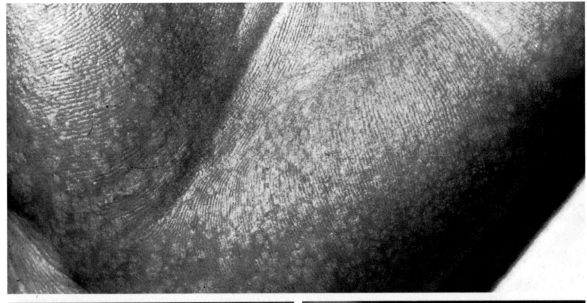

2.50

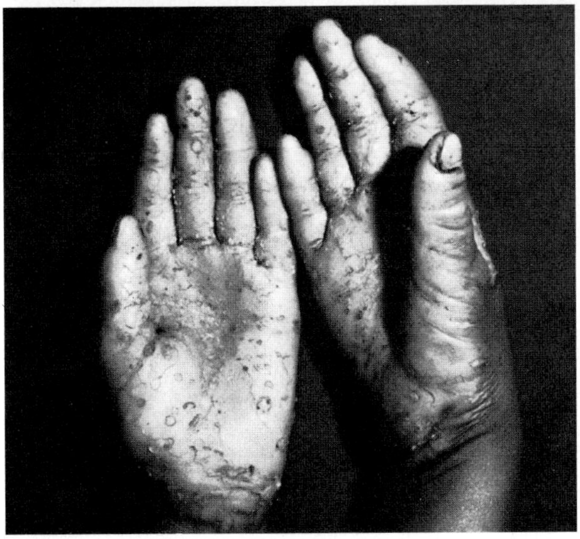

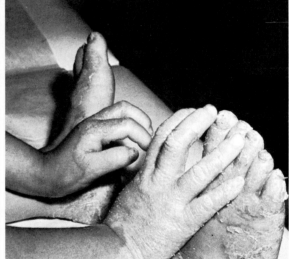

2.51   2.52

Fig. 2.50. Papulotranslucent acrokeratodermia. Note the smooth, translucent papules. (From Onwukwe, M.F., et al.: Arch. Derm. *108*, 108–110, 1973)

Fig. 2.51. Keratoma hereditaria mutilans

Fig. 2.52. Mal de Meleda. The well-delineated keratodermia involves the palms and soles and extends to the dorsal aspects of the hands and feet

Other Keratodermias

There are many hereditary palmoplantar keratodermias that show variations in age of onset, severity, and associated abnormalities. Many of these fit in well-characterized syndromes already discussed. Others seem to be distinctive but the reports are too few to delineate the disorders into specific syndromes. Some of these will be mentioned briefly. Two sisters were reported with palmoplantar keratosis, hypodontia, hypotrichosis, and cysts of the eyelids [24] (Figs. 2.53–2.56). The milk teeth were lost early and the permanent dentition was greatly reduced. The alopecia was universal. These patients also developed onychodystrophy [24].

Several pedigrees have been reported in which the palmoplantar keratodermia varies considerably within a family; it may be striate, diffuse, or disseminate [25]. The inheritance is of the autosomal dominant type.

Another rare form of keratodermia, referred to as "circumscribed palmoplantar keratodermia," is characterized by tender callosities at pressure points on the soles (Fig. 2.57), fingertips, and hypothenar eminences, associated with mental deficiency, leukoplakia of the buccal mucosa, corneal dystrophies, and occasional nail dystrophies.

A pedigree, with probable autosomal dominant mode of inheritance, has been described in which palmoplantar keratodermia is associated with congenital alopecia and fingernail dystrophy [26]. (See also Sclero-atrophic and Keratotic Dermatosis of the Limbs, p. 128.)

References

1. Klintworth, G.K., Anderson, I.F.: Tylosis palmaris et plantaris familiaris associated with clinodactyly. S. Afr. med. J. *35*, 170–175 (1960)
2. Wigley, J.E.M.: A case of hyperkeratosis palmaris et plantaris associated with ainhum-like constriction of the fingers. Brit. J. Derm. *41*, 188–191 (1929)
3. Šalamon, T., Bogdanović, B., Lazović-Tepavac, O.: Die Krankheit von Mljet. Dermatologica (Basel) *138*, 433–443 (1969)
4. Klaus, S., Weinstein, G.D., Frost, P.: Localized epidermolytic hyperkeratosis. A form of keratoderma of the palms and soles. Arch. Derm. *101*, 272–275 (1970)
5. Orbaneja, J.G., Lozano de Sosa, J.L.S., Huarte, P.S.: Hiperqueratosis palmoplantar difusa y circunscrita (tipo Thost-Unna) con degeneración reticular del cuerpo mucoso. Int. J. Derm. *11*, 96–105 (1972)
6. Heiss, H.B., Gross, P.R.: Keratosis palmaris et plantaris treatment with topically applied vitamin A acid. Arch. Derm. *101*, 100–103 (1970)
7. Günther, S.H.: Vitamin A acid in the treatment of palmoplantar keratoderma. Arch. Derm. *106*, 854–857 (1972)
8. Wynn-Williams, D.: Plantar keratodermia treated by split-skin grafts. Brit. J. plast. Surg. *6*, 123–129 (1953–1954)
9. Dencer, D.: Tylosis. Brit. J. plast. Surg. *6*, 130–140 (1953–1954)
10. Landazuri, H.F.: Keratosis palmaris et plantaris and its new surgical treatment. Acta Chir. plast. (Praha) *5*, 289–292 (1963)
11. Howell-Evans, W., McConnell, R.B., Clarke, C.A., Sheppard, P.M.: Carcinoma of the oesophagus with keratosis palmaris et plantaris (tylosis). Quart. J. Med. *27*, 413–429 (1958)
12. Shine, I., Allison, P.R.: Carcinoma of the oesophagus with tylosis (keratosis palmaris et plantaris). Lancet *1966 I*, 951–953
13. Grayson, M.: Corneal manifestations of keratosis plantaris and palmaris. Amer. J. Ophthal. *59*, 483–486 (1965)
14. Buchanan, R.N., Jr.: Keratosis punctata palmaris et plantaris. Arch. Derm. *88*, 644–650 (1963)
15. Stone, O.J., Mullins, J.F.: Nail changes in keratosis punctata. Arch. Derm. *92*, 557–558 (1965)
16. Onwukwe, M.F., Mihm, M.C., Jr., Toda, K.: Hereditary papulotranslucent acrokeratoderma: a new variant of familial punctate keratoderma? Arch. Derm. *108*, 108–110 (1973)
17. Brown, F.C.: Punctate keratoderma. Arch. Derm. *104*, 682–683 (1971)
18. Gibbs, R.C., Frank, S.B.: Keratoma hereditaria mutilans (Vohwinkel). Differentiating features of conditions with constriction of digits. Arch. Derm. *94*, 619–625 (1966)
19. Žmegač, Z.J., Sarajlić, M.V.: A rare form of an inheritable palmar and plantar keratosis. Dermatologica (Basel) *130*, 40–52 (1964)
20. Greither, A.: Keratosis extremitatum hereditaria progrediens mit dominantem Erbgang. Hautarzt *3*, 198–203 (1952)
21. Schnyder, U.W., Franceschetti, A.T., Ceszarovic, B., Segedin, J.: La maladie de Meleda autochtone. Ann. Derm. Syph. (Paris) *96*, 517–530 (1969)
22. Gorlin, R.J., Sedano, H., Anderson, V.E.: The syndrome of palmar-plantar hyperkeratosis and premature periodontal destruction of the teeth. A clinical and genetic analysis of the Papillon-Lefèvre syndrome. J. Pediat. *65*, 895–908 (1964)
23. Haim, S., Munk, J.: Keratosis palmo-plantaris congenita, with periodontosis, arachnodactyly and a peculiar deformity of the terminal phalanges. Brit. J. Derm. *77*, 42–54 (1965)
24. Schöpf, E., Schulz, H.-J., Passarge, E.: Syndrome of cystic eyelids, palmo-plantar keratosis, hypodontia and hypotrichosis as a possible autosomal recessive trait. In: The clinical delineation of birth defects. Bergsma, D. (ed.). Vol. VII, No. 8, pt. XII, pp. 219–221. Baltimore: Williams & Wilkins Co. 1971
25. Baes, H., de Beukelaar, L., Wachters, D.: Kératodermie palmo-plantaire variante. Ann. Derm. Syph. (Paris) *96*, 45–50 (1969)
26. Stevanovic, D.V.: Alopecia congenita. The incomplete dominant form of inheritance with varying expressivity. Acta Genet. Statist. med. *9*, 127–132 (1959)

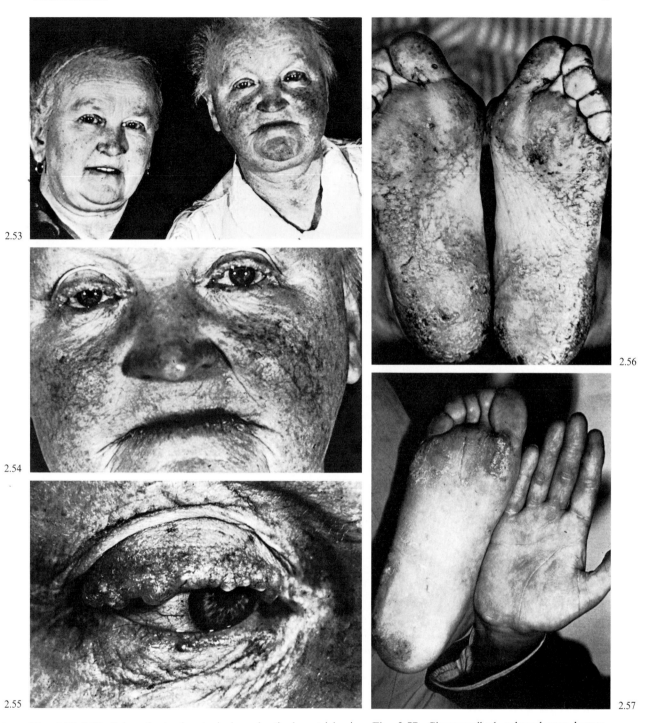

2.53

2.54

2.55

2.56

2.57

Figs. 2.53–2.56. Palmoplantar keratosis, hypodontia, hypotrichosis, and cysts of eyelids. (Courtesy of Dr. E. Schöpf)

Fig. 2.57. Circumscribed palmoplantar keratodermia

Porokeratoses

Even though it is generally believed that this disorder was independently described by Mibelli [1] and Resphigi [2] in 1893, it seems that Mibelli was actually the first to describe it in 1889 [3]. Porokeratosis may assume several clinical forms in which the lesions may be scanty or numerous, faint or prominent, small or extensive [4].

Porokeratosis (Mibelli)

Clinical Presentation. Onset is usually during early childhood. The primary lesion is a 1-mm, keratotic, crateriform papule. The papule slowly and gradually extends peripherally to form an annular or circinate plaque, several millimeters or centimeters in diameter (Fig. 2.58). The elevated firm ridge which forms the border of this plaque may be white, gray, brown, or skin-colored. Frequently this ridge has a longitudinal furrow from which protrude horny plugs (Fig. 2.59). The center of the plaque is depressed and atrophic but occasionally may be hypertrophic. The eruption may be composed of one or several such lesions. The sites of predilection are the extremities, especially the hands and feet, as well as the face, neck, and genitalia. Other areas may also be involved including the mucous membranes. The mucosal lesions may appear as small, slightly depressed opalescent rings with hyperemic borders [4]. The nails are occasionally involved and show splitting, ridging, and partial destruction.
Squamous cell carcinoma may arise at sites of lesions of porokeratosis.

Pathology and Pathophysiology. The distinctive histologic feature of porokeratosis is the cornoid lamella. This corresponds to the central furrow of the raised ridge and appears as a keratin-filled invagination of the epidermis. In the center of this invagination there is a column of parakeratosis, the base of which is made up of degenerating cells with pyknotic nuclei [5, 6]. The granular layer is absent where the cornoid lamella rises. Dyskeratotic cells, singly or in clusters, may appear in the prickle cell layer beneath the lamella [3]. The epidermis overlying the central portion of the lesion may be atrophic or acanthotic, accompanied by liquefaction degeneration of the basal cells [3]. A mild inflammatory dermal infiltrate is seen. Ultrastructurally, it has been demonstrated that the cornoid lamella is made up of degenerate cells with pyknotic nuclei [6].

Initially, the disease was considered to be essentially a disorder of the sweat pore [1]. However, even though the cornoid lamella may involve a sweat pore or a pilosebaceous follicle, recent evidence supports the concept that porokeratosis is a mutant clonal disease of the epidermis [3].

Inheritance. Autosomal dominant, probably with some reduction in penetrance in females [7].

Treatment. For localized, nonextensive lesions, surgical excision or destruction by electrodesiccation or cryosurgery can be attempted. Topical application of 5% 5-fluorouracil ointment has been found helpful [8]. Surgical excision of the carcinomas is indicated.

Linear Porokeratosis

This is a variant of the classic plaque type of porokeratosis of Mibelli. The eruption, which usually appears in early childhood, assumes a linear distribution. Often it simulates a linear verrucous epidermal nevus [9] (Fig. 2.60).

Plantar, Palmar, and Disseminate Porokeratosis

This is another variant characterized by onset in the late teens or early twenties, with early appearance of palmoplantar lesions. Subsequently there is symmetric involvement of other areas. The lesions are more superficial than in the classic type [10].

Disseminated Superficial Actinic Porokeratosis

Clinical Presentation. The eruption is characterized by numerous superficial lesions affecting the sun-exposed areas of the skin [11]. The distinctive feature of the lesions is the slight elevation of the ridges which also lack furrows. The sites of involvement are usually the extensor surfaces of the extremities and no lesions appear in areas not exposed to sunlight. The center of the plaque is skin-colored. Keratotic papules with delling may be seen and simulate lichen sclerosus et atrophicus [11]. Most lesions are small and superficial, and are accentuated during summer.

Fig. 2.58. Porokeratosis (Mibelli). Typical annular plaque

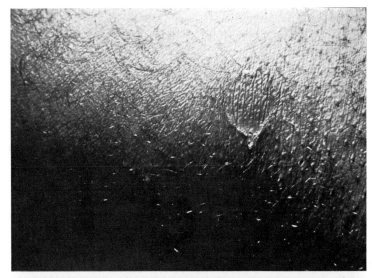

Fig. 2.59. Porokeratosis (Mibelli). Close view showing the longitudinal furrow at the peripheral ridge

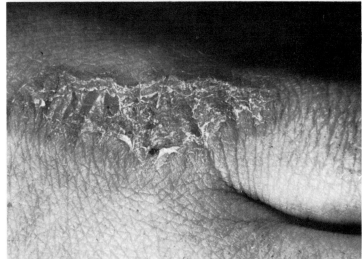

Fig. 2.60. Linear porokeratosis

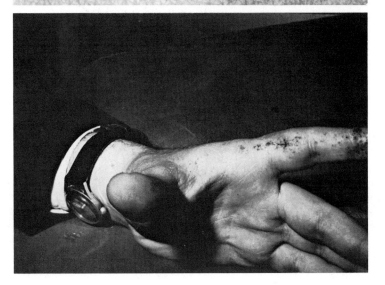

Pathology and Pathophysiology. The histologic features are essentially those of porokeratosis of Mibelli but of a milder degree.

Inheritance. Autosomal dominant. Penetrance becomes almost complete by 30 or 40 years of age [7].

Treatment. Superficial cryotherapy, mild keratolytics, and intralesional corticosteroids give symptomatic relief. Topical sunscreens are also recommended.

References

1. Mibelli, V.: Contributo allo studio della ipercheratosi dei canali sudoriferi (porokeratosis). G. ital. Mal. vener. *28*, 313–355 (1893)
2. Resphigi, E.: Di una ipercheratosi non ancora descritta. G. ital. Mal. vener. *28*, 356–386 (1893)
3. Reed, R.J., Leone, P.: Porokeratosis – a mutant clonal keratosis of the epidermis. I. Histogenesis. Arch. Derm. *101*, 340–347 (1970)
4. Mikhail, G.R., Wertheimer, F.W.: Clinical variants of porokeratosis (Mibelli). Arch. Derm. *98*, 124–131 (1968)
5. Braun-Falco, O., Balsa, R.E.: Zur Histochemie der cornoiden Lamelle. Ein Beitrag zur Pathogenese der Porokeratosis Mibelli. Hautarzt *20*, 543–550 (1969)
6. Mann, P.R., Cort, D.F., Airburn, E.A., Abdel-Aziz, A.: Ultrastructural studies on two cases of porokeratosis of Mibelli. Brit. J. Derm. *90*, 607–617 (1974)
7. McKusick, V.A.: Mendelian inheritance in man, 5th ed., pp. 326–327. Baltimore: Johns Hopkins University Press 1978
8. Gonçalves, J.C.A.: Fluorouracil ointment treatment of porokeratosis of Mibelli. Arch. Derm. *108*, 131–132 (1973)
9. Rahbari, H., Cordero, A.A., Mehregan, A.H.: Linear porokeratosis. A distinctive clinical variant of porokeratosis of Mibelli. Arch. Derm. *109*, 526–528 (1974)
10. Guss, S.B., Osbourn, R.A., Lutzner, M.A.: Porokeratosis plantaris, palmaris et disseminata. A third type of porokeratosis. Arch. Derm. *104*, 366–373 (1971)
11. Chernosky, M.E., Freeman, R.G.: Disseminated superficial actinic porokeratosis (DSAP). Arch. Derm. *96*, 611–624 (1967)

Other Abnormalities of Keratinization

Hyperkeratosis Lenticularis Perstans (Flegel Disease)

Flegel was the first to describe this disorder in 1958 [1]; Bean documented its genetic basis in 1969 [2].

Clinical Presentation. The onset is between the fourth and seventh decades, with initial lesions on the dorsa of the feet. Involvement of the lower legs is most common, but other affected areas are the thighs, buttocks, arms, dorsa of hands, and trunk [2]. The lesions are discrete, 1–5 mm, irregular, slightly infiltrated scaly papules, yellow-brown or reddish brown in color [2] (Figs. 2.61 and 2.62). The palms and soles may show punctate keratoses.
In one of the reported families, there was a high incidence of skin tumors, mainly squamous cell carcinomas [3]. These tumors did not necessarily arise at sites of lesions of hyperkeratosis lenticularis perstans. Furthermore, there was a high incidence of lung cancer in the affected family [3].

Pathology and Pathophysiology. There is hyper- and parakeratosis, and acanthosis or atrophy. In the dermis, the superficial vessels are dilated and surrounded by an inflammatory infiltrate [2, 3]. In well-developed lesions, however, the findings are characteristic. There is marked parakeratotic hyperkeratosis; absent granular cell layer; atrophy of the prickle cell layer; a well-circumscribed, bandlike, lymphohistiocytic upper dermal infiltrate hugging the epidermis; and thickened capillary walls [4].

Inheritance. Probably autosomal dominant [3, 5].

Treatment. There is no available treatment. Patients should be observed to detect any development of neoplasms.

References

1. Flegel, H.: Hyperkeratosis lenticularis perstans. Hautarzt *9*, 362–364 (1958)
2. Bean, S.F.: Hyperkeratosis lenticularis perstans. A clinical, histopathologic, and genetic study. Arch. Derm. *99*, 705–709 (1969)
3. Beveridge, G.W., Langlands, A.O.: Familial hyperkeratosis lenticularis perstans associated with tumours of the skin. Brit. J. Derm. *88*, 453–458 (1973)
4. Kocsard, E., Bear, C.L., Constance, T.J.: Hyperkeratosis lenticularis perstans (Flegel). Dermatologica (Basel) *136*, 35–42 (1968)
5. Bean, S.F.: The genetics of hyperkeratosis lenticularis perstans. Arch. Derm. *106*, 72 (1972)

Kyrle Disease (Hyperkeratosis Follicularis et Parafollicularis in Cutem Penetrans)

This uncommon disease was first described by Kyrle in 1916 [1].

Clinical Presentation. The age of onset ranges from 20–63 years and both sexes are affected [2]. The lesions are symmetrically distributed, especially on the legs and arms, less so on the trunk, head, and neck. Palms, soles, and mucous membranes are not

Fig. 2.61. Hyperkeratosis perstans. Discrete scaly papules on the foot.
(Courtesy of Dr. S. F. Bean)

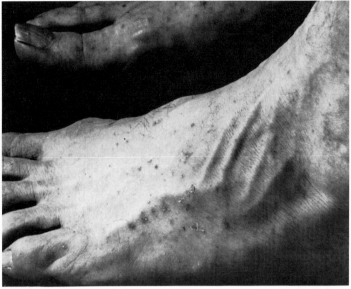

Fig. 2.62. Hyperkeratosis lenticularis perstans. Close-up view of papules on the
foot. (Courtesy of Dr. S. F. Bean)

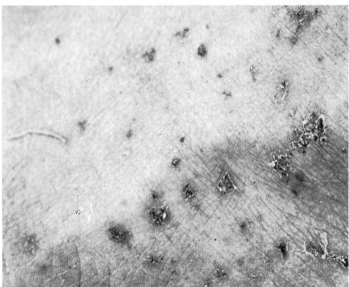

involved. The eruption is made up of papules, 1–8 mm in diameter, with a central hyperkeratotic plug [2] (Figs. 2.63 and 2.64). These papules may be follicular or parafollicular. In some areas, a Köbner-like picture is seen, unrelated to trauma, in which lesions form a circinate or linear arrangement [2] (Fig. 2.65). Other lesions may coalesce into plaques or verrucous streaks. Such streaks are usually seen in flexural regions of the ankle, popliteal, and antecubital surfaces [2]. The lesions are asymptomatic and of chronic duration.

Associated disorders include diabetes mellitus, and possibly renal insufficiency and heart failure [2]. Ocular findings include multiple, minute, yellow-brown anterior stromal corneal opacities and possibly posterior subcapsular cataracts [3].

Pathology and Pathophysiology. The diagnostic histologic features are a hyperkeratotic and parakeratotic plug filling an epithelial invagination; basophilic cellular debris, not of elastic tissue, within the plug; and parakeratotic keratinization in at least one region deep in the plug where epidermal disruption occurs. Such a disruption allows keratinized cells to reach the dermis where a granulomatous reaction sets in. Neutrophils and lymphocytes also participate in this reaction [4]. Around the plug, the epidermis may be acanthotic or atrophic. In the upper dermis there is a mild perivascular infiltrate [4].

Inheritance. Probably autosomal dominant [3]. However, no male-to-male transmission is described.

Treatment. The oral administration of vitamin A (100,00 units daily) for at least 1 month has been of help [2]. Keratolytics are palliative.

References

1. Kyrle, J.: Hyperkeratosis follicularis et parafollicularis in cutem penetrans. Arch. Derm. Syph. (Berl.) *123*, 466–493 (1916)
2. Carter, V.H., Constantine, V.S.: Kyrle's disease. I. Clinical findings in five cases and review of literature. Arch. Derm. *97*, 624–632 (1968)
3. Tessler, H.H., Apple, D.J., Goldberg, M.F.: Ocular findings in a kindred with Kyrle disease. Hyperkeratosis follicularis et parafollicularis in cutem penetrans. Arch. Ophthal. *90*, 278–280 (1973)
4. Constantine, V.S., Carter, V.H.: Kyrle's disease. II. Histopathologic findings in five cases and review of the literature. Arch. Derm. *97*, 633–639 (1968)

Acrokeratoelastoidosis (Collagenous Plaques of the Hands)

Costa was the first to draw attention to this disorder in 1953 [1]. Confusion has arisen as to the relation of this entity to degenerative elastotic collagenous plaques of the hands and feet [2].

Clinical Presentation. The eruption affects elderly individuals. The palms and soles are primarily involved and secondarily the dorsa of the hands and feet [3]. The skin appears thickened with yellowish or grayish, oval or polygonal papules arranged in lines along the sides of the hands and feet, as well as the dorsal aspects of the feet and the anterior surfaces of the lower legs [4]. The eruption is asymptomatic.

Pathology and Pathophysiology. The main histologic changes are hyperkeratosis, acanthosis, ectasia of the upper dermal capillaries, and elastotic changes in the dermis [4].

Inheritance. Autosomal dominant.

Treatment. No treatment is available.

References

1. Costa, O.G.: Acrokerato-elastoidosis (a hitherto undescribed skin disease). Dermatologica (Basel) *107*, 164–168 (1953)
2. Burks, J.W., Wise, L.J., Jr., Clark, W.H., Jr.: Degenerative collagenous plaques of the hands. Arch. Derm. *82*, 362–366 (1960)
3. Jung, E.G., Beil, F.U.: Acrokeratoelastoides mimicking palmo-plantar xanthomata. Nutr. Metab. *15*, 124–127 (1973)
4. Costa, O.G.: Acrokerato-elastoidosis. Arch. Derm. Syph. *70*, 228–231 (1954)

Familial Continual Skin Peeling (Keratolysis Exfoliativa Congenita, Deciduous Skin)

Clinical Presentation. This rare disorder is characterized by peeling of the skin which starts in infancy and continues throughout life [1–3]. The exfoliation is generalized but spares the palms and soles. It is constant and not accompanied by erythema. Sheets of keratin, of various sizes, are shed simulating postsunburn peeling. There are no other associated symptoms or signs [1–3].

Pathology and Pathophysiology. There is loose hyperkeratosis overlying an otherwise normal epidermis. Autoradiographic, histochemical, and electron microscopic studies point to a rapid proliferation of the epidermis [3].

Inheritance. Probably autosomal recessive [3].

Treatment. The use of keratolytics and emollients may be of symptomatic help.

References

1. Fox, H.: Skin shedding (keratolysis exfoliativa congenita). Report of case. Arch. Derm. Syph. *3*, 202 (1921)
2. Bechet, P.E.: Deciduous skin. Arch. Derm. Syph. *37*, 267–271 (1938)
3. Kurban, A.K., Azar, H.A.: Familial continual skin peeling. Brit. J. Derm. *81*, 191–195 (1969)

Pityriasis Rubra Pilaris

This chronic, mildly inflammatory exfoliative disorder was first described by Tarral in 1828 [1].

Clinical Presentation. According to the age of onset, there seem to be two distinct groups of patients with pityriasis rubra pilaris (PRP): a childhood group (up to the age of 20 years) and an adult group (26 years and older) [2]. The familial type of PRP has its onset usually in childhood, whereas the acquired type is found in adults. The relationship, if any, between the familial and acquired types is not clear.

Even in the hereditary type, the disease does not appear at birth [3] but usually in early childhood. The characteristic lesions are fine, firm acuminate papules that appear at the follicular openings. The papules are pierced by a hair. Together with these papules there may be well-defined erythematous plaques with, characteristically, islands of normal

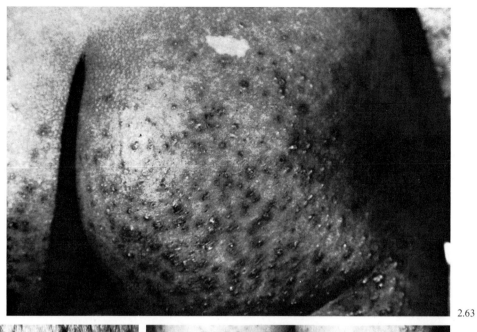

2.63

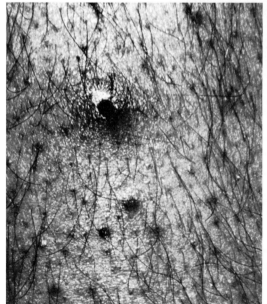

2.64

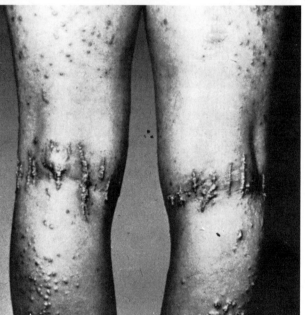

2.65

Figs. 2.63–2.65. Kyrle disease

Fig. 2.63. Papules with central keratotic plugs on buttocks. (Courtesy of Dr. I. Zeligman)

Fig. 2.64. Papules with central keratotic plugs. Close-up view. (Courtesy of Dr. I. Zeligman)

Fig. 2.65. Köbner-like phenomenon at popliteal area. (Courtesy of Dr. I. Zeligman)

skin (Figs. 2.66 and 2.67). Palmoplantar keratoder-mia with a yellow horny cast (keratodermic sandal) appears frequently. Fissuring and secondary infection may ensue. The sites of involvement are usually the palms and soles, arms, and dorsa of hands [4] (Figs. 2.68 and 2.69). Other sites are the scalp (with diffuse scaliness), face (with scaliness and erythema), and the trunk. Ectropion of the eyelids may result. When present, the papular lesions over the dorsal surface of the proximal phalanges of the fingers are quite characteristic [3, 5]. The scales vary in size and thickness. The eruption may progress to generalized exfoliative erythrodermia. Pruritus is uncommon.

The hair and teeth show no abnormalities. The nails may be dystrophic with subungual accumulation of keratinous material, simulating psoriasis. Oral mucosal lesions are variable and infrequent. Similarly, systemic associations seem to be fortuitous, pending confirmation. In some patients the disease seems to be exacerbated by exposure to sunlight [3].

Pathology and Pathophysiology. The histologic features in PRP are fairly characteristic when fully developed. Hyperkeratosis with focal parakeratosis, especially around the follicular openings, and follicular plugging are present. Irregular acanthosis and liquefaction degeneration of the basal cell layer are seen. In the dermis there is a mild chronic inflammatory infiltrate [5]. There is a rapid epidermal turnover [6].

The resemblance between PRP and the follicular eruption of hypovitaminosis A (phrynoderma) has stirred conjecture as to their possible relationship. However, the variable and inconstant findings from the measurement of serum vitamin A levels, vitamin A tolerance test, and dark-adaptation threshold test negate any definite relationship [5].

Inheritance. Autosomal dominant [3].

Treatment. Oral vitamin A (100,000–200,000 units daily) is beneficial to most patients. The use of topical vitamin A (250,000–500,000 units per ounce of lotion base) under occlusive dressing has also given good results [5]. Corticosteroids are especially helpful in the erythrodermic phase. Methotrexate is efficacious, especially when administered orally for a long period [7].

References

1. Tarral, C.: Communication in Rayer, P.: A theoretical and practical treatise on the diseases of the skin, 2nd ed., p. 648. London: Bailliere, J.B. 1835
2. Davidson, C.L., Jr., Winkelmann, R.K., Kierland, R.R.: Pityriasis rubra pilaris. A follow-up study of 57 patients. Arch. Derm. *100*, 175–178 (1969)
3. Beamer, J.E., Newman, S.B., Reed, W.B., Cram, D.: Pityriasis rubra pilaris. Cutis *10*, 419–423 (1972)
4. Gross, D.A., Landau, J.W., Newcomer, V.D.: Pityriasis rubra pilaris. Report of a case and analysis of the literature. Arch. Derm. *99*, 710–716 (1969)
5. Lamar, L.M., Gaethe, G.: Pityriasis rubra pilaris. Arch. Derm. *89*, 515–522 (1964)
6. Porter, D., Shuster, S.: Epidermal renewal and amino acids in psoriasis and pityriasis rubra pilaris. Arch. Derm. *98*, 339–343 (1968)
7. Knowles, W.R., Chernosky, M.E.: Pityriasis rubra pilaris. Prolonged treatment with methotrexate. Arch. Derm. *102*, 603–612 (1970)

Psoriasis

In 1808 Wilan presented what seems to be the first accurate clinical description of psoriasis [1]. Since this is a common disorder that is adequately covered in most textbooks of dermatology, only a very brief clinical discussion will be given here.

The primary lesion of psoriasis is an erythematous, scaly papule. These papules coalesce to form plaques that may vary in configuration and distribution; however, the elbows and knees are probably involved with greater frequency than any other area. Characteristically, the erythema is a rich red color and the scales are silvery (Figs. 2.70–2.72).

Discrete punctate pits in the nail surface are part of the psoriatic picture. Arthritis associated with psoriasis is variable in incidence and severity. In addition to the usual sites of involvement, psoriatic skin lesions also appear at sites of trauma (physical injuryty, overexposure to UV, allergic damage) – the Köbner reaction.

The disease is classified into two main types: psoriasis vulgaris and pustular psoriasis.

Pathology and Pathophysiology. The essential histopathologic features are the following: parakeratotic hyperkeratosis, acanthosis, Monroe microabscesses, elongation of dermal papillae, thinning of the suprapapillary epidermal plates, and engorgement of the dermal capillaries. There is increased mitotic activity and a more rapid turnover of the epidermis, an absent or diminished stratum granulosum, and an inflammatory infiltrate within the subpapillary dermis.

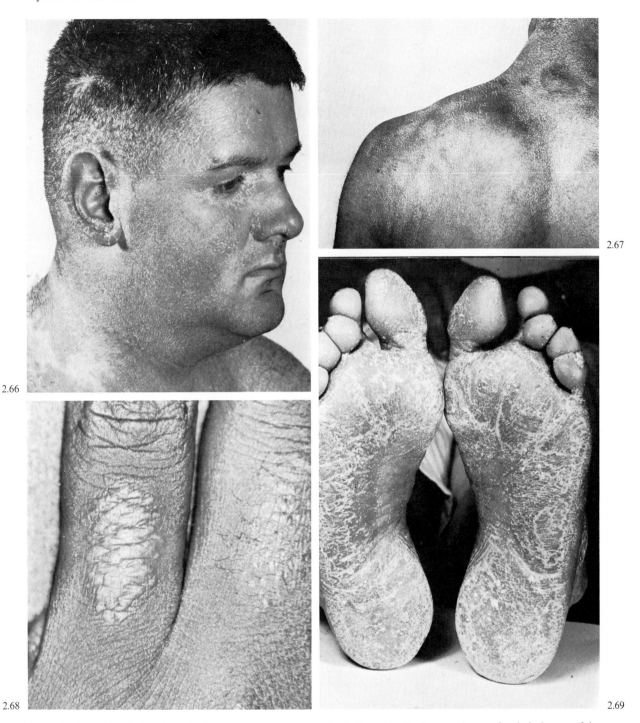

2.66

2.67

2.68

2.69

Figs. 2.66–2.69. Pityriasis rubra pilaris

Fig. 2.66. Diffuse scaliness and erythema of the face and scalp. (Courtesy of Dr. W. Frain-Bell)

Fig. 2.67. Disseminate fine papules

Fig. 2.68. Typical lesions on the proximal phalanges of the fingers. (Courtesy of Dr. I. Zeligman)

Fig. 2.69. Plantar keratodermia. (Courtesy of Dr. W. Frain-Bell)

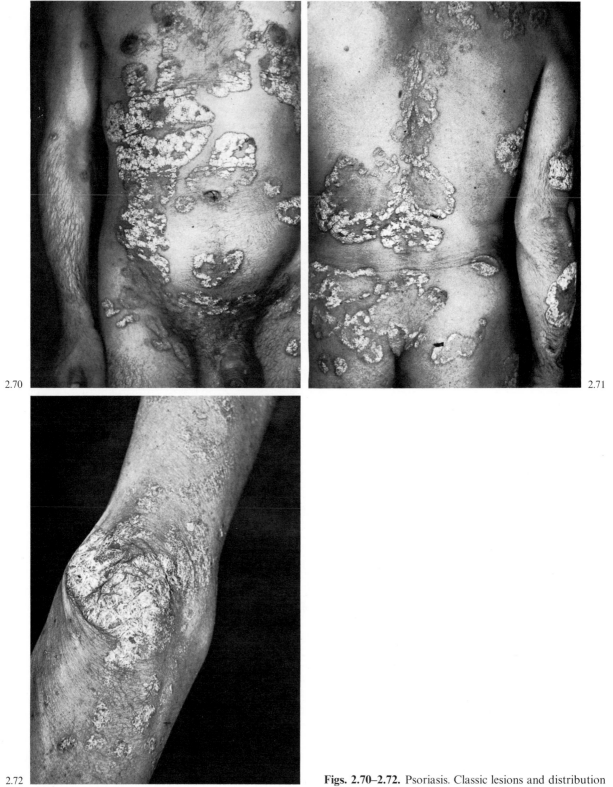

2.70

2.71

2.72

Figs. 2.70–2.72. Psoriasis. Classic lesions and distribution

Highly significant increases in HL-A13 and HL-A17 are found in psoriasis vulgaris: about half of the patients carry either of these antigens as compared to about 12% of the controls. The effect of HL-A13 and HL-A17 is almost exclusively confined to psoriasis with onset before the age of 35 years. According to some recent investigations, psoriasis vulgaris and pustular psoriasis are probably different etiologic entities, since none of the above antigens is increased in pustular psoriasis [2]. It is thought that psoriasis vulgaris is a polygenic threshold disease and HL-A13 and HL-A17 decrease the threshold, making the expression of psoriasis more likely in individuals carrying these determinants. In psoriatic arthritis the frequencies of HL-A13 and HL-A17 are not significantly increased; however, HL-A27 may show an increase in frequency [2].

Inheritance. Psoriasis has long been suspected of having a genetic etiology but its precise mode of inheritance remains uncertain. It is possible that this disease is genetically heterogeneous [3]. This is suggested by the apparently different modes of inheritance (autosomal dominant with 60% penetrance or multigenic) seen in families in different studies [4, 5].

Treatment. Numerous modalities have been used and these include topical coal tar with UV irradiation, topical corticosteroids, 8-methoxypsoralen with UVA (long ultraviolet), and immunosuppressants such as systemic methotrexate.

References

1. Shelley, W. B., Crissey, J. T.: Classics in clinical dermatology, p. 10. Springfield: Charles C Thomas 1970
2. Svejgaard, A., Nielsen, L., Svejgaard, E., Kissmeyer-Nielsen, F., Hjortshøj, A., Zachariae, H.: HL-A in psoriasis vulgaris and in pustular psoriasis – population and family studies. Brit. J. Derm. *91*, 145–153 (1974)
3. Kimberling, W., Dobson, R. L.: The inheritance of psoriasis. J. invest. Derm. *60*, 538–540 (1973)
4. Abele, D. C., Dobson, R. L., Graham, J. B.: Heredity and psoriasis. Study of a large family. Arch. Derm. *88*, 38–47 (1963)
5. Watson, W., Cann, H. M., Farber, E. M., Nall, M. L.: The genetics of psoriasis. Arch. Derm. *105*, 197–207 (1972)

Familial Dyskeratotic Comedones

Rodin et al. described familial comedones in 1967 [1]. In 1972 Carneiro et al. described another family with this disorder [2].

Clinical Presentation. The eruption appears around puberty in the form of papules topped by hard, blackish keratotic plugs resembling true comedones [2]. The lesions involve the face, trunk, and extremities but not the palms, soles, and scalp. The central plug can be extracted but re-forms. There are no associated inflammatory changes.

Pathology and Pathophysiology. The dilated follicular openings are filled with keratinous material. Focal areas of dyskeratosis (cells with eosinophilic cytoplasm and pyknotic nuclei and others showing individual cell keratinization) are evident [2].

Inheritance. Probably autosomal dominant [2].

Treatment. No treatment has been reported. Vitamin A acid may be helpful.

References

1. Rodin, H. H., Blankenship, M. L., Bernstein, G.: Diffuse familial comedones. Arch. Derm. *95*, 145–146 (1967)
2. Carneiro, S. J. C., Dickson, J. E., Knox, J. M.: Familial dyskeratotic comedones. Arch. Derm. *105*, 249–251 (1972)

Chapter 3   Abnormalities of Pigmentation

Contents

Hypo- and Amelanosis

Vitiligo

This is a rather common disorder affecting all races.

Clinical Presentation. The age of onset varies from infancy to late adulthood, but usually the disease is manifested by the second or third decade. Precipitating factors may be sunburn and emotional stress. The sites most often involved early in the course of the disease are the sun-exposed areas, the groin, and axillae. In fully developed cases, the sites most often affected are the dorsa of hands, the forearms, face, and neck. The involved skin is white or hypopigmented, but otherwise shows no abnormalities in texture (Figs. 3.1–3.4). Hairs growing in a vitiliginous patch may or may not be depigmented. The borders of the vitiliginous macules are usually convex, hyperpigmented, and may be slightly erythematous at the onset. Extension of already existing patches may be rapid or slow, while new patches may appear. Depending on the extent of involvement of the skin, vitiligo may be classified as localized, generalized, or universal. Usually, the patches are symmetric. Sites of repeated trauma may also be involved, while segmental distribution of the lesions can occur. In light-skinned individuals, Wood's light may help in detecting the involved skin.

The vitiliginous macules are asymptomatic, but on exposure to sunlight become painful and erythematous. One of the main problems in this disorder is the emotional trauma due to the cosmetic disfigurement. Spontaneous repigmentation may occur, but only rarely.

The association of vitiligo with organ-specific autoimmune disorders like hyperthyroidism, adrenocortical insufficiency, pernicious anemia, diabetes [1–3], and especially alopecia areata is frequent. Vitiligo may be associated with poliosis, uveitis, alopecia, meningeal irritation, and dysacousia in the Vogt-Koyanagi-Harada syndrome [4] (Fig. 3.5). A rare association of vitiligo with unilateral impairment of vision due to a degenerative retinitis,

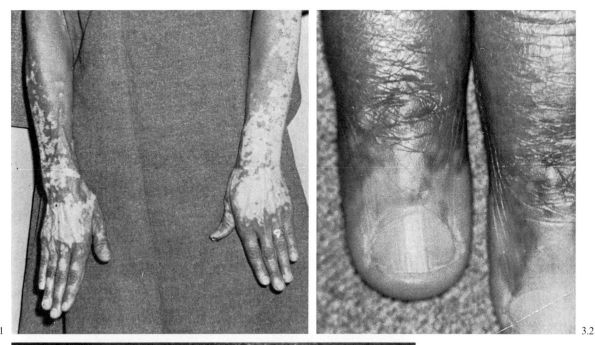

3.1   3.2

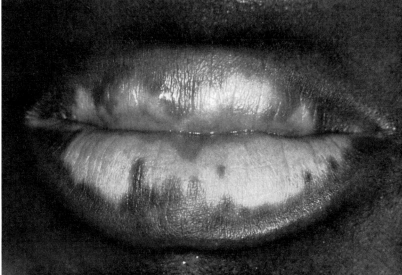

Figs. 3.1–3.3. Vitiligo. Sharply demarcated depigmented macules. (Courtesy of Dr. I. Zeligman)

3.3

poliosis, and perceptive deafness is known as Alezzandrini syndrome [5]. More frequently, vitiligo is associated with halos of leukodermas around diverse neuroectodermally derived tumors (halo nevus) [6, 7] (Fig. 3.6).

Pathology and Pathophysiology. The early lesions may show an inflammatory reaction in the epidermis and dermis. Gradually the melanocytes in the basal cell layer become scanty, abnormal, or may be completely absent [8].

Many theories have been presented to explain vitiligo (e.g., autoimmunity, neurochemical factors), but to date no convincing proof is available.

Inheritance. Autosomal dominant suspected [9].

Treatment. The best available treatment is the use of 8-methoxypsoralen (or other psoralen derivatives) and sunlight or long UV light (UVA). A daily oral dose of 40–80 mg psoralen, followed 2 h later by gradual exposure to light, is helpful when continued for several weeks. Repigmentation usually starts

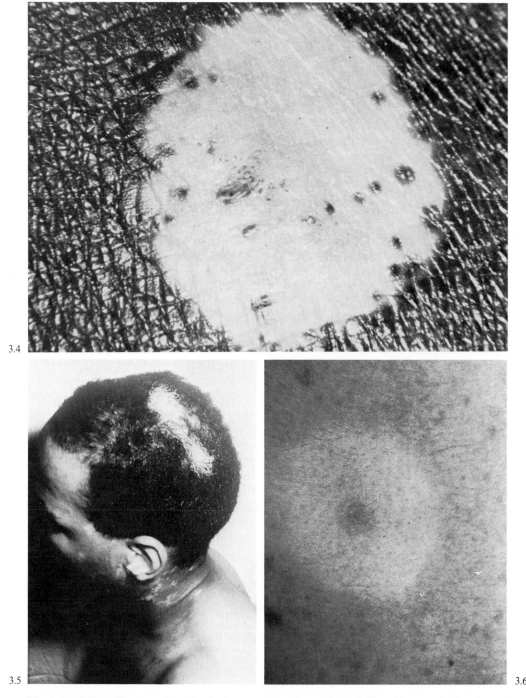

3.4

3.5

3.6

Fig. 3.4. Vitiligo. Close-up view of a depigmented macule in a black

Fig. 3.5. Vogt-Koyanagi-Harada syndrome

Fig. 3.6. Halo nevus

around the hair follicles and gradually spreads. After treatment is stopped loss of this pigmentation may occur. When vitiligo is extensive one may consider depigmenting what remains of the pigmented skin by topical application of monobenzyl ether of hydroquinone.

Albinism

Albinism is found throughout the animal kingdom and affects all races. In certain isolated communities, like the Cuna Indians of the San Blas Islands off Panama, the incidence is quite high [10]. The following classification is proposed [11].
1. Oculocutaneous albinism
    Tyrosinase-negative
    Tyrosinase-positive
2. Ocular albinism

Oculocutaneous Albinism

Clinical Presentation. The affected individuals have white skin and hair in the tyrosinase-negative type and·dilution of the normal skin color in the tyrosinase-positive type [11, 12]. In the eyes, the iris is light gray and translucent, the pupils red, and the retina not pigmented (Figs. 3.7–3.9). In the tyrosinase-negative variety, the skin and hair color as well as the eye changes persist throughout life. In the tyrosinase-positive variety, on the other hand, there is a tendency for pigmentation of the skin, hair, and eyes to increase with age [11, 12]. Freckles and pigmented nevi may develop. In a third variant, affected individuals resemble tyrosinase-negative albinos at birth. By 6 months to 1 year of age they develop yellow-red hair, a moderate red reflex, nystagmus, photophobia, and defect in visual acuity. Such individuals are designated as *yellow mutant (ym)* [12].

In all albinos, but less so in those of the tyrosinase-positive type, there is photophobia, nystagmus, decreased visual acuity, and iris translucency (Fig. 3.9). The severity of these features bears an inverse relationship to the amount of pigment produced [12]. Similarly there are chronic effects of solar radiation on the skin such as thickening and development of keratoses and squamous cell carcinomas (Fig. 3.10).

Albinism with a hemorrhagic diathesis has been described [13] (Hermansky-Pudlak syndrome). The bleeding seems to be due to a decreased amount of nonmetabolic adenine nucleotide in the platelet and, ultrastructurally, a virtual absence of platelet-dense bodies [12].

Oculocutaneous albinism with giant peroxidase-positive lysosomal granules in leukocytes and a marked susceptibility to infection is better known as the Chédiak-Higashi syndrome (see p. 65).

The association of albinism and congenital perceptive deafness has also been reported [14, 15].

The reports of deaf-mutism with dominant albinism [16] and with X-linked albinism [17, 18] probably represent the association of deaf-mutism with generalized piebaldism, since there is no ocular involvement.

Ocular Albinism

Clinical Presentation. The skin and hair are normally pigmented; however, the ocular findings are similar to those of oculocutaneous albinism. The fundus is depigmented and there is nystagmus, head-nodding, and impaired vision. Inheritance follows the X-linked recessive pattern. In carrier females the fundus shows a mosaic of pigmentation ("lyonization," see p. 9) (Nettleship variety).

Another form of ocular albinism, the Forsius-Eriksson type (Åland Island disease), is characterized by hypoplasia of the fovea, vision impairment, nystagmus, protanomalous color blindness, myopia, and astigmatism, in addition to the depigmentation of the fundus. The inheritance is also X-linked recessive. However, female carriers lack the characteristic fundus mosaic pigmentary pattern [19, 20]. A third rare form of ocular albinism, observed in four kindreds, is inherited as an autosomal recessive trait [11].

Pathology and Pathophysiology. In albinos, melanocytes are present in normal numbers. In the tyrosinase-positive type, the presence of tyrosinase is indicated by the darkening of the hair bulbs when incubated in tyrosine solution. In the tyrosinase-negative type, the hair bulbs fail to darken [11]. In the *yellow mutants*, the hair bulbs do not darken in L-tyrosine solution, but in L-tyrosine plus cysteine there is intensification of yellow or red pheomelanin [12].

Ultrastructurally, premelanosomes are seen in all cases of albinism, but progression of these to mature melanosomes is not seen in the tyrosinase-negative type. In this latter type the defect is the deficiency of tyrosinase. In the tyrosinase-positive type, it is postulated that the failure of melanogenesis results from a restriction in the amount of tyrosine in the melanosomes [11].

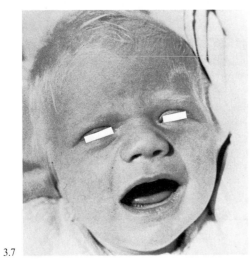

Fig. 3.7. Albinism in an infant. (Courtesy of Dr. F.C. Fraser)

Fig. 3.8. Albinism in a black. Note pigmented nevi and freckles

Fig. 3.9. Albinism. Note translucent iris

Fig. 3.10. Actinic keratoses in an albino. (Courtesy of Dr. V. A. McKusick, from Ward, W.Q., Hambrick, G.W., Jr.: In: The clinical delineation of birth defects. Bergsma, D. (ed.), Vol. VII, No. 8, pt. XII, pp. 224–226. Baltimore: Williams & Wilkins Co. 1971

Fig. 3.11. Albinoidism. Note mild pigmentation of skin, hair, and iris. (Courtesy of Dr. V. A. McKusick, from Char, F.: In: The clinical delineation of birth defects. Bergsma, D. (ed.), Vol. VII, No. 8, pt. XII, pp. 227–228. Baltimore: Williams & Wilkins Co. 1971

3.7

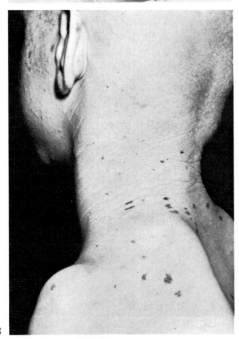

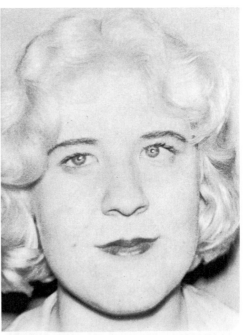

3.8

3.9

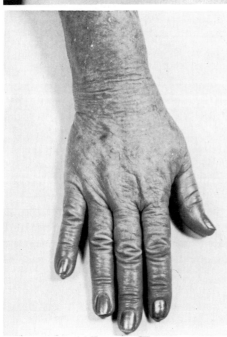

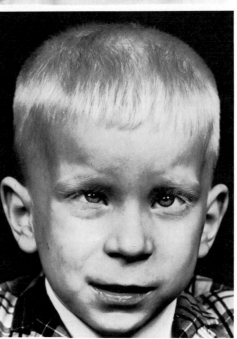

3.10

3.11

In ocular albinism the mechanism is not completely known.

Inheritance. All types of oculocutaneous albinism are inherited as autosomal recessive, but are nonallelic. There has been a recent report of a dominant type of oculocutaneous albinism with moderate dilution of skin and hair color and iris translucency [21]. With rare exceptions, patients do not have associated nystagmus, photophobia, or markedly decreased visual acuity. Hair bulbs from these patients incubated in L-tyrosine form increased pigment. The condition has also been called oculocutaneous albinoidism [11] (Fig. 3.11). Two types of ocular albinism are inherited as X-linked recessive and one type as autosomal recessive (see above).

Treatment. The only available treatment is the use of sunscreens. Albinos should be screened regularly for the development of keratoses and skin cancer and treated accordingly.

Piebaldism (White Spotting, White Forelock)

Clinical Presentation. The disease is manifested at birth with the appearance of patches of hypomelanosis, in a distinctive pattern, that persist throughout life. Often these are associated with a white forelock, although occasionally the latter may occur alone. The usually involved sites are the forehead, chin, chest, abdomen, forearms, and lower extremities. The hands, feet, and back are usually uninvolved. Islands of normally pigmented skin may be present within the hypomelanotic macules. A white lock of occipital hair may be a variety of piebaldism.

A possible variant of piebaldism is Tietz syndrome. This is an autosomal dominantly inherited defect characterized by lack of pigment in the skin and hair, normal eyes, severe deafness, and hypoplasia of the eyebrows [16]. The association of piebaldism and deafness has been reported in several patients [15–18]. Piebaldism may also be associated with neurologic defects (cerebellar ataxia, impaired motor coordination, mental retardation) [22].

Pathology and Pathophysiology. In the affected area, electron microscopic studies show absence of melanocytes and presence of Langerhans cells [23, 24] or reduction in the number of melanocytes that appear abnormal and are dissociated from flanking

keratinocytes [25]. Thus, the mechanism of hypopigmentation seems to be similar to that of vitiligo.

Inheritance. Autosomal dominant. The occipital white lock is probably transmitted as X-linked recessive [23]. Some of the syndromes of piebaldism with deafness [17, 18] are transmitted as X-linked recessive [26].

Treatment. There is no treatment.

Premature Canities (Early Graying of Hair)

This condition affects both sexes. In childhood there may be a few scattered gray hairs, but during the teens the number of gray hairs increases so that all the hair is white by 25–30 years. The eyebrows and eyelashes usually retain their color [27]. Premature canities is a feature of Book syndrome (premolar aplasia, hyperhidrosis, premature canities – PHC syndrome) as well as Waardenburg syndrome. Inheritance is probably autosomal dominant.

Cross-McKusick-Breen Syndrome (Oculocerebral Syndrome with Hypopigmentation)

This syndrome was described by Cross et al. in 1967 [28].

Clinical Presentation. Affected individuals are hypopigmented and have microphthalmia, small opaque cornea, coarse nystagmus, athetosis, severe oligophrenia, and gingival fibromatosis [28, 29] (Fig. 3.12).

Pathology and Pathophysiology. Ultrastructurally, melanocytes are present, but they have scanty melanosomes. In vitro, incubation in L-tyrosine or L-dopa results in increased pigmentation [29].

Inheritance. Autosomal recessive.

Treatment. There is no treatment.

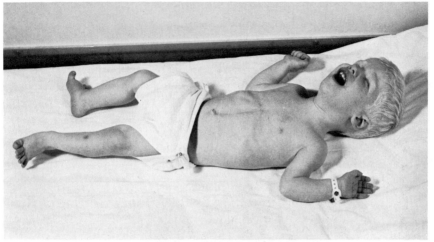

3.12

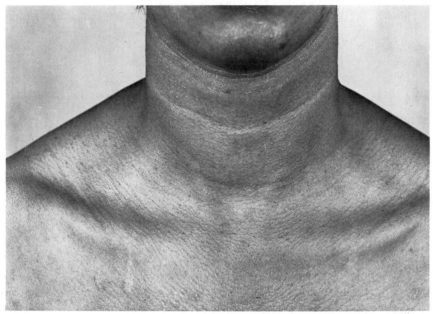

3.13

Fig. 3.12. Cross-McKusick-Breen syndrome. Note hypopigmentation and microphthalmia. (Courtesy of Dr. V. A. McKusick)

Fig. 3.13. Raindrop hypopigmentation. Note characteristic appearance of depigmentation on the anterior chest, near the clavicle. (Courtesy of Dr. V. A. McKusick)

Raindrop Hypopigmentation

Two Negro families have been described with a distinctive bilateral and sharply localized hypopigmentation of the upper chest [30, 31]. The hypopigmented areas are about 0.5–1.0 cm, just below the inner third of the clavicles, and have the appearance of raindrops (Fig. 3.13). No other abnormalities have been detected. Either X-linked or autosomal dominant inheritance is possible.

Waardenburg Syndrome (Klein-Waardenburg Syndrome)

In 1951 Waardenburg [32] described this syndrome characterized by lateral displacement of the medial canthi, partial albinism, and deafness. A few years prior to Waardenburg's report, Klein reported a deaf-mute child with pronounced partial albinism of the entire body [33]. More than 180 patients have been reported [15].

Clinical Presentation. The different characteristic signs occur with the following percentages: (a) dystopia canthorum, 99%; (b) broad and high nasal bridge, 78%; (c) synophrys, 45%; (d) heterochromia iridis, 25%; (e) deafness, 20%; and (f) a white forelock, 17% [34]. Areas of vitiligo may be present on the skin and patches of white hair other than the forelock may be present on the scalp. The white forelock may be present at birth and later disappear [35]. Premature graying of the hair is an effect of the gene. Congenital deafness, when present, is usually bilateral and severe. Occasionally, the following abnormalities may be noted: hypoplastic iris, hypopigmentation of the fundi [36], flattened alae nasi, cleft palate with harelip, and defects of the limbs (Figs. 3.14–3.16).

Pathology and Pathophysiology. The pigmentary abnormalities are of the type seen in vitiligo, i.e., absence of melanocytes with presence of Langerhans cells.

The deafness is due to abnormalities in the organ of Corti, with atrophic changes in the spinal ganglion and nerve.

Inheritance. Autosomal dominant. Many patients represent fresh mutations [34]. Skipped generations are documented, suggesting reduced penetrance [37].

Treatment. Corrective surgery is advised when indicated; otherwise treatment is symptomatic.

Chédiak-Higashi Syndrome

In 1943 Beguez Cesar [38] described this lethal disorder characterized by partial albinism, neutropenia, and cytoplasmic inclusions. Later, Chédiak [39] and Higashi [40] recognized the syndrome which carries their eponym.

Clinical Presentation. The disease is characterized by oculocutaneous albinism with very light skin and light-colored hair. The retinas are pale and the irides translucent. There is associated photophobia and nystagmus (Figs. 3.17 and 3.18). Hepatosplenomegaly and lymphadenopathy may be present. The disease appears in infancy and is manifested by infections which may resemble pyoderma gangrenosum [41].

Occasionally, the following abnormalities may be found: corneal opacity, buccal ulcerations, hyperhidrosis, peripheral neuropathy, seizures, and mental retardation.

Laboratory findings include neutropenia with a mild lymphocytosis, anemia, and thrombocytopenia. Pancytopenia occurs in the terminal stages with hypersplenism. There are large, eosinophilic, peroxidase-positive cytoplasmic inclusions in the leukocytes, promyeloblasts, and myeloblasts of the bone marrow. Occasionally, hyperlipemia may be present.

Most patients die in early childhood of recurrent infections or a peculiar malignant lymphoma. Rarely, patients may survive to adulthood [42].

Pathology and Pathophysiology. Light microscopic examination of the skin shows an irregularly shaped epidermis with large melanin granules scattered through its lower portion. Similar large, irregularly shaped melanin granules are seen scattered through the upper dermis within melanophages. The hairs also contain large, clumped, and sparse melanin granules [43].

Electron microscopy reveals [44, 45] that the cytoplasmic granules of the leukocytes are swollen lysosomes. Giant melanosomes are also found in the melanocytes. The hypopigmentation is caused by the fact that within keratinocytes the melanosomes, rather than being dispersed, lie within relatively few large phagolysosomes [43–45]. The presence of swollen lysosomes and giant melanosomes suggests an abnormality in the function of limiting membranes [46].

Several possibilities by which the structural abnormality could lead to a decrease in pigmentation have been suggested [41]: either the number of melanosomes, the amount of tyrosinase, or the ability of the melanosomes to be transferred to keratinocytes could be affected, or the giant melanosome may be more readily autolyzed by the melanocyte.

Moreover, glycolipid inclusions were described in histiocytes, renal tubular epithelium, and neurons [47]. Heterozygotes are identifiable by the presence of a granular anomaly in the lymphocytes.

The polymorphonuclear leukocyte function is impaired and leads to severe pyogenic infections. This impairment of the leukocyte function seems to be related to abnormal microtubular assembly and, subsequently, to delayed delivery of lysosomal contents to phagosomes. These abnormalities may be related to decreased cyclic guanosine monophosphate levels. Such an abnormality may be corrected by cholinergic agonists or ascorbate [48].

Inheritance. Autosomal recessive. Heterozygotes may have enlarged cytoplasmic inclusions in the lymphocytes.

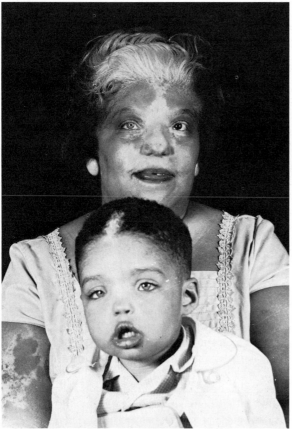

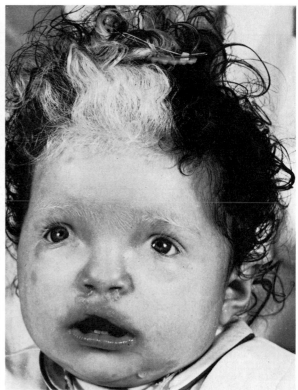

3.14

3.16

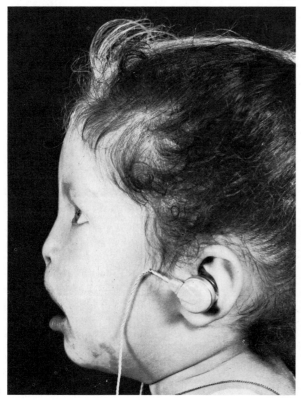

Figs. 3.14–3.16. Mother and children affected with the Waardenburg syndrome. Note heterochromia of the iris (in the mother), broad nasal bridge, dystopia canthorum, and synophrys. (Courtesy of Dr. V. A. McKusick)

Fig. 3.17. Chédiak-Higashi syndrome. Note light skin, hair color, and photophobia. (Courtesy of Dr. O.C. Stegmaier)

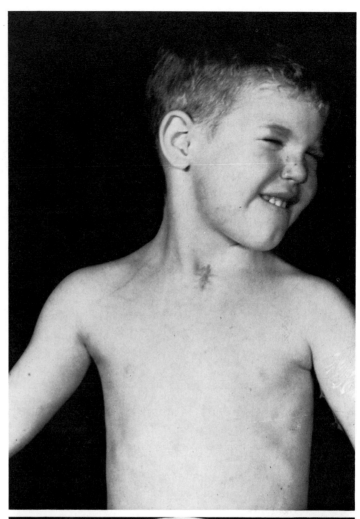

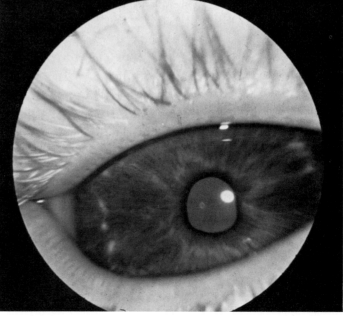

Fig. 3.18. Chédiak-Higashi syndrome. Translucent iris. (Courtesy of Dr. O.C. Stegmaier)

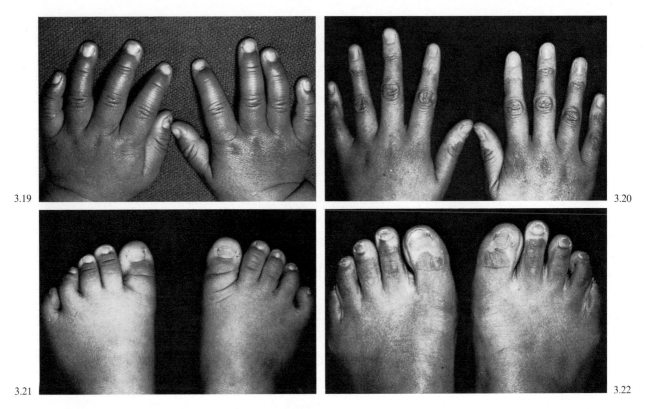

Figs. 3.19–3.22. Symmetric acroleukopathy. Depigmentation around the nails of mother and daughter. (From Sugai, T., et al.: Arch. Derm. *92*, 172–173, 1965)

Treatment. Treatment is symptomatic. Administration of prednisone results in a significant increase in circulating granulocytes, concomitantly with correction of manifest hypersplenism and reduction in splenomegaly [49].

Symmetric Acroleukopathy

A Japanese mother and daughter have been described with symmetric periungual depigmentation [50]. The depigmentation is noticed in infancy or childhood, gradually progresses from the nail folds to involve the interphalangeal joints, and remains constant (Figs. 3.19–3.22). Histologically, the involved skin is deficient in melanin, with dopanegative melanocytes. Inheritance is probably autosomal dominant.

Red Skin Pigment Anomaly of New Guinea

Several pedigrees have been described in which the color of the skin is reddish brown rather than black [51]. The patients are all from New Guinea. The hair color is unremarkable and varies from the usual black to white. Nystagmus and photophobia are present in some of the affected individuals. Histologically, melanin is present and its deposition increases with age. The exact nature of the pigment that contributes to the "red" color is not known. Inheritance is autosomal recessive.

Hypermelanosis

Ephelides

Clinical Presentation. The onset is usually in childhood. The lesions are light brown macules in the sun-exposed areas that darken and increase in number during the summer months and tend to fade in the winter. Melanocytic nevi are more abundant in individuals with freckles. The lesions are asymptomatic, but may be cosmetically disfiguring.

Pathology and Pathophysiology. The melanocytes in freckled areas are larger and more dendritic than in normal skin [52]. Freckle melanocytes produce large numbers of fully melanized granules [53].

Inheritance. Mode of inheritance is not definitely established.

Treatment. For cosmetic reasons, sunscreens are advised.

Lentigines

Lentigines and Multiple Lentigines Syndrome (Leopard Syndrome, Lentiginosis Profusa Syndrome, Cardiocutaneous Syndrome)

Clinical Presentation. Lentigines, which are dark brown macules (1–3 mm), appear at birth or in infancy and increase in number until puberty. These are more numerous over the trunk and neck, but involve all parts of the body including the palms and soles. There is a tendency for lentigines to fade slightly in color after puberty (Figs. 3.23 and 3.24). Lentigines as an isolated trait is probably inherited as autosomal dominant.

The main associated abnormalities are included in the mnemonic designation "leopard syndrome": *l*entigens, *e*lectrocardiographic abnormalities, *o*cular hypertelorism, *p*ulmonary stenosis, *a*bnormalities of genitalia, *r*etardation of growth, and *d*eafness [54] (Figs. 3.25–3.27). The cardiac abnormalities include cardiomyopathy, conduction defects, and pulmonic and subaortic stenoses. Skeletal abnormalities include mandibular prognathism, chest and vertebral anomalies, hypermotility of joints, and winging of the scapulae [54]. Hypogonadism, small stature, and sensorineural deafness are frequently present. Less frequent associations are granular cell schwannomas, interdigital webs of the hands, nail dystrophies, and abnormal dermatoglyphics [55].

A possible variant has been reported in a kindred in which freckling of the face and iris was associated with short stature, deafness (congenital perceptive), congenital mitral regurgitation, and fusion of cervical vertebrae and of carpal and tarsal bones [56]. Inheritance is probably autosomal dominant.

Pathology and Pathophysiology. The classic histologic picture of lentigines is that of elongated, clubbed epidermal ridges with increased melanocytes and melanin in the basal cell layer. Packets of melanosomes are frequently seen within the melanocytes [57]. It is postulated that the basic defect in this syndrome is of neuroectodermal origin with secondary or pleiotropic changes in the organs derived from the mesoderm [57].

Inheritance. Autosomal dominant with varying expressivity.

Treatment. A good cosmetic result has been obtained with facial dermabrasion [55].

Centrofacial Lentiginosis

Clinical Presentation. This rare syndrome is characterized by a band of lentigines across the center of the face, appearing during the first year of life. Associated defects include coalescence of eyebrows, high-arched palate, absent upper median incisors, pectus carinatum, sacral hypertrichosis, spina bifida, cervicodorsal scoliosis, kyphosis, mental retardation, epilepsy, emotional instability, disturbances of character and behavior, endocrine abnormalities, and vegetative dysfunctions [58, 59].

Inheritance. Most probably autosomal dominant [59, 60].

Treatment. No treatment is advocated except for cosmetic improvement of the facial eruption and management of the associated defects.

Peutz-Jeghers Syndrome

In 1921 Peutz [61] described three generations of a family in which there were seven proven and three suspected cases of intestinal polyposis associated

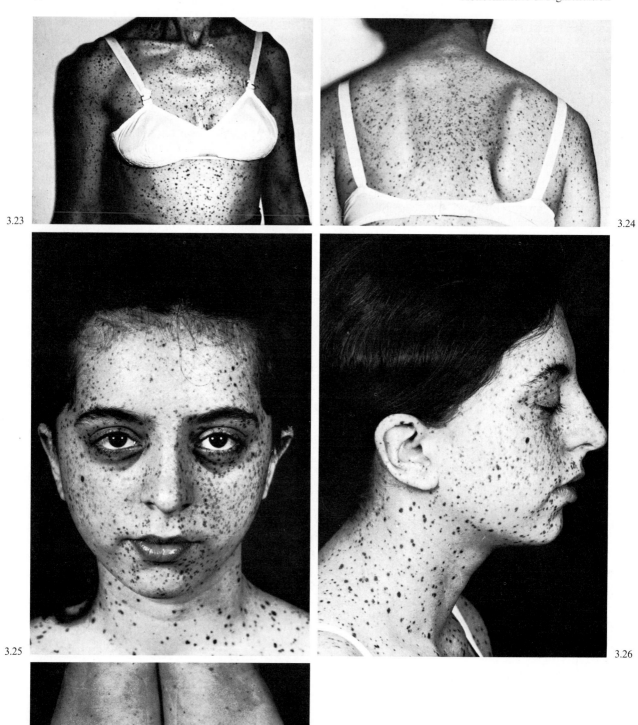

Figs. 3.23 and 3.24. Lentigenes over the chest and the back

Figs. 3.25–3.27. Leopard syndrome. Note numerous lentigenes over the face and the feet. (Courtesy of Dr. V.A. McKusick. Fig. 25 from Char, F.: In: The clinical delineation of birth defects. Bergsma, D. (ed.), Vol. VII, No. 8, pt. XII, pp. 234–235. Baltimore: Williams & Wilkins Co. 1971

with melanotic pigmentation of the lips and oral mucosa. In 1944 Jeghers [62] commented on two patients with the syndrome and in 1949 Jeghers et al. [63] demonstrated that this "hereditary peculiarity" was carried as a mendelian dominant characteristic.

Clinical Presentation. Melanotic pigmentary lesions described as "black freckles" may be present at birth and persist throughout life. The lesions on the lips are discrete macules, brown, black, or dark blue in color; rarely they coalesce to cover the entire surface of the lips. Round, oval, or irregular macules are found on the buccal mucosa (Figs. 3.28 and 3.29). They occur less often on the gums and hard palate and only rarely on the tongue. Sometimes the pigmentation may cover the circumoral area, the cheeks, and the nose in a "butterfly" configuration, with much smaller individual lesions. Infrequently, the palms, soles, and interdigital web spaces may be affected. The cutaneous lesions may not be present at birth, but appear during adolescence and may disappear with advancing age. The mucosal lesions persist. The macules of Peutz-Jeghers syndrome (PJS) do not change color on exposure to sunlight. The intestinal polyposis is rarely encountered in infants, but appears during puberty. The polyps are generally found in the jejunum, less frequently in the ileum, occasionally in the duodenum, and rarely in the stomach or colon. The common symptoms are diarrhea, borborygmi, bleeding due to ulceration, and frequent intussusception. The lesions of the jejunum and ileum are not malignant and there is no evidence of increased incidence of rectal cancer. The gastric or duodenal polyps may undergo malignant transformation and metastasis [64]. Moreover, individuals with this syndrome appear to have a greater tendency to develop colonic carcinoma than normal persons [65]. Finally, PJS is associated with a distinctive ovarian tumor [66] and sometimes ureteral polyps [67].

Pathology and Pathophysiology. The pigmented macules show an increase in melanocytes and melanin in the basal layer. In some, there may be junctional nervus cells.

The polyps range in size from microadenomas too small to be seen to lesions 5 cm or more in diameter. They are most numerous in the jejunum. These hamartomatous polyps characteristically contain all of the elements normally found at the level of the intestinal mucosa including columnar, goblet, Paneth, and argentaffine cells. The presence of Paneth cells is one differentiating feature between PJS

polyps and adenomatous polyps of the small bowel [68].

Inheritance. Autosomal dominant.

Treatment. The gastric and duodenal polyps require diagnosis and prompt surgical treatment to avoid malignant transformation and metastasis.

Neurocutaneous Melanosis

This rare syndrome of cutaneous and meningeal pigmentation is potentially highly malignant and usually causes death in early childhood [69]. To date, there is no evidence of its familial occurrence. The condition may be considered as a congenital dysplasia of the neural crest [69].

Melanocytic Nevi (Pigmented Moles)

Common moles are usually present at birth, but may appear in childhood or early adulthood. They vary in color from skin color to dark brown or black. Morphologically, moles may have one of eight forms: flat, slightly elevated with pigmented halos, verrucoid, polypoid, elevated, dome-shaped, sessile, and papillomatous [70]. Moles may be found anywhere on the body surface (Figs. 3.30–3.32). Histologically, moles are due to proliferation of melanocytes (nevus cells) and the aggregates of these cells could be at the epidermodermal junction (junctional nevi), in the dermis (dermal nevi), or at both sites (compound nevi). Inheritance is autosomal dominant.

Universal Melanosis

During the first year of life there is a gradual darkening of the skin. This is later followed by the appearance of white patches in the hyperpigmented areas. The trunk shows most of the hyperpigmentation [71]. There may be brownish patches in the oral mucosa. The process is asymptomatic. Muscular weakness may be an associated finding.

Histologically, there is increased pigment in the epidermis (basal and malpighian layers) and incontinence of pigment in the dermis [71]. The pathogenesis of this pigmentation is not clear. Inheritance is autosomal dominant.

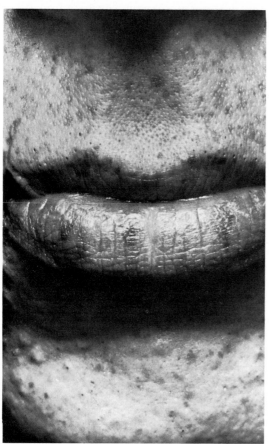

Fig. 3.28. Peutz-Jeghers syndrome. Note pigmentation over the lips and the perioral area. (Courtesy of Dr. W. Frain-Bell)

Fig. 3.29. Peutz-Jeghers syndrome. Pigmentation of the lip and the buccal mucosa. (Courtesy of Dr. W. Frain-Bell)

3.28

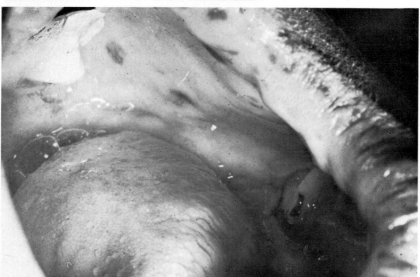

3.29

Figs. 3.30–3.32. Melanocytic nevi on the trunk, the dorsum of the foot, and the sole. (Courtesy of Dr. I. Zeligman)

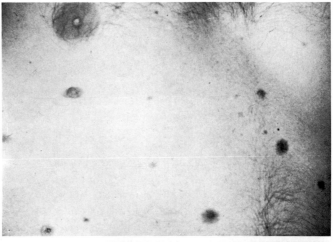

3.30

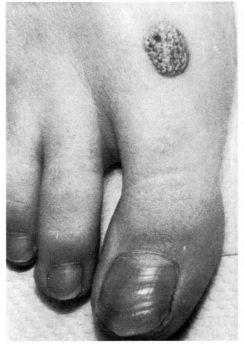

3.31

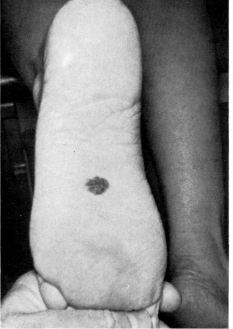

3.32

Symmetric Dyschromatosis of the Extremities (Acropigmentation of Dohi)

During infancy mottled pigmentation and depigmentation appear on the dorsa of the hands and feet and sometimes on the arms and legs. The disorder is common among the Japanese. The mode of inheritance is not definitely established [72].

Dyschromatosis Universalis

This syndrome occurs predominantly among the Japanese and is characterized by the appearance in early childhood of pigmented macules over the body, most prominent on the abdomen and sparing the face. Depigmented macules give the affected areas a mottled appearance. There are no associated defects [73]. Inheritance may be autosomal dominant or autosomal recessive and only quasi-dominant in view of the high inbreeding in some families.

Acropigmentation (Acromelanosis Progressiva)

There is diffuse hyperpigmentation of the dorsal aspects of the fingers and toes, beginning in infancy and gradually increasing [74]. The mode of inheritance is not definitely established.

Incontinentia Pigmenti
(Bloch-Sulzberger Syndrome)

This comparatively rare disorder was described by Bloch [75] and Sulzberger [76] in 1926 and 1927, respectively. Since then, over 653 cases have been reported, all but 16 of which are females [77].

Clinical Presentation. Onset is commonly soon after birth with an erythematous and vesiculobullous eruption of a linear pattern which involves mainly the extremities. The trunk and head may also be affected. The lesions may be persistent or recurrent over a period of several months, to be replaced by verrucous growths (Fig. 3.33). In a few months these verrucous bands disappear, leaving either mild atrophy or remnants of the papules. About this time a bizarre type of slate-colored macular pigmentation in whorls and splashes appears (Figs. 3.34 and 3.35). Occasionally, the other skin changes are minimal or absent and the pigmentary lesions may be the only abnormality. The pigmentary lesions do not follow the pattern, shape, or location of the bullous and verrucous lesions [78]. The pigmentation gradually fades after many years and tends to be minimal by the second or third decade.
Associated findings include poorly formed and missing dentition (Fig. 3.36), partial alopecia of the vertex, strabismus, microphthalmia, and retrolental fibroplasia [78]. Microcephaly, mental retardation, spastic tetraplegia, and epilepsy may also be associated with incontinentia pigmenti [79].

Pathology and Pathophysiology. The vesicles seen in the first stage of the disease are intraepidermal and are associated with spongiosis. Numerous eosinophils are present within and around the vesicles. In between the vesicles the epidermis contains large dyskeratotic cells. In the dermis, an infiltrate of round cells and eosinophils is present [80]. In the second stage, the epidermis is acanthotic and hyperkeratotic. Intraepidermal keratinization is seen as scattered dyskeratotic cells [80]. In the pigmentary stage, the findings are essentially those of extensive deposits of melanin within macrophages and decreased melanin in the basal cell layer.
Ultrastructurally, all three stages show dyskeratosis, phagocytosis of dyskeratotic cells and melanosomes by macrophages, and the presence of melanophages in the upper dermis [81]. These findings point to the relationship among all three stages of incontinentia pigmenti and suggest that pigmentary incontinence is a phagocytic phenomenon [81].

Inheritance. Although there is controversy as to the exact mode of inheritance [82], the X-linked dominant pattern is favored. Affected males die in utero.

Treatment. Symptomatic treatment and control of secondary infections are recommended.

Incontinentia Pigmenti Achromians (Ito)
(Hypomelanosis of Ito)

Since Ito described this condition in 1952 [83] over 20 cases have been reported [84].

Clinical Presentation. The eruption appears at or shortly after birth as asymmetric, hypopigmented, bizarre whorls and streaks which occur unilaterally or bilaterally [84]. Any part of the body may be involved except the scalp, palms, and soles. There is no preceding inflammation. The hypopigmentation may regress.
The associated abnormalities that have been reported to date include diminution of capillary resistance, decreased sweating, diffuse alopecia, facial hypertrichosis, verrucous epidermal nevus, dysplastic teeth, strabismus and other ocular abnormalities, various musculoskeletal defects, mental retardation, auditory conduction defect, and other neural defects [84].

Pathology and Pathophysiology. The main histopathologic feature is the decrease of melanin in the basal cell layer in the involved areas without any dermal inflammation or incontinence of pigment [85-87]. The dopa reaction is weak in hypopigmented areas [87]. In one study, dyskeratotic cells, similar to those of incontinentia pigmenti, have been identified [85].
It is generally accepted that incontinentia pigmenti and incontinentia pigmenti achromians are two separate entities [84, 86], despite the report of a mother with incontinentia pigmenti achromians and daughter with incontinentia pigmenti [88].

Inheritance. Autosomal dominant [84, 86].

Treatment. There is no specific treatment.

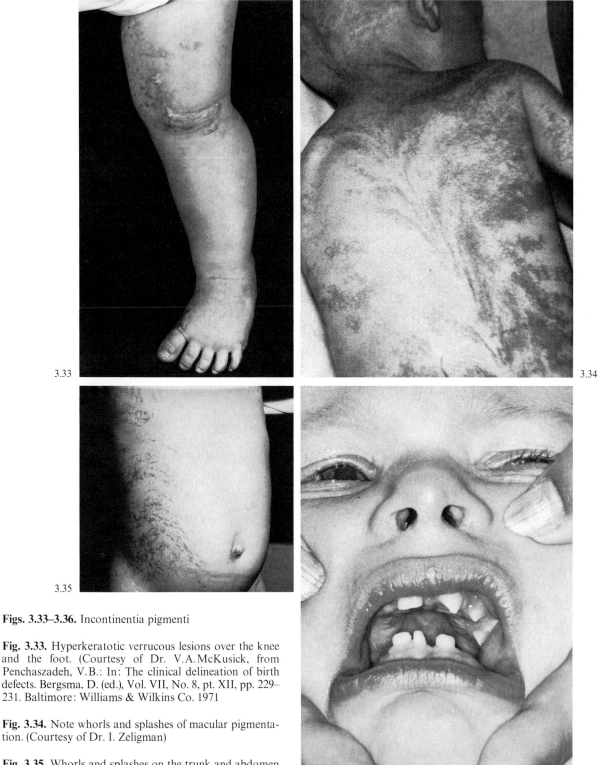

3.33

3.34

3.35

Figs. 3.33–3.36. Incontinentia pigmenti

Fig. 3.33. Hyperkeratotic verrucous lesions over the knee and the foot. (Courtesy of Dr. V.A.McKusick, from Penchaszadeh, V.B.: In: The clinical delineation of birth defects. Bergsma, D. (ed.), Vol. VII, No. 8, pt. XII, pp. 229–231. Baltimore: Williams & Wilkins Co. 1971

Fig. 3.34. Note whorls and splashes of macular pigmentation. (Courtesy of Dr. I. Zeligman)

Fig. 3.35. Whorls and splashes on the trunk and abdomen

Fig. 3.36. Missing and dysplastic teeth in a 4-year-old child. (Courtesy of Dr. V.A.McKusick, from Penchaszadeh, V.B.: In: The clinical delineation of birth defects. Bergsma, D. (ed.), Vol. VII, No. 8, pt. XII, pp. 229–231. Baltimore: Williams & Wilkins Co. 1971

3.36

Franceschetti-Jadassohn Syndrome (Naegeli Type of Incontinentia Pigmenti, Melanophoric Nevus Syndrome)

This very rare disorder was first described by Naegeli in 1927 [89] and was confused with incontinentia pigmenti. Later, the two conditions were separated [90].

Clinical Presentation. Reticular pigmentation, starting around the age of 2 years, is characteristic and is not preceded by any inflammatory signs. There are no associated findings in the eyes or hair, although the teeth may show yellow spotting. Hypo- or anhidrosis and palmoplantar thickening may occur.

Pathology and Pathophysiology. The main finding is incontinence of pigment. It has been suggested that this phenomenon is due to fragility of the epidermal melanin unit with subsequent loading of discharged pigment in a network along the veins [91]. The relationship between this disorder and incontinentia pigmenti (Bloch-Sulzberger) is not clear. "Transitional" cases showing a mixture of symptoms of both diseases have been reported [92].

Inheritance. Autosomal dominant.

Treatment. No treatment is needed.

Hyperpigmentation of Eyelids

This unique syndrome is characterized by periorbital hyperpigmentation. The lower eyelids are first involved and pigmentation progresses with age to the upper eyelids [93]. The pigmentation starts in childhood and is asymptomatic. Histologically, there is increased melanin pigment in the dermis [93]. Inheritance is autosomal dominant.

Familial Progressive Hyperpigmentation

One kindred (four individuals in two generations of a Negro family) has been described with this condition [94]. The syndrome is characterized by the appearance of patches of hyperpigmentation at birth. These patches increase in size and number with age, resulting in marked hyperpigmentation of extensive areas of skin and mucous membrane [94].

Histologically, there is an increase in number and average size of melanin granules and seemingly more premelanosomes in the hyperpigmented skin [94]. The syndrome is probably inherited as autosomal dominant.

Hyperpigmentation of Fuldauer and Kuijpers

A Dutch family has been described with a peculiar pattern of hyperpigmentation which involves predominantly the hands, wrists, and neck, and less often the axillae [95]. Inheritance is probably autosomal dominant.

References

1. Cunliffe, W.J., Hall, R., Newell, D.J., Stevenson, C.J.: Vitiligo, thyroid disease and autoimmunity. Brit. J. Derm. *80*, 135–139 (1968)
2. Bor, S., Feiwel, M., Chanarin, I.: Vitiligo and its aetiological relationship to organ-specific autoimmune disease. Brit. J. Derm. *81*, 83–88 (1969)
3. Dawber, R.P.R.: Integumentary associations of pernicious anemia. Brit. J. Derm. *82*, 221–223 (1970)
4. Johnson, W.C.: Vogt-Koyanagi-Harada syndrome. Arch. Derm. *88*, 146–149 (1963)
5. Alezzandrini, A.A.: Manifestation unilatérale de dégénérescence tapéto-rétinienne de vitiligo, de poliose, de cheveaux blancs et d'hypoacousie. Ophthalmologica (Basel) *147*, 409–419 (1964)
6. Kopf, A.W., Morrill, S.D., Silberberg, I.: Broad spectrum of leukoderma acquisitum centrifugum. Arch. Derm. *92*, 14–35 (1965)
7. Swanson, J.L., Wayte, D.M., Helwig, E.B.: Ultrastructure of halo nevi. J. invest. Derm. *50*, 434–437 (1968)
8. Birbeck, M.S., Breathnach, A.S., Everall, J.D.: An electron microscope study of basal melanocytes and high-level clear cells (Langerhans cells) in vitiligo. J. invest. Derm. *37*, 51–64 (1961)
9. Lerner, A.B.: Vitiligo. J. invest. Derm. *32*, 285–310 (1959)
10. McFadden, A.W.: Skin disease in the Cuna Indians. Dermatology and geography of the San Blas Coast of Panama. Arch. Derm. *84*, 1013–1023 (1961)
11. Witkop, C.J., Jr., Quevedo, W.C., Jr., Fitzpatrick, T.B.: Albinism. In: The metabolic basis of inherited disease. Stanbury, J.B., Wyngaarden, J.B., Fredrickson, D.S. (eds.), 4th ed., pp. 283–316. New York: McGraw-Hill Book Co. 1978
12. Witkop, C.J., Jr., Hill, C.W., Desnick, S., Thies, J.K., Thorn, H.L., Jenkins, M., White, J.G.: Ophthalmologic, biochemical, platelet, and ultrastructural defects in the various types of oculocutaneous albinism. J. invest. Derm. *60*, 443–456 (1973)
13. Hermansky, F., Pudlak, P.: Albinism associated with hemorrhagic diathesis and unusual pigmented reticular cells in the bone marrow. Report of two cases with histochemical studies. Blood *14*, 162–169 (1959)
14. Ziprkowski, L., Adam, A.: Recessive total albinism and congenital deaf-mutism. Arch. Derm. *89*, 151–155 (1964)
15. Reed, W.B., Stone, V.M., Boder, E., Ziprkowski, L.: Pigmentary disorders in association with congenital deafness. Arch. Derm. *95*, 176–186 (1967)

16. Tietz, W.: A syndrome of deaf-mutism associated with albinism showing dominant autosomal inheritance. Amer. J. hum. Genet. 15, 259–264 (1963)

17. Ziprkowski, L., Krakowski, A., Adam, A., Costeff, H., Sade, J.: Partial albinism and deaf mutism. Due to a recessive sex-linked gene. Arch. Derm. 86, 530–539 (1962)

18. Woolf, C.M., Dolowitz, D.A., Aldous, H.E.: Congenital deafness associated with piebaldism. Arch. Otolaryng. 82, 244–250 (1965)

19. Warburg, M.: Ocular albinism and protanopia in the same family. Acta ophthal. (Kbh.) 42, 444–451 (1964)

20. Waardenburg, P.J.: Some notes on publications of Professor Arnold Sorsby and Åland eye disease (Forsius-Eriksson syndrome). J. med. Genet. 7, 194–199 (1970)

21. Fitzpatrick, T.B., Jimbow, K., Donaldson, D.D.: Dominant oculocutaneous albinism. Brit. J. Derm. 91, Suppl. 10, 23 (1974)

22. Telfer, M.A., Sugar, M., Jaeger, E.A., Mulcahy, J.: Dominant piebald trait (white forelock and leukoderma) with neurological impairment. Amer. J. hum. Genet. 23, 383–389 (1961)

23. Comings, D.E., Odland, G.F.: Partial albinism. J. Amer. med. Ass. 195, 519–523 (1966)

24. Grupper, C., Pruniéras, M., Hincky, M., Garelly, E.: Albinisme partiel familial (piebaldisme): étude ultrastructurale. Ann. Derm. Syph. (Paris) 97, 267–286 (1970)

25. Breathnach, A.S., Fitzpatrick, T.B., Wyllie, L.M.A.: Electron microscopy of melanocytes in human piebaldism. J. invest. Derm. 45, 28–37 (1965)

26. McKusick, V.A.: Mendelian inheritance in man, 4th ed., p. 648. Baltimore: Johns Hopkins University Press 1975

27. Hare, H.J.H.: Premature whitening of hair. J. Heredity 20, 31–32 (1929)

28. Cross, H.E., McKusick, V.A., Breen, W.: A new oculocerebral syndrome with hypopigmentation. J. Pediat. 70, 398–406 (1967)

29. Witkop, C.J., Jr.: Albinism. In: Advances in human genetics. Harris, H., Hirschhorn, K. (eds.), Vol. 2, pp. 61–142. New York: Plenum Press 1971

30. Weary, P.E., Behlen, C.H.: Unusual familial hypopigmentary anomaly. Arch. Derm. 92, 54–55 (1965)

31. Scott, C.I.: Raindrop hypopigmentation. In: The clinical delineation of birth defects. Bergsma, D. (ed.), Vol. VII, No. 8, pt. XII, pp. 236–237. Baltimore: Williams & Wilkins Co. 1971

32. Waardenburg, P.J.: A new syndrome combining developmental anomalies of the eyelids, eyebrows and nose root with pigmentary defects of the iris and head hair and with congenital deafness. Amer. J. hum. Genet. 3, 195–253 (1951)

33. Klein, D.: Albinisme partiel (leucisme) accompagné de surdimité, d'ostéomyodysplasie, de raideurs articulaires congénitales multiples et d'autres malformations congénitales. Arch. Julius Klaus. Stift. Vererbungsforsch. 22, 336–342 (1947)

34. Waardenburg, P.J.: Merkwaardige nieuwe gegevens over de erfelijkheid van bepaalde vormen van albinisme en leukisme bij de mens. Ned. T. Geneesk. 109, 1057–1065 (1965)

35. Feingold, M., Robinson, M.J., Gellis, S.S.: Waardenburg's syndrome during the first year of life. J. Pediat. 71, 874–876 (1967)

36. Goldberg, M.F.: Waardenburg's syndrome with fundus and other anomalies. Arch. Ophthal. 76, 797–810 (1966)

37. Giacoia, J.P., Klein, S.W.: Waardenburg's syndrome with bilateral cleft lip. Amer. J. Dis. Child. 117, 344–348 (1969)

38. Beguez Cesar, A.: Neutropenia cronica maligna familar con granulaciones atipicas de los leucocitos. Bol. Soc. Cub. Pediat. 15, 900–922 (1943)

39. Chédiak, M.: Nouvelle anomalie leucocytaire de caractère constitutionel et familial. Rev. Hematol. 7, 362–367 (1952)

40. Higashi, O.: Congenital gigantism of peroxidase granules. Tôhoku J. exp. Med. 59, 315–322 (1954)

41. Fitzpatrick, T.B., Mihm, M.C., Jr.: Abnormalities of the melanin pigmentary system. In: Dermatology in general medicine. Fitzpatrick, T.B., Arndt, K.A., Clark, W.H., Jr., Eisen, A.Z., Van Scott, E.J., Vaughan, J.H. (eds.), p. 1613. New York: McGraw-Hill Book Co. 1971

42. Stegmaier, O.C., Schneider, L.A.: Chédiak-Higashi syndrome. Dermatologic manifestations. Arch. Derm. 91, 1–9 (1965)

43. Lever, W.F., Schaumburg-Lever, G.: Histopathology of the skin, p. 421. Philadelphia: Lippincott, J.B. Co. 1975

44. Windhorst, D.B., Zelickson, A.S., Good, R.A.: Chédiak-Higashi syndrome: hereditary gigantism of cytoplasmic organelles. Science 151, 81–83 (1966)

45. Windhorst, D.B., Zelickson, A.S., Good, R.A.: A human pigmentary dilution based on a heritable subcellular structural defect – the Chédiak-Higashi syndrome. J. invest. Derm. 50, 9–18 (1968)

46. White, J.G.: The Chédiak-Higashi syndrome: a possible lysosomal disease. Blood 28, 143–156 (1966)

47. Kritzler, R.A., Terner, J.Y., Lindenbaum, J., Magidson, J., Williams, R., Preisig, R., Phillips, G.B.: Chédiak-Higashi syndrome. Cytologic and serum lipid observations in a case and family. Amer. J. Med. 36, 583–594 (1964)

48. Boxer, L.A., Watanabe, A.M., Rister, M., Besch, H.R., Allen, J., Baehner, R.L.: Correction of leukocyte function in Chédiak-Higashi syndrome by ascorbate. New Engl. J. Med. 295, 1041–1045 (1976)

49. Blume, R.S., Bennett, J.M., Yankee, R.A., Wolff, S.M.: Defective granulocyte regulation in the Chédiak-Higashi syndrome. New Engl. J. Med. 279, 1009–1015 (1968)

50. Sugai, T., Saito, T., Hamada, T.: Symmetric acroleukopathy in mother and daughter. Arch. Derm. 92, 172–173 (1965)

51. Walsh, R.J.: A distinctive pigment of the skin in New Guinea indigenes. Ann. hum. Genet. 34, 379–388 (1971)

52. Breathnach, A.S.: Melanocyte distribution in forearm epidermis of freckled human subjects. J. invest. Derm. 29, 253–261 (1957)

53. Breathnach, A.S., Wyllie, L.M.: Electron microscopy of melanocytes and melanosomes in freckled human epidermis. J. invest. Derm. 42, 389–394 (1964)

54. Gorlin, R.J., Anderson, R.C., Blaw, M.: Multiple lentigenes syndrome. Complex comprising multiple lentigenes, electrocardiographic conduction abnormalities, ocular hypertelorism, pulmonary stenosis, abnormalities of genitalia, retardation of growth, sensorineural deafness, and autosomal dominant hereditary pattern. Amer. J. Dis. Child. 117, 652–662 (1969)

55. Selmanowitz, V.J., Orentreich, N., Felsenstein, J.M.: Lentiginosis profusa syndrome (multiple lentigines syndrome). Arch. Derm. 104, 393–401 (1971)

56. Forney, W.R., Robinson, S.J., Pascoe, D.J.: Congenital heart disease, deafness, and skeletal malformation; a new syndrome? J. Pediat. 68, 14–26 (1966)

57. Nordlund, J.J., Lerner, A.B., Braverman, I.M., McGuire, J.S.: The multiple lentigines syndrome. Arch. Derm. 107, 259–261 (1973)

58. Touraine, A.: Lentiginose centro-faciale et dysplasies associées. Bull. Soc. franç. Derm. Syph. 48, 518–521 (1941)

59. Dociu, I., Galaction-Niţelea, O., Şirjiţa, N., Murgu, V.: Centrofacial lentiginosis. A survey of 40 cases. Brit. J. Derm. 94, 39–43 (1976)

60. McKusick, V.A.: Mendelian inheritance in man, 5th ed., p. 239. Baltimore: Johns Hopkins University Press 1978

61. Peutz, J.L.A.: Over een zeer Merkwaardige, gecombineerde familiare polyposis van de slijmvliezen van den tractus intestinalis met die van de neuskeelholte en gepaard met eignnaardige pigmentaties van huid en slijmvlisen. Ned. T. Geneesk. *10*, 134–146 (1921)
62. Jeghers, H.: Medical progress. Pigmentation of the skin. New Engl. J. Med. *231*, 122–136 (1944)
63. Jeghers, H., McKusick, V.A., Katz, K.H.: Generalized intestinal polyposis and melanin spots of the oral mucosa, lips and digits. A syndrome of diagnostic significance. New Engl. J. Med. *241*, 993–1005 (1949)
64. McAllister, A.J., Hicken, N.F., Latimer, R.G., Condon, V.R.: Seventeen patients with Peutz-Jeghers syndrome in four generations. Amer. J. Surg. *114*, 839–843 (1967)
65. Dodds, W.J., Schulte, W.J., Hensley, G.T., Hogan, W.J.: Peutz-Jeghers syndrome and gastrointestinal malignancy. Amer. J. Roentgenol. *115*, 374–377 (1972)
66. Scully, R.E.: Sex cord tumor with annular tubules – a distinctive ovarian tumor of the Peutz-Jeghers syndrome. Cancer *25*, 1107–1121 (1970)
67. Sommerhaug, R.G., Mason, T.: Peutz-Jeghers syndrome and ureteral polyposis. J. Amer. med. Ass. *211*, 120–122 (1970)
68. McKittrick, J.E., Lewis, W.M., Doane, W.A., Gerwig, W.H.: The Peutz-Jeghers syndrome. Report of two cases, one with 30 year follow-up. Arch. Surg. *103*, 57–62 (1971)
69. Fox, H., Emery, J.L., Goodbody, R.A., Yates, P.O.: Neurocutaneous melanosis. Arch. Dis. Child. *39*, 508–516 (1964)
70. Shaffer, B.: Pigmented nevi. A clinical appraisal in the light of present-day histopathologic concepts. Arch. Derm. *72*, 120–132 (1955)
71. Pegum, J.S.: Diffuse pigmentation in brothers. Proc. roy. Soc. Med. *48*, 179–180 (1955)
72. Siemens, H.W.: Acromelanosis albo-punctata. Dermatologica (Basel) *128*, 86–87 (1964)
73. Suenaga, M.: Genetical studies on skin diseases. VII. Dyschromatosis universalis hereditaria in five generations. Tôhoku J. exp. Med. *55*, 373–376 (1952)
74. Furuya, T., Mishima, Y.: Progressive pigmentary disorder in Japanese child. Arch. Derm. *86*, 412–418 (1962)
75. Bloch, B.: Eigentümliche bisher nicht beschriebene Pigmentaffektion (Incontinentia Pigmenti). Schweiz. med. Wschr. *56*, 404–405 (1926)
76. Sulzberger, M.B.: Über eine bisher nicht beschriebene congenitale Pigmentanomalie (Incontinentia pigmenti). Arch. Derm. Syph. (Berlin) *154*, 19–32 (1927)
77. Carney, R.G., Jr.: Incontinentia pigmenti: world statistical analysis. Arch. Derm. *112*, 535–542 (1976)
78. Carney, R.G., Carney, R.G.,Jr.: Incontinentia pigmenti. Arch. Derm. *102*, 157–162 (1970)
79. Reed, W.B., Carter, C., Cohen, T.M.: Incontinentia pigmenti. Dermatologica (Basel) *134*, 243–250 (1967)
80. Epstein, S., Vedder, J.S., Pinkus, H.: Bullous variety of incontinentia pigmenti (Bloch-Sulzberger). Arch. Derm. Syph. *65*, 557–567 (1952)
81. Schamburg-Lever (sic), G., Lever, W.F.: Electron microscopy of incontinentia pigmenti. J. invest. Derm. *61*, 151–158 (1973)
82. Curth, H.O., Warburton, D.: The genetics of incontinentia pigmenti. Arch. Derm. *92*, 229–235 (1965)
83. Ito, M.: Studies on melanin. XI. Incontinentia pigmenti achromians? A singular case of nevus depigmentosus systematicus bilateralis. Tôhoku J. exp. Med. *55*, Suppl. 1, 57–59 (1952)
84. Jelinek, J.E., Bart, R.S., Schiff, G.M.: Hypomelanosis of Ito ("incontinentia pigmenti achromians"). Report of three cases and review of the literature. Arch. Derm. *107*, 596–601 (1973)
85. Grosshans, E.M., Stoebner, P., Bergoend, H., Stoll, C.: Incontinentia pigmenti achromians (Ito). Étude clinique et histo-pathologique. Dermatologica (Basel) *142*, 65–78 (1971)
86. Rubin, M.B.: Incontinentia pigmenti achromians. Multiple cases within a family. Arch. Derm. *105*, 424–425 (1972)
87. Aram, H.: Incontinentia pigmenti achromians (Ito). Cutis *6*, 197–201 (1970)
88. Piñol, J., Mascaro, J.M., Romaguera, C.,Jr., Asprer, J.: Considérations sur l'*incontinentia pigmenti achromians* de Ito. A propos de deux nouveaux cas. Bull. Soc. franç. Derm. Syph. *76*, 553–555 (1969)
89. Naegeli, O.: Familiärer Chromatophorennävus. Schweiz. med. Wschr. *57*, 48 (1927)
90. Franceschetti, A., Jadassohn, W.: A propos de l'incontinentia pigmenti, délimitation de deux syndromes différents figurant sous le même terme. Dermatologica (Basel) *108*, 1–28 (1954)
91. Whiting, D.A.: Naegeli's reticular pigmented dermatosis. Brit. J. Derm. *85*, Suppl. 7, 71–72 (1971)
92. Greither, A., Haensch, R.: Anhydrotische retikuläre Pigmentdermatose mit blasig-erythematösem Anfangsstadium. Ein Beitrag zu den Übergangsfällen zwischen Incontinentia pigmenti Bloch-Sulzberger und der retikulären Pigmentdermatose Naegeli-Franceschetti-Jadassohn. Schweiz. med. Wschr. *100*, 228–233 (1970)
93. Goodman, R.M., Belcher, R.W.: Periorbital hyperpigmentation. An overlooked genetic disorder of pigmentation. Arch. Derm. *100*, 169–174 (1969)
94. Chernosky, M.E., Anderson, D.E., Chang, J.P., Shaw, M.W., Romsdahl, M.M.: Familial progressive hyperpigmentation. Arch. Derm. *103*, 581–598 (1971)
95. Fuldauer, M.L., Kuijpers, P.B.: Een erfelijke pigmentanomalie (incontinentia pigmenti?). Ned. T. Geneesk. *108*, 1613–1623 (1964)

Chapter 4   Bullous Eruptions

Contents

Acrodermatitis Enteropathica

In 1942 Danbolt and Closs [1] described a rare disease which manifests itself with erosive skin lesions of the scalp, eyebrows and eyelashes, alopecia, and intractable diarrhea.

Clinical Presentation. The children appear normal at birth. The onset of the cutaneous and intestinal symptoms coincides frequently with weaning from breast feeding. The cutaneous manifestations consist of irregular plaques of vesicles and bullae on erythematous bases. Satellite vesicles, bullae, and pustules may occur on the skin around the plaques. The lesions are characteristically localized at the mucocutaneous orifices and on the peripheral parts of the extremities (mouth, eyelids, elbows, knees, nails, anogenital areas) (Figs. 4.1 and 4.2). Resolution of the skin lesions leaves no scarring or atrophy. Hair loss occurs early in the disease and involves the scalp, eyebrows, and eyelashes (Fig. 4.3). Paronychia and dystrophic changes of the nails are usual. The cutaneous and intestinal symptoms follow simultaneous exacerbations and remissions. *Candida albicans* may be recovered from the stools, oral cavity, skin, and nails. The general health of the patient is greatly affected. There is tissue wasting, growth retardation, listlessness, anorexia, apathy, and sometimes schizoid changes. In most cases the disease is fatal [2].

Pathology and Pathophysiology. Histologic examination of a bullous lesion shows acanthosis with large intraepidermal vesicles containing single and clumped acantholytic cells [3], many neutrophils, and a few eosinophils. The dermis exhibits dilated blood vessels with a mild perivascular round cell infiltration in the middermis and a marked diffuse infiltration in the pars papillaris and upper dermis. The quiescent plaques show acanthosis and hyperkeratosis and there are signs of inflammation in the dermis.

Several hypotheses have been suggested to explain the pathophysiology of the disease. Defects in the metabolism of essential unsaturated fatty acids found in cow's milk [4] or abnormalities in the metabolism of essential amino acids have been suspected.

Successful treatment with the oral administration of zinc sulfate was reported in 1974 [4]. Since then, other reports [5] have confirmed the excellent results of zinc sulfate therapy. Thus, although the basic pathophysiology of this disease is still unclear, there is sufficient evidence to suspect that the defect is somewhere in zinc metabolism or zinc absorption from the small intestine.

Inheritance. Autosomal recessive.

Treatment. The treatment with diiodohydroxyquinoline (Diodoquin) or iodochlorhydroxyquin (Entero-Vioform) gives inadequate results and is highly toxic, especially to the eyes. The standard, effective, simple, and innocuous treatment at present consists of the oral administration of zinc sulfate, 50 mg three times daily, in the form of tablets or powder dissolved in fruit juice (Figs. 4.4 and 4.5).

References

1. Danbolt, N., Closs, K.: Acrodermatitis enteropathica. Acta derm.-venereol. (Stockh.) 23, 127–169 (1943)
2. Idriss, Z.H., Der Kaloustian, V.M.: Acrodermatitis enteropathica. Clin. Pediat. 12, 393–395 (1972)
3. Juljulian, H.H., Kurban, A.K.: Acantholysis: a feature of acrodermatitis enteropathica. Arch. Derm. 103, 105–106 (1971)
4. Moynahan, E.J.: Acrodermatitis enteropathica. A lethal inherited human zinc deficiency disorder. Lancet 1974 II, 399
5. Der Kaloustian, V.M., Musallam, S.S., Sanjad, S.A., Murib, A., Hammad, W.D., Idriss, Z.H.: Treatment of acrodermatitis enteropathica with oral zinc sulfate. Amer. J. Dis. Child. 130, 421–424 (1976)

Epidermolysis Bullosa

Epidermolysis bullosa (EB) is a group of genetically determined, chronic, noninflammatory disorders characterized by blistering of the skin and certain mucosae. The blisters frequently result from minor mechanical trauma or may arise spontaneously. Since the blistering is not due to epidermal lysis in all types of EB, the term "epidermolysis" may be inappropriate [1]. The term "mechanobullous disease" has been suggested for this group of disorders [1]. However, we are retaining the old term because of its constant usage since it was first introduced in 1886 [2].

The various syndromes that comprise EB are genetically distinct diseases with characteristic clinical manifestations. They can be classified according to the mode of inheritance and the presence or absence of scarring (Table 4.1).

Nonscarring EB

Epidermolysis Bullosa Simplex (Köbner)

Clinical Presentation. The severity of this condition varies considerably even though it is uniform in any one kindred. The general development and health of affected individuals are normal. The disease becomes manifest usually in early childhood, rarely at birth or in early infancy. Occasionally, the trauma of parturition results in bullae and denuded areas which are apparent at birth, especially involving the lower extremities. In this connection the cases reported with congenital localized absence of the skin [3] that may be considered as suffering from EB will be discussed separately (see p. 127). More often the bullae appear when the child starts to crawl or walk. The bullae, ranging in size from a few millimeters to several centimeters, are tense and clear, although occasionally they are hemorrhagic (Figs. 4.6 and 4.7). They rupture easily and heal without scarring although there may be temporary hypo- or hyperpigmentation. Secondary bacterial infection may ensue in the eroded areas. The most commonly affected areas are those exposed to trauma, like hands, feet, elbows, and knees, and sites of pressure with clothing. The disease is worse in warm weather, especially if the patients have hyperhidrosis. Occasionally, the oral mucous membrane may be involved. The severity of the blistering tends to decrease after puberty. The hair, nails, and teeth are normal.

Table 4.1. Classification of epidermolysis bullosa syndromes

Nonscarring EB	
Epidermolysis bullosa simplex (Köbner)	Autosomal dominant
Epidermolysis bullosa simplex (Ogna)	Autosomal dominant
Epidermolysis bullosa simplex of the hands and feet (Weber-Cockayne) (recurrent bullous eruption of the hands and feet)	Autosomal dominant
Epidermolysis bullosa letalis (Herlitz) (junctional bullous epidermatosis)	Autosomal recessive
Scarring EB	
Epidermolysis bullosa dystrophica (Cockayne-Touraine) (dermolytic bullous dermatosis-dominant)	Autosomal dominant
Epidermolysis bullosa dystrophica albopapuloidea (Pasini) (dermolytic bullous dermatosis-dystrophic)	Autosomal dominant
Epidermolysis bullosa dystrophica polydysplastica (Hallopeau-Siemens) (dermolytic bullous dermatosis-recessive)	Autosomal recessive
Other variants	

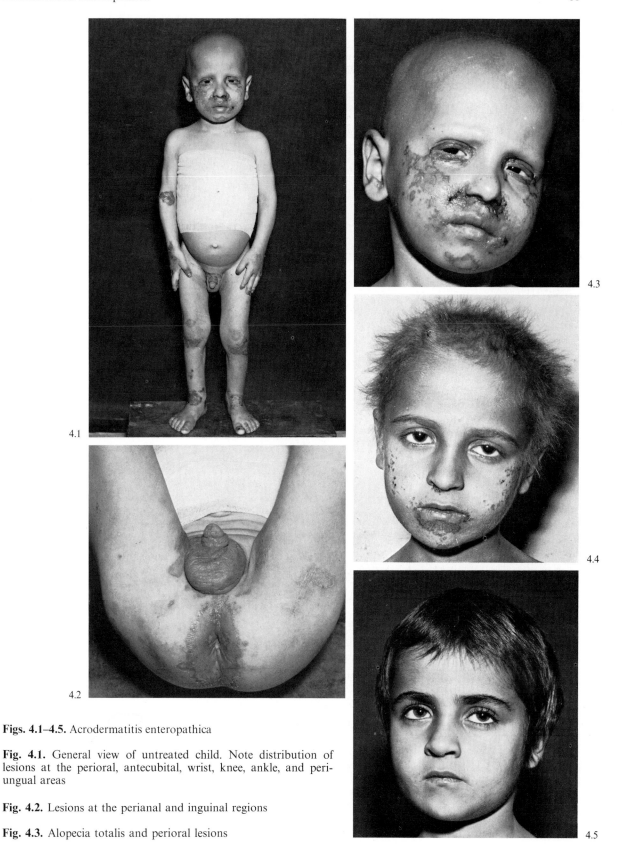

Figs. 4.1–4.5. Acrodermatitis enteropathica

Fig. 4.1. General view of untreated child. Note distribution of lesions at the perioral, antecubital, wrist, knee, ankle, and periungual areas

Fig. 4.2. Lesions at the perianal and inguinal regions

Fig. 4.3. Alopecia totalis and perioral lesions

Figs. 4.4 and 4.5. A 7-year-old child before and 1 month after oral zinc sulfate treatment. (From Der Kaloustian, V.M., et al.: Am. J. Dis. Child. *130*, 421–424, 1976)

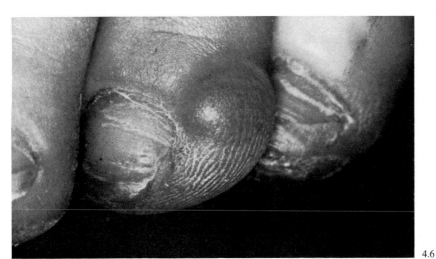

Figs. 4.6 and 4.7. Epidermolysis bullosa simplex. Note tense bullae

4.6

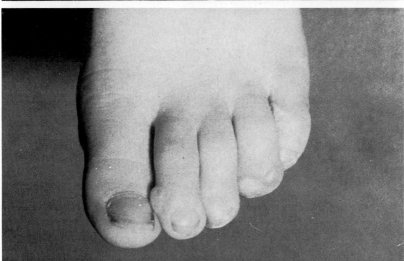

4.7

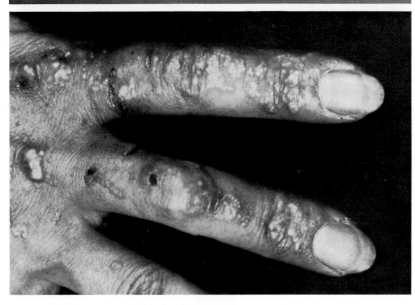

Fig. 4.8. Epidermolysis bullosa simplex of the hands and feet. (Courtesy of Dr. I. Zeligman)

Pathology and Pathophysiology. Bullae are formed by vacuolation of the basal and suprabasal cells [4]. The PAS-positive basement membrane is intact and remains on the dermal side. The elastic tissue is normal [4]. Ultrastructurally, there is perinuclear edema, degenerative changes in the mitochondria, and dissolution of tonofilaments followed by destruction of organelles and disintegration of the cytoplasm [5]. It is postulated that the defect in this disorder is "activation" of cytolytic enzymes within the epidermal cells by mechanical trauma [1].

Inheritance. Autosomal dominant.

Treatment. General measures are important in the management of EB and include protection from trauma, avoidance of excessive heat, and the use of antibiotics and chemotherapeutic agents to control secondary infections.

Epidermolysis Bullosa Simplex (Ogna)

This is a variant of epidermolysis bullosa simplex (Köbner) that has been identified only in a Norwegian kindred [6]. This syndrome differs from the Köbner type in its association with a congenital generalized bruising tendency. This latter feature may be related to red cell-soluble glutamate-pyruvate transaminase [7].

Epidermolysis Bullosa Simplex of the Hands and Feet (Weber-Cockayne) (Recurrent Bullous Eruption of the Hands and Feet)

Clinical Presentation. The bullae may appear in childhood or adult life, are worse in summer, and affect predominantly the feet. Both the plantar and dorsal surfaces of the feet are involved. The hand lesions are usually few and occasionally other sites are involved. Healing is without scarring (Fig. 4.8).

Pathology and Pathophysiology. The characteristic finding is the cytolysis of the epidermal cells similar to that of epidermolysis bullosa simplex, but sparing the basal cells. Cleavage is usually in the midsquamous level. Dyskeratosis is also present [1].

Inheritance. Autosomal dominant.

Treatment. The general management encompasses protection of the patients from trauma. In particular, specially cushioned shoes should be used.

Epidermolysis Bullosa Letalis (Junctional Bullous Epidermatosis, Herlitz Syndrome)

Clinical Presentation. The disease is usually manifest at birth with erosions and bullae over the lower extremities, around the bases of the nails, and at other sites (Figs. 4.9–4.11). The palms and soles are rarely involved. The nails may be absent. Mucous membranes and the eyes [8] may be involved. The teeth may be small, deformed, discolored, or have early caries. The erosions tend to heal slowly, but without scarring or milia. Fluid loss and secondary infections may lead to early death because of the large areas involved. In mild cases, the disease runs a chronic course with periods of amelioration and exacerbation.

Pathology and Pathophysiology. The bullae are formed by a complete dermal-epidermal separation with a PAS-positive basement membrane on the dermal side [9]. Ultrastructurally, the separation is shown to be between the basement and plasma membranes (intermembrane space) [1,9].

Inheritance. Autosomal recessive.

Treatment. In addition to the general measures mentioned above, corticosteroid therapy should be instituted early. Infections should be combated and fluid loss replaced.

Scarring EB

Epidermolysis Bullosa Dystrophica (Cockayne-Touraine) (Dermolytic Bullous Dermatosis – Dominant)

Clinical Presentation. The affected individuals are usually of normal stature and good health, with normal hair and teeth. Bulla formation usually appears at birth at sites of trauma. The most affected sites are the limbs, especially at sites of pressure, and occasionally the oral and anogenital mucosa (Figs. 4.12 and 4.13). Healing results in scars that often are atrophic, but occasionally hypertrophic and keloidal. Hyper- and hypopigmentation may be present at healed sites. Milia are frequent.
Other associated findings are palmoplantar keratoses, hyperhidrosis, thick dystrophic nails, and keratosis pilaris.

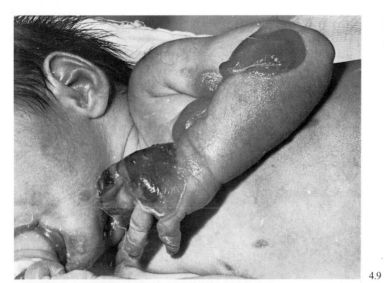

Figs. 4.9–4.11. Epidermolysis bullosa letalis. Bullae and denuded areas at sites of pressure

4.9

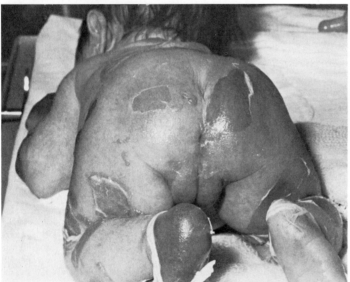

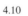

4.10

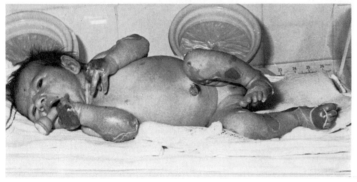

4.11

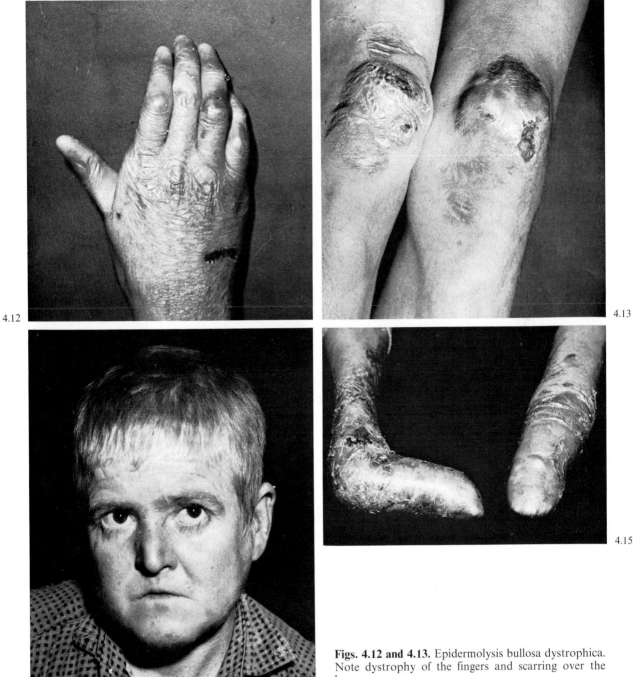

4.12

4.13

4.15

4.14

Figs. 4.12 and 4.13. Epidermolysis bullosa dystrophica. Note dystrophy of the fingers and scarring over the knees

Figs. 4.14 and 4.15. Epidermolysis bullosa dystrophica polydysplastica. Note the puckered face and the fusion of the fingers in the scarred tissue

Pathology and Pathophysiology. The bullae are subepidermal with a normal overlying epidermis. The PAS-positive basement membrane is poorly defined [1,4]. Ultrastructurally, the characteristic findings are a sharp separation beneath the basement membrane, varying degrees of degeneration of the connective tissue, and absence of anchoring fibers [1].

The pathogenetic role of increased collagenolytic activity at the sites of the bullae is controversial [10,11].

Inheritance. Autosomal dominant.

Treatment. Other than the general measures referred to above, corticosteroids may be of limited help. It has been claimed that vitamin E, in a daily dose of 1600 IU, decreases blister formation effectively [12–14]. A controlled study, however, has shown no significant effect with vitamin E [15]. Esophageal dilatation and plastic surgical repair of deformities, especially of the hand, may be helpful.

Epidermolysis Bullosa Dystrophica Albopapuloidea (Pasini) (Dermolytic Bullous Dermatosis – Dystrophic)

This is a variant of epidermolysis bullosa dystrophica (dominant) characterized by the development of small, firm, white papules. These appear on the trunk, especially the lower back, are often perifollicular, and enlarge slowly to reach a diameter of 1.5 cm [16,17]. A disturbance in the catabolism of acid mucopolysaccharides in the lesions in this disorder is suggested [17]. In all other respects, the findings are identical with those of the dominant dystrophic form.

Epidermolysis Bullosa Dystrophica Polydysplastica (Hallopeau-Siemens) (Dermolytic Bullous Dermatosis – Recessive)

Clinical Presentation. Onset is usually at birth or in early infancy with bullae and erosions, especially on the feet. The bullae are large, flaccid, occasionally hemorrhagic, and occur on any part of the skin surface. Nikolsky's sign is positive. Healing is rather slow and results in atrophic scars, although there may be repeated cycles of blistering and erosion. In the hands and feet this may result in fusion of the fingers and toes by pseudowebbing of scar tissue to form a clublike useless appendage. The face may have a puckered appearance (Figs. 4.14 and 4.15).

Mucosal involvement is usual and results in chronic erosions in the mouth, binding down of the tongue, esophageal strictures, and mild conjunctival scarring. These complications interfere with feeding and nutrition.

Other associated findings are dry, atrophic, wrinkled skin, dystrophic nails, and malformed carious teeth. There is marked retardation of growth and development.

It is well-established that the scar tissue in this type of EB is prone to develop epidermal neoplasms. The squamous cell carcinomas that develop are usually of a low-grade malignancy, affecting the skin and less commonly the mouth or esophagus. The onset of the neoplasm is usually after the age of 30 years. It is postulated that abnormal collagen scarring predisposes the epidermis to the neoplastic change [18, 19].

Pathology and Pathophysiology. The basic changes are similar to those of the dominant dystrophic EB.

Inheritance. Autosomal recessive.

Treatment. General management is outlined above. For the neoplasms arising in the scar tissue, surgical treatment is indicated despite its limitations [18].

Other Variants

There are several reports in the literature of a number of variants of EB. In the majority of these, however, their nosologic identity and independent status are questionable. Such variants include:
1. Localized absence of the skin with blistering and nail dystrophy [3].
2. Epidermolysis bullosa dystrophica–macular type of Mendes da Costa (X-linked recessive inheritance) [20]. The main features are the appearance of depigmented spots on the hands and feet and later the face, pigmented spots on the trunk, cyanosis, and bullae with scar formation, especially in summer. The hands are short, the fingers tapered, the nails short and smooth, and the skin hypotrichotic. Death usually occurs before adulthood.
3. Acantholytic bullous epidermatosis (dominant inheritance) [1].
4. Epidermolysis bullosa vegetans (dominant inheritance). There is persistent secondary infection, ulceration, and exuberant granulation tissue, complicated by anemia and amyloidosis.
5. Epidermolysis bullosa dystrophica neurotrophica (recessive inheritance). There is congenital, progressive perceptive deafness in addition to the traumatic skin blistering.

6. Epidermolysis bullosa dystrophica associated with pyloric atresia (recessive inheritance) [21].

References

1. Pearson, R.W.: The mechanobullous diseases (epidermolysis bullosa). In: Dermatology in general medicine. Fitzpatrick, T.B., Arndt, K.A., Clark, W.C., Jr., Eisen, A.Z., Van Scott, E.J., Vaughan, J.H. (eds.), pp. 621–643. New York: McGraw-Hill Book Co. 1971
2. Köbner, H.: Hereditäre Anlage zur Blasenbildung (Epidermolysis bullosa hereditaria). Dtsch. med. Wschr. 12, 21–22 (1886)
3. Bart, B.J.: Epidermolysis bullosa and congenital localized absence of skin. Arch. Derm. 101, 78–81 (1970)
4. Lowe, L.B., Jr.: Hereditary epidermolysis bullosa. Arch. Derm. 95, 587–595 (1967)
5. Pearson, R.W.: Some observations on epidermolysis bullosa and experimental blisters. In: The epidermis. Montagna, W., Lobitz, W.C. (eds.), pp. 613–626. New York: Academic Press 1964
6. Gedde-Dahl, T., Jr.: Epidermolysis bullosa. A clinical, genetic and epidemiological study. Baltimore: Johns Hopkins University Press 1971
7. Olaisen, B., Gedde-Dahl, T., Jr.: GPT-epidermolysis bullosa simplex (EBS Ogna) linkage in man. Hum. Heredity 23, 189–196 (1973)
8. Aurora, A.L., Madhavan, M., Rao, S.: Ocular changes in epidermolysis bullosa letalis. Am. J. Ophthal. 79, 464–470 (1975)
9. Pearson, R.W., Potter, B., Strauss, F.: Epidermolysis bullosa hereditaria letalis. Clinical and histological manifestations and course of the disease. Arch. Derm. 109, 349–355 (1974)
10. Eisen, A.Z.: Human skin collagenase: relationship to the pathogenesis of epidermolysis bullosa dystrophica. J. invest. Derm. 52, 449–453 (1969)
11. Lazarus, G.S.: Collagenase and connective tissue metabolism in epidermolysis bullosa. J. invest. Derm. 58, 242–248 (1972)
12. Seghal, V.N., Vadiraj, S.N., Rege, V.L., Beohar, P.C.: Dystrophic epidermolysis bullosa in a family. Response to vitamin E (tocopherol). Dermatologica (Basel) 144, 27–34 (1972)
13. Smith, E.B., Michener, W.M.: Vitamin E treatment of dermolytic bullous dermatosis. Arch. Derm. 108, 254–256 (1973)
14. Michaelson, J.D., Schmidt, J.D., Dresden, M.H., Duncan, W.C.: Vitamin E treatment of epidermolysis bullosa. Changes in tissue collagenase levels. Arch. Derm. 109, 67–69 (1974)
15. Adams, R.H., Main, R.A., Marsden, R.A.: A controlled study of vitamin E in epidermolysis bullosa. Brit. J. Derm. 93, Suppl. 11, 10 (1975)
16. Schnyder, U.W., Jung, E.G., Salamon, T.: Zur Klassifizierung, Histogenetik, Gerinnungsphysiologie und Therapie der hereditären Epidermolysen. Arch. klin. exp. Derm. 220, 38–59 (1964)
17. Sasai, Y., Saito, N., Seiji, M.: Epidermolysis bullosa dystrophica et albo-papuloidea. Report of a case and histochemical study. Arch. Derm. 108, 554–557 (1973)
18. Wechsler, H.L., Krugh, F.J., Domonkos, A.N., Schneen, S.R., Davidson, C.L., Jr.: Polydysplastic epidermolysis bullosa and development of epidermal neoplasms. Arch. Derm. 102, 374–380 (1970)
19. Reed, W.B., College, J., Jr., Francis, M.J.O., Zachariae, H., Mohs, F., Sher, M.A., Sneddon, I.B.: Epidermolysis bullosa dystrophica with epidermal neoplasms. Arch. Derm. 110, 894–902 (1974)
20. Mendes da Costa, S., van der Valk, J.W.: Typhus maculatus der bullosen hereditären Dystrophie. Arch. Derm. Syph. (Wien–Leipz.) 91, 3–8 (1908)
21. De Groot, W.G., Postuma, R., Hunter, A.G.W.: Familial pyloric atresia associated with epidermolysis bullosa. J. Pediat. 92, 429–431 (1978)

Benign Familial Chronic Pemphigus (Hailey-Hailey Disease)

The disease was first described by the brothers Hailey in 1939 [1].

Clinical Presentation. The usual age of onset is the second or third decade. The primary lesions are grouped vesicles appearing in areas of friction, particularly the sides of the neck, axillae, and groin (Figs. 4.16 and 4.17). Other infrequently involved sites are the periumbilical and perianal areas, cubital and popliteal fossae, and scalp. The vesicles initially have clear fluid that soon becomes turbid. They rupture producing erosions covered by crusts. The plaques extend peripherally and have circinate active borders while the centers heal (Figs. 4.18 and 4.19). There are intervals of exacerbation and remission. In a warm, humid environment the lesions may show vegetations and have a fetid odor. Itching and pain are common complaints.

Mucosal lesions are infrequently observed [2, 3]. Atypical cases have been reported with hyperkeratotic verrucous lesions, papulovesicles and papulopustules, and neurodermatitic features [4].

Pathology and Pathophysiology. The characteristic histologic features are suprabasal vesiculation with protrusions into the vesicles by villi lined with a single layer of cells. Individual and groups of acantholytic cells are present, but there is incomplete loss of intercellular bridges allowing some loose adherence between the cells ("dilapidated brick wall"). *Corps ronds* and grains, similar to those in Darier disease (see p. 22), are seen.

Ultrastructurally, acantholysis and abnormal keratinization occur together or independently. The co-occurrence of the bizarre microvillar changes and abnormal tonofilament configurations is said to be pathognomonic of this disease [5]. It is generally believed that the genetically determined epidermal defect may lead to acantholysis either spontaneously or, more often, in response to external physical stimuli (candidal or bacterial infection). The role of infection in the pathogenesis of this disease seems to be important [6].

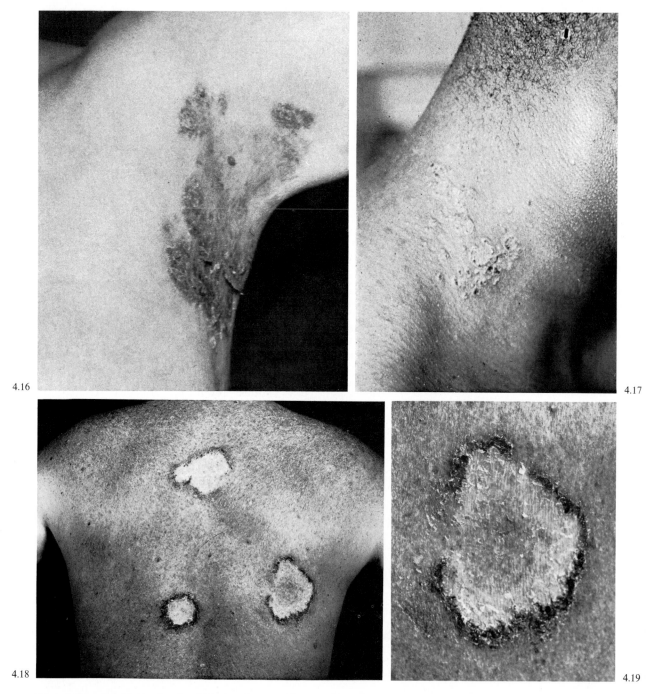

4.16

4.17

4.18

4.19

Figs. 4.16 and 4.17. Benign familial chronic pemphigus. Usual sites of involvement (axilla and neck)

Figs. 4.18 and 4.19. Benign familial chronic pemphigus. Circinate erosions over the back

Inheritance. Autosomal dominant.

Treatment. Topical and systemic antibiotics are effective in controlling the eruption. Bacteriologic examination determines the choice of antibiotic. Dapsone [7] and grenz-ray treatment [8] have been reported to be helpful. In certain cases, excision of the affected area and grafting give good results [9].

References

1. Hailey, H., Hailey, H.: Familial benign chronic pemphigus. Arch. Derm. Syph. *39*, 679–685 (1939)
2. Botvinick, I.: Familial benign pemphigus with oral mucous membrane lesions. Cutis *12*, 371–373 (1973)
3. Kahn, D., Hutchinson, E.: Esophageal involvement in familial benign chronic pemphigus. Arch. Derm. *109*, 718–719 (1974)
4. Lyles, T.W., Knox, J.M., Richardson, J.B.: Atypical features in familial benign chronic pemphigus. Arch. Derm. *78*, 446–453 (1958)
5. Gottlieb, S.K., Lutzner, M.A.: Hailey-Hailey disease – an electron microscopic study. J. invest. Derm. *54*, 368–376 (1970)
6. Montes, L.F., Narkates, A.J., Hunt, D., Pittilo, R.F., Noojin, R.O., Sherer, R.J.: Microbial flora in familial benign chronic pemphigus. Arch. Derm. *101*, 140–159 (1970)
7. Sire, D.J., Johnson, B.L.: Benign familial chronic pemphigus treated with dapsone. Arch. Derm. *103*, 262–265 (1971)
8. Sarkany, I.: Grenz-ray treatment of familial benign chronic pemphigus. Brit. J. Derm. *71*, 247–252 (1959)
9. Bitar, A., Giroux, J.-M.: Treatment of benign familial pemphigus (Hailey-Hailey) by skin grafting. Brit. J. Derm. *83*, 402–404 (1970)

Chapter 5 Hyperplasias, Aplasias, Dysplasias, and Atrophies

Contents

Dermal Hypoplasias and Dysplasias

Aplasia Cutis Congenita (Congenital Skin Defect)

Campbell was the first to describe this rare condition in 1826 [1]. To date, some 375 cases have been reported [2].

Clinical Presentation. The disorder is apparent from birth due to the presence of a sharply defined skin defect. The most frequent site of involvement is the midline of the scalp, but the trunk and extremities may be affected as well. The defect is usually 1–2 cm, oval or circular, with a glistening red base. Occasionally, multiple defects are present [3]. Healing occurs with atrophic or hypertrophic scar formation (Figs. 5.1 and 5.2). In deep defects, secondary bacterial infections and hemorrhage are troublesome and may lead to death.

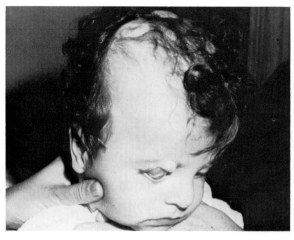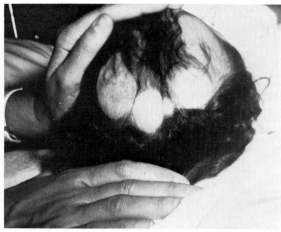

5.1   5.2

Figs. 5.1 and 5.2. Aplasia cutis congenita. Localized defects of the scalp

Associated abnormalities include peculiar facies [3], constricting rings, hydrocephalus, cleft palate [4], focal dermal hypoplasia, tracheoesophageal fistula, and patent ductus arteriosus [2].

Pathology and Pathophysiology. The epidermis and dermis may be absent and the defect may extend to the subcutaneous tissues. With healing the scar is devoid of appendages.
This condition should be differentiated from epidermolysis bullosa (see p. 80) and congenital localized absence of the skin (see p. 127).

Inheritance. There seems to be more than one genotype. Both autosomal dominant [5] and autosomal recessive [4] forms exist.

Treatment. Initially, nursing care and combating secondary infections are recommended. Surgical intervention is indicated for extensive lesions and cosmetic defects.

References

1. Campbell, W.: Case of congenital ulcer on the cranium of a foetus, terminating in fatal hemorrhage on the 18th day after birth. Edinb. J. med. Sci. *5*, 82–83 (1826)
2. Deeken, J.H., Caplan, R.M.: Aplasia cutis congenita. Arch. Derm. *102*, 386–389 (1970)
3. Rudolph, R.I., Schwartz, W., Leyden, J.J.: Bitemporal aplasia cutis congenita. Occurrence with other cutaneous abnormalities. Arch. Derm. *110*, 615–618 (1974)
4. Pers, M.: Congenital absence of the skin: pathogenesis and relation to ring constriction. Acta. chir. scand. *126*, 388–396 (1963)
5. Fisher, M., Schneider, R.: Aplasia cutis congenita in three successive generations. Arch. Derm. *108*, 252–253 (1973)

Focal Dermal Hypoplasia (Goltz Syndrome)

Cases of this syndrome have been presented since 1921 as examples of several different disorders. In 1962 Goltz et al. were the first to recognize the disorder as a distinct entity [1].

Clinical Presentation. The disease has its onset in childhood, is progressive, and encompasses cutaneous, skeletal, ocular, dental, and other defects. It affects predominantly females (45:3) [2]. The cutaneous lesions are characterized by reticular, vermiform, cribriform, frequently linear areas of thin skin which are dark in color or erythematous [1, 2] (Figs. 5.3 and 5.4). In a few cases, there may be at birth areas of total absence of skin. A rather pathognomonic finding is the presence of soft, yellow, baggy herniations of subcutaneous fat covered by very thin skin [1]. In addition, there are linear or reticular areas of hyper- or hypopigmentation [2]. Papillomas frequently develop on the lips, gums, base of tongue, circumoral area, anogenital and inguinal regions (Fig. 5.5), axillae, and around the umbilicus [2]. Inconstant features are an initial inflammatory, scaly, or blistering process that subsides before the other characteristic lesions appear [1]. The scalp hair may be sparse and brittle [1] or there may be small areas where hair is lacking [1, 2]. Absent, dystrophic, spooned, grooved, or hypopigmented fingernails and toenails frequently occur [1, 2].
Skeletal defects include rounded skull, pointed chin, and thin, deviated nasal septum [1]; kyphosis, scoliosis, and vertebral anomalies [2]; asymmetric

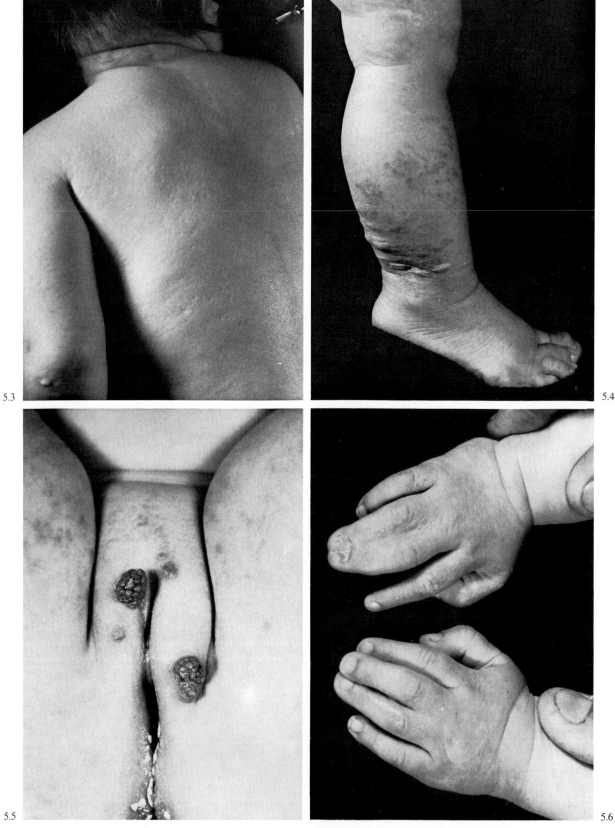

Figs. 5.3–5.6. Focal dermal hypoplasia

Fig. 5.3. Reticular cribriform areas of depressed skin

Fig. 5.4. Reticular hyperpigmentation over the leg with baggy herniations of subcutaneous fat

Fig. 5.5. Papillomas in the genital area

Fig. 5.6. Syndactyly

5.3

5.4

5.5

5.6

development of face, trunk, or extremities [2]; absence of part of an extremity [2]; anomalies of hands and feet (hypoplasia or absence of digits, polydactyly, claw or split hand, fusion of phalanges (Fig. 5.6) camptodactyly, clinodactyly, anomalies of the small bones of the hands and feet) [2]; and striate osteopathy [3].

Ocular defects include anophthalmia [4], strabismus, [1, 2], nystagmus [1, 2], colobomas of iris [1, 2], and patchy hypo- or hyperpigmentation of the retina [1, 2]. Oral and dental defects include dysplasia of teeth [1, 2], enamel defects with caries [1, 4], and notching of incisors [2]. Other defects include protrusion and asymmetry of ears [1], thenar and hypothenar hypoplasia [1], and mental deficiency [4]. Dermatoglyphic patterns are abnormal, notably localized areas of ridge dysplasia or hypoplasia [2].

Pathology and Pathophysiology. The main feature is a defect in the dermis and the presence of accumulations of normal fat cells in the dermis in some areas extending almost to, but separated by a thin connective tissue band from, the epidermis [1]. The epidermis shows no abnormalities. Ultrastructurally, the collagen fibers are small, but normally striated, and the fibroblasts appear normal [2]. The syndrome is considered to be a widespread dysplasia of mesodermal and ectodermal structures [2].

Inheritance. The possibilities of X-linked dominance with lethality in males, autosomal dominance with sex limitation [2], or environmental factors affecting development [5] have been considered.

Treatment. Plastic surgery may have to be resorted to for correction of some of the deformities.

References

1. Goltz, R.W., Peterson, W.C., Gorlin, R.J., Ravits, H.G.: Focal dermal hypoplasia. Arch. Derm. *86*, 708–717 (1962)
2. Goltz, R.W., Hendersen, R.R., Hitch, J.M., Ott, J.E.: Focal dermal hypoplasia syndrome. A review of the literature and report of two cases. Arch. Derm. *101*, 1–11 (1970)
3. Larrègue, M., Michel, Y., Maroteaux, J., Degos, R., Stewart, W.-M.: L'hypoplasie dermique en aires: considérations sur l'ostéopathie striée et sur le problème génétique. Ann. Derm. Syph. (Paris) *98*, 491–499 (1971)
4. Gottlieb, S.K., Fisher, B.K., Violin, G.A.: Focal dermal hypoplasia. A nine-year follow up study. Arch. Derm. *108*, 551–553 (1973)
5. Ishibashi, A., Kurihara, Y.: Goltz's syndrome: focal dermal dysplasia syndrome (focal dermal hypoplasia). Report of a case and on its etiology and pathogenesis. Dermatologica (Basel) *144*, 156–167 (1972)

Progressive Hemifacial Atrophy (Parry-Romberg Syndrome)

This syndrome was described in 1825 by Parry and in 1846 by Romberg [1].

Clinical Presentation. There is slow, progressive atrophy of the soft tissues of half of the face, accompanied by Jacksonian epilepsy, trigeminal neuralgia, and changes in the eyes and hair [2, 3] (Figs. 5.7 and 5.8).

Pathology and Pathophysiology. There is thickening of collagenous bundles in the corium, lymphocytic perivascular infiltration, absent skin appendages, and marked thickening of the vessels [4].

Inheritance. Probably autosomal dominant with reduced penetrance.

Treatment. No special treatment is available.

References

1. McKusick, V.A.: Mendelian inheritance in man, 5th ed., p. 144. Baltimore: Johns Hopkins University Press 1978
2. Wartenberg, R.: Progressive facial hemiatrophy. Arch. Neurol. Psychiat. *54*, 75–96 (1945)
3. Franceschetti, A., Koenig, H.: L'importance du facteur hérédodégénératif dans l'hémiatrophie faciale progressive (Romberg). Étude des complications oculaires dans ce syndrome. J. Génét. hum. *1*, 27–64 (1952)
4. Harper, P.S.: Hemifacial atrophy (the Romberg syndrome). In: The clinical delineation of birth defects. Bergsma, D. (ed.), Vol. VII, No. 8, pt. XII, pp. 293–294. Baltimore: Williams & Wilkins Co. 1971

Striae Distensae

Transverse striae of the lumbar area have been observed in a father and two sons [1]. The inheritance is probably autosomal dominant.

Reference

1. McKusick, V.A.: Transverse striae distensae in the lumbar area in father and two sons. In: The clinical delineation of birth defects. Bergsma, D. (ed.), Vol. VII, No. 8, pt. XII, pp. 260–261. Baltimore: Williams & Wilkins Co. 1971

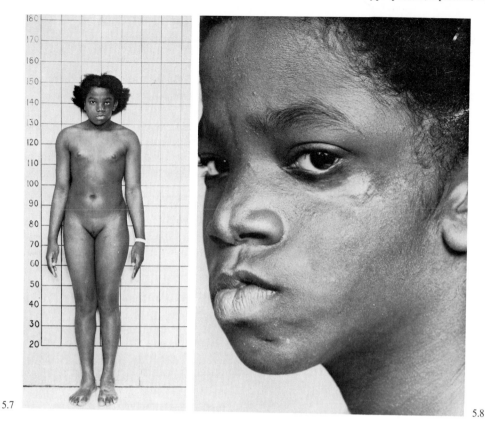

5.7

5.8

Figs. 5.7 and 5.8. Progressive hemifacial atrophy. Note asymmetry of the face and atrophic skin. (Courtesy of Dr. V. A. McKusick)

Flynn-Aird Syndrome

In 1965 Flynn and Aird [1] reported a family in which 15 members in five generations were affected by a disorder characterized by nerve deafness, ocular anomalies, cerebral deficits, and atrophy of the skin.

Clinical Presentation. The initial symptoms usually develop in the second decade, although bilateral nerve deafness, which is the earliest defect observed, may appear as early as 7 years of age. Myopia also has a relatively early onset [1].
Cerebral deficits include possible mental retardation and atypical convulsive phenomena with EEG dysrhythmias. Severe muscular wasting, ataxia, peripheral neuritic pain, and stiffness of the joints occur in the second decade. Kyphoscoliosis follows the muscle wasting and peripheral neuritis. Cystic disease of bone is found in some patients. Dental caries is severe and widespread. Diabetes mellitus was found in two patients.
Of the 15 patients studied, 13 had atrophy of the skin and subcutaneous tissue similar to that found

in scleroderma. Skin ulceration is frequent. Baldness is a late manifestation.
Eye defects include retinitis pigmentosa, bilateral cataracts, severe myopia, and total blindness.
Life is not shortened, but the physical defects are severely crippling.

Pathology and Pathophysiology. Histologically, there is evidence of skin atrophy and changes characteristic of peripheral neuritis. The brain was atrophic in three patients, with changes typical of ischemia. One case had diffuse and bilateral adrenal hypertrophy and pituitary basophilic hyperplasia. Two cases had atrophic adrenals. Thyroid enlargement was present in one case.

Inheritance. Autosomal dominant [1].

Treatment. The treatment is only symptomatic.

Reference

1. Flynn, P., Aird, R. B.: A neuroectodermal syndrome of dominant inheritance. J. neurol. Sci. *2*, 161–182 (1965)

Freeman-Sheldon Syndrome (Whistling Face–Windmill Vane Hand Syndrome, Cranio-Carpo-Tarsal Dysplasia)

This disorder was described in two patients by Freeman and Sheldon in 1938 [1].

Clinical Presentation. The most striking feature of the syndrome is the masklike facies with small mouth and pursed lips, giving a "whistling" appearance. Associated findings include deep-sunken eyes, hypertelorism or dystopia canthorum, a small nose, hypoplastic alae nasi, and a long philtrum. A fibrous band or elevation extends from the middle of the lower lip to the chin. It is demarcated by two paramedian grooves, forming an H- or V-shaped scarlike structure (Figs. 5.9–5.12). The hands have an ulnar deviation with thick skin over the flexor surfaces of the proximal phalanges. There may also be an equinovarus deformity with contracted toes [2–4]. The striated muscles are generally flabby, leading to a protuberant abdomen and hernias in some patients.
Occasional associated abnormalities include blepharophimosis, ptosis, convergent strabismus, small stature, scoliosis, and low weight.
The intelligence of all reported patients has been normal.

Pathology and Pathophysiology. There is marked atrophy of the buccinator muscle with sparse fibers and degenerated cells [3].

Inheritance. Autosomal dominant [5].

Treatment. Treatment is surgical [3].

References

1. Freeman, E.A., Sheldon, J.H.: Cranio-carpo-tarsal dystrophy. An undescribed congenital malformation. Arch. Dis. Child. *13*, 277–283 (1938)
2. Otto, F.M.G.: Die "Cranio-carpo-tarsal Dystrophie" (Freeman and Sheldon). Ein kasuistischer Beitrag. Z. Kinderheilk. *737*, 240–250 (1953)
3. Burian, F.: The "whistling face" characteristic in a compound cranio-facio-corporal syndrome. Brit. J. plast. Surg. *16*, 140–143 (1963)
4. Weinstein, S., Gorlin, R.J.: Cranio-carpo-tarsal dysplasia or the whistling face syndrome. I. Clinical considerations. Amer. J. Dis. Child. *117*, 427–433 (1969)
5. McKusick, V.A.: Mendelian inheritance in man, 5th ed., pp. 391–392. Baltimore: Johns Hopkins University Press 1978

Familial Transverse Nasal Groove

The main feature of this disorder is a wide groove (1–3 mm) across the nose just proximal to the alae nasi [1, 2]. It is about 1 mm deep and is not effaced by stretching the skin. It appears in childhood and may become minimally noticeable after the third or fourth decade [2]. In young adults, acne lesions may be clustered within the groove and, as the acne clears, scales and large follicles may persist for a while [2]. In one family, hyperelasticity of the joints was an associated finding, while in another family there was early, severe dental caries [2]. Inheritance is autosomal dominant. No treatment is needed because of spontaneous improvement.

References

1. Cornbleet, T.: Transverse nasal stripe at puberty (stria nasi transversa). Arch. Derm. *63*, 70–72 (1951)
2. Anderson, P.C.: Familial transverse nasal groove. Arch. Derm. *84*, 316–317 (1961)

Ainhum

Ainhum is said to be common among Negroes. Familial occurrence has been reported in a few instances [1–4]. The disease usually appears around the age of 40 years, and affects the fifth toe, unilaterally or bilaterally, and less so the other toes [5]. A constricting ring around the toe gradually deepens to form a groove. This may progress to cause spontaneous amputation. The sites most frequently affected by the groove are over the first or second interphalangeal joints. The distal part of the phalanx becomes edematous with increased or decreased sensations. The constricting band is of fibrous tissue and produces atrophy, phalangeal bone rarefaction, and ultimately fragmentation and absorption of the distal end. Inheritance is not clear, but is probably autosomal dominant [3].

References

1. DaSilva Lima, J.F.: On ainhum. Arch. Derm. Syph. *6*, 367–376 (1880)
2. Simon, K.M.B.: Ainhum, a family disease. J. Amer. med. Ass. *76*, 590 (1921)
3. Maass, E.: Beobachtungen über Ainhum. Arch. Schiffs- u. Tropenhyg. *30*, 32–34 (1926)
4. Kean, B.H., Tucker, H.A.: Etiologic concepts and pathologic aspects of ainhum. Arch. Path. *41*, 639–644 (1946)
5. Horwitz, M.T., Tunick, I.: Ainhum. Report of six cases in New York. Arch. Derm. Syph. *36*, 1058–1063 (1937)

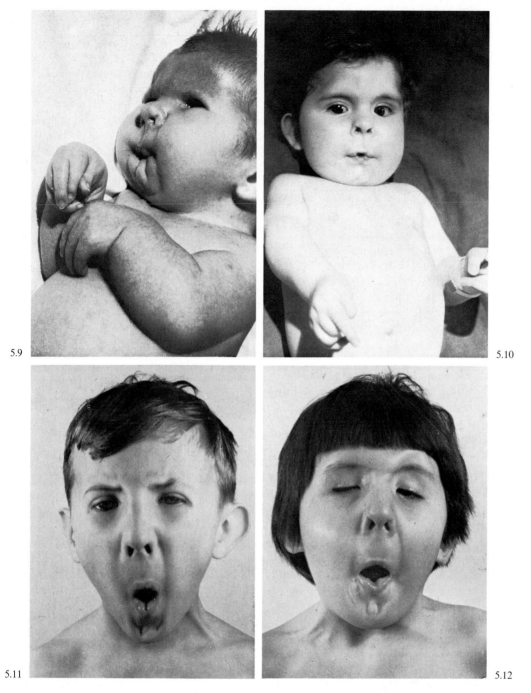

5.9

5.10

5.11

5.12

Figs. 5.9–5.12. Freeman-Sheldon syndrome

Fig. 5.9. Note sunken eyes, pursed lips, long philtrum, fibrous band from lower lip to chin demarcated by two grooves, and ulnar deviation of the hands. (Courtesy of Dr. F.C. Fraser)

Fig. 5.10. Note small mouth with a whistling appearance. (Courtesy of Dr. F.C. Fraser)

Figs. 5.11 and 5.12. Note masklike facies. (From Cervenka, J., et al.: Amer. J. Dis. Child. *117*, 434–435, 1969)

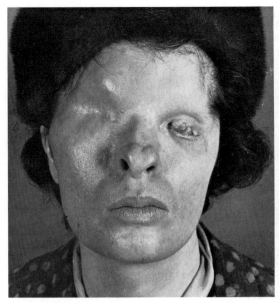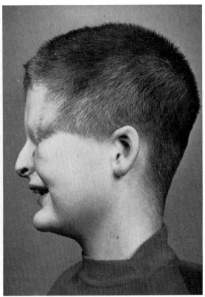

5.13   5.14

Fig. 5.13. Cryptophthalmos. Note absence of palpebral fissure, eyelids, and eyelashes. (From Sugar, S.: Amer. J. Ophthal. *66*, 897–899, 1968)

Fig. 5.14. Cryptophthalmos. Note hairline extending down toward the orbit and the deformity of the nostrils. (From Ide, C. H., Wollschlaeger, P. B.: Arch. Ophthal. *81*, 638–644, 1969)

Cryptophthalmos Syndrome

The term cryptophthalmos – "hidden eye" – was first used by Zehender [1] in 1872.

Clinical Presentation. The most striking characteristic of this syndrome is the absence of the palpebral fissure which may be unilateral or bilateral. There are no eyelids and no eyelashes. The lacrimal ducts may be absent or malformed. Small eyeballs are usually palpable beneath the skin covering and may enable the patient to perceive light and occasionally even colors [2, 3] (Figs. 5.13 and 5.14).
Deformities of the nose may be present, such as lateral cleft of the nostril. The ears may have abnormally shaped pinnae, atretic external auditory canals, and malformed middle ear ossicles. The hairline may extend from the temporal area toward the orbit; syndactyly may be present in about 40% of cases (Figs. 5.15 and 5.16). Subnormal intelligence is relatively frequent [2, 3]. Cerebral defects, meningomyeloceles, kidney malformations, bicornuate uterus, and malformed fallopian tubes have been reported.

Inheritance. Autosomal recessive [2, 3].

Treatment. Reconstructive surgery of the middle ear may result in marked improvement in hearing. There is no special treatment for the eyes.

References

1. Zehender, W.: Eine Mißgeburt mit hautüberwachsenen Augen oder Kryptophthalmus. Klin. Mbl. Augenheilk. *10*, 225–249 (1872)
2. Fraser, G. R.: Our genetical "load". A review of some aspects of genetical variation. Ann. hum. Genet. *25*, 387–415 (1962)
3. Ide, C. H., Wollschlaeger, P. B.: Multiple congenital abnormalities associated with cryptophthalmia. Arch. Ophthal. *81*, 638–644 (1969)

Hallermann-Streiff Syndrome (Oculomandibulodyscephaly with Hypotrichosis)

Hallermann [1] in 1948 and Streiff [2] in 1950 independently described this syndrome consisting of craniofacial anomalies, proportionate nanism, hypotrichosis, atrophy of the skin, and congenital cataracts. More than 60 cases have been reported.

Clinical Presentation. The disease manifests itself early in life. The skull is characteristically brachycephalic with frontal and parietal bossing, a thin calvarium, and delayed ossification of the sutures. There is malar hypoplasia, micrognathia, and temporomandibular joint anomalies. The nose is thin, small, and pointed, with hypoplasia of the cartilage, giving, in older patients, a parrotlike profile. The mouth is small and the palate is high and narrow-

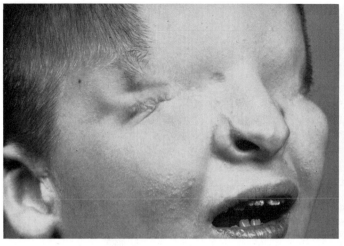

5.15

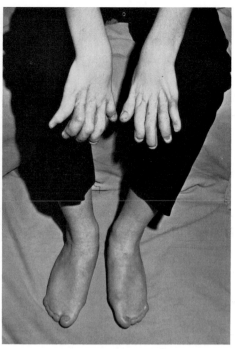

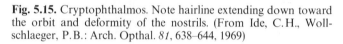

Fig. 5.15. Cryptophthalmos. Note hairline extending down toward the orbit and deformity of the nostrils. (From Ide, C.H., Wollschlaeger, P.B.: Arch. Opthal. *81*, 638–644, 1969)

Fig. 5.16. Cryptophthalmos. Syndactyly of the toes. (From Ide, C.H., Wollschlaeger, P.B.: Arch. Ophthal *81*, 638–644, 1969)

5.16

arched. There is dental hypoplasia and malimplantation with partial anodontia. Some teeth may be present at birth. Most patients present with microphthalmia and bilateral congenital cataracts [3] (Figs. 5.17–5.20).

Atrophy of the skin is present, usually limited to the head, where it is white, thin, dry, soft, and marked by prominent veins. The last finding is most striking over the anterior surface of the nose. Hypotrichosis occurs in all cases and involves mainly the anterior part of the scalp. The eyebrows and eyelashes are scanty and frequently absent [4].

Osteoporosis, hypogenitalism, claw hands, syndactyly, malformations of the spine, glaucoma, and slight mental retardation may be part of the syndrome [5].

Pathology and Pathophysiology. The majority of the literature is concerned with the ocular anomalies and there are insufficient data on the natural history of the growth defect and the development of the abnormalities of the skin and hair.

Inheritance. The reported patients did not have similarly affected family members. Only one report [6] mentions an affected father and daughter. It is possible that a single dominant gene is causing the disease and most patients represent fresh mutations.

Treatment. Treatment is symptomatic. Eye surgery is unsuccessful.

References

1. Hallermann, W.: Vogelgesicht und Cataracta congenita. Klin. Mbl. Augenheilk. *113*, 315–318 (1948)
2. Streiff, E.B.: Dysmorphie mandibulo-faciale (tête d'oiseau) et altérations oculaires. Ophthalmologica (Basel) *120*, 79–83 (1950)
3. François, J.: A new syndrome. Dyscephalia with bird face and dental anomalies, nanism, hypotrichosis, cutaneous atrophy, microphthalmia and congenital cataract. Arch. Ophthal. *60*, 842–862 (1958)
4. Falls, H.F., Schull, W.J.: Hallermann-Streiff syndrome. A dyscephaly with congenital cataracts and hypotrichosis. Arch. Ophthal. *63*, 409–420 (1960)
5. Caspersen, I., Warburg, M.: Hallermann-Streiff syndrome. Acta ophthal. (Kbh.) *46*, 385–390 (1968)
6. Guyard, M., Perdriel, G., Ceruti, F.: Sur deux cas de syndrome dyscéphalique a téte d'oiseau. Bull. Soc. Opthal. (Paris) *62*, 443–447 (1962)

Ear Malformations

Ear Pits (Auricular Fistulas)

Ear pits are not an uncommon finding [1]. The pits may be uni- or bilateral and usually occur on the margin of the helix just above the tragus, or elsewhere on the pinna [2]. The pit is circular or elliptical, may be inconspicuous and asymptomatic, or may intermittently discharge a milky fluid of cell debris. Secondary infection and suppuration may

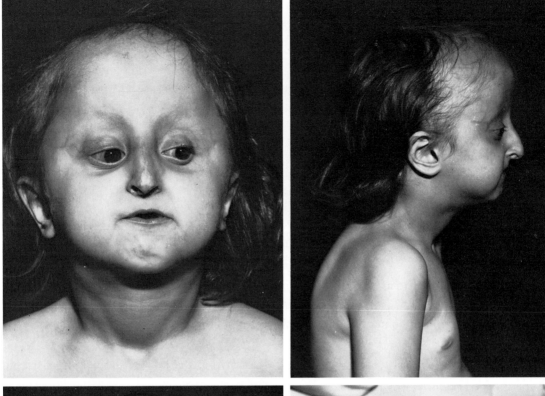

5.17

5.18

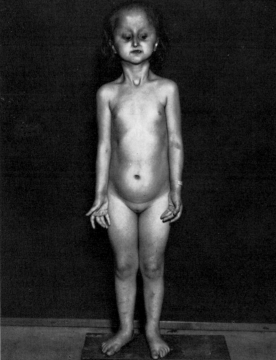

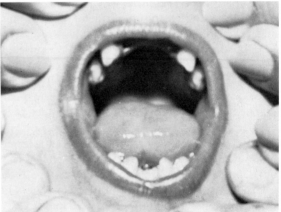

5.20

5.19

Figs. 5.17–5.20. Hallermann-Streiff syndrome

Fig. 5.17. Note scanty hair over the anterior part of the skull, absence of eyebrows, scanty eyelashes, dilated veins over the nose, and cataract of the left eye

Fig. 5.18. Lateral view. Note parrotlike profile

Fig. 5.19. General view of the body

Fig. 5.20. Note partial anodontia

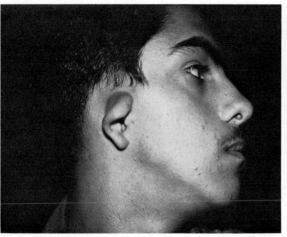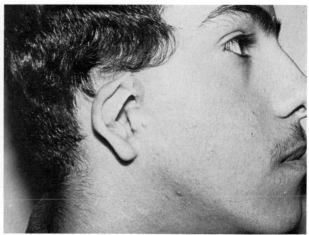

5.21

Figs. 5.21 and 5.22. "Cup ear" before and after corrective surgery. (From Abu-Jamra, F.: Lebanese med. J. *23*, 213–217, 1970)

be a complication. Association with branchial fistulas or other developmental anomalies of the branchial clefts may occur [2]. The inheritance of ear pits is probably autosomal dominant.

Ear pits are associated with deafness in a distinct syndrome [2, 3]. The deafness is of the hereditary perceptive type [2]. In some patients with ear pits and deafness, branchial pits or fistulas are present [2]. In one pedigree, cervical and preauricular branchial fistulas are associated with congenital deafness (conductive and sensorineural) [4]. In three generations of another family, deformed ears (flapped) and preauricular pits and appendages occur [3]. Conductive deafness is an associated feature in 2 of the 14 affected members of the family [3]. Since the deafness in the various pedigrees is not identical, it is possible that there may be more than one type of this syndrome (ear pits and deafness). Inheritance in the reported pedigrees is autosomal dominant.

References

1. Ewing, M.R.: Congenital sinuses of the external ear. J. Laryng. *61*, 18–23 (1946)
2. Fourman, P., Fourman, J.: Hereditary deafness in family with earpits (fistula auris congenita). Brit. med. J. *1955 II*, 1354–1356
3. Wildervanck, L.S.: Hereditary malformations of the ear in three generations. Marginal pits, pre-auricular appendages, malformations of the auricle, and conductive deafness. Acta otolaryng. (Stockh.) *54*, 553–560 (1962)
4. Rowley, P.T.: Familial hearing loss associated with branchial fistulas. Pediatrics *44*, 978–985 (1969)

"Cup Ear"

Potter [1] described this abnormality in 1937. It consists of a congenital malformation of the pinna which is curled up like a cup, concealing the external auditory meatus (Figs. 5.21 and 5.22). The inheritance follows the autosomal dominant pattern. Plastic surgery is very rewarding [2].

References

1. Potter, E.L.: A hereditary ear malformation transmitted through five generations. J. Heredity *28*, 255–258 (1937)
2. Erich, J.B., Abu-Jamra, F.N.: Congenital cup-shaped deformity of the ears transmitted through four generations. Mayo Clin. Proc. *40*, 597–602 (1965)

Branchial Cleft Anomalies, Cup-Shaped Ear, and Deafness

A mutation combining branchial cleft anomalies with "cup ear" and deafness has been observed in an autosomal dominant pedigree pattern [1].

Reference

1. Karmody, C., Feingold, M.: Autosomal dominant first and second branchial arch syndrome. A new inherited syndrome? In: The clinical delineation of birth defects. Bergsma, D. (ed.), Vol. X, No. 1, pp. 31–40. Baltimore: Williams & Wilkins Co. 1974

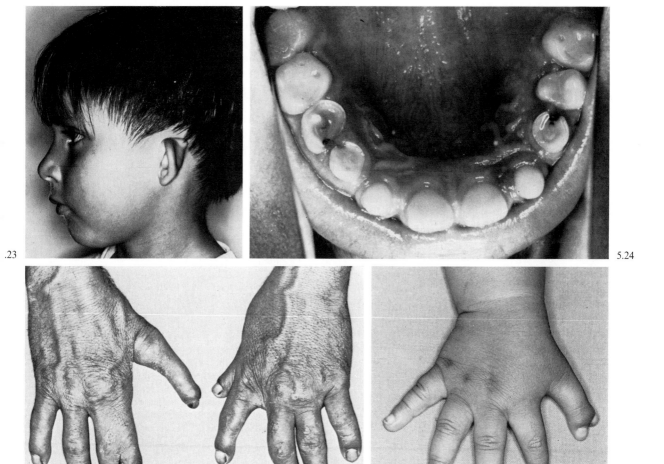

.23

5.24

.25

5.26

Figs. 5.23–5.26. LADD

Fig. 5.23. Cup-shaped pinna. (From Hollister, D.W., et al.: J. Pediat. *83*, 438–444, 1973)

Fig. 5.24. Small and peg-shaped lateral maxillary incisors. (From Hollister, D.W., et al.: J. Pediat. *83*, 438–444, 1973)

Figs. 5.25 and 5.26. Syndactyly. (From Hollister, D.W., et al.: J. Pediat. *83*, 438–444, 1973)

Lacrimo-Auriculo-Dento-Digital Syndrome (LADD)

In 1967 Levy [1] described this syndrome for the first time in a sporadic case. In 1973 Hollister et al. [2] described the syndrome in a family.

Clinical Presentation. There is aplasia or hypoplasia of the lacrimal puncta with obstruction of the nasolacrimal ducts. The pinnae are cup-shaped with mixed hearing deficit (Fig. 5.23). The lateral maxillary incisors are small and peg-shaped and have mild enamel dysplasia (Fig. 5.24). The digital features are variable (fifth finger clinodactyly, duplication of the distal phalanx of the thumb, triphalangeal thumb, syndactyly) [1, 2] (Figs. 5.25 and 5.26). Although each individual feature may be inherited as an autosomal dominant trait, their association in this distinct syndrome is quite definite.

Pathology and Pathophysiology. The pathogenesis of this syndrome is not known.

Inheritance. Autosomal dominant.

Treatment. No special treatment is available.

References

1. Levy, W.J.: Mesoectodermal dysplasia. A new combination of anomalies. Amer. J. Ophthal. *63*, 978–982 (1967)
2. Hollister, D.W., Klein, S.H., De Jager, H.J., Lachman, R.S., Rimoin, D.L.: The lacrimo-auriculo-dento-digital syndrome. J. Pediat. *83*, 438–444 (1973)

Facioauriculovertebral Anomalad (Goldenhar Syndrome, Oculoauriculovertebral Dysplasia)

The symptom complex was first noted in 1845 by Von Arlt [1]. It was first established as a distinct entity in 1952 by Goldenhar [2], who reported three patients with epibulbar dermoids, auricular appendages, and mandibular anomalies. With the addition of the vertebral anomalies, the descriptive term "oculoauriculovertebral" (OAV) dysplasia was suggested in 1963 [3]. Later, because hemifacial microsomia was found in many patients [4], the appellation of "facioauriculovertebral anomalad" was introduced.

Clinical Presentation. The main features of this association of defects include malar, maxillary, and mandibular hypoplasia; unilateral macrostomia (enlargement and lateral extension of one corner of the mouth); microtia with preauricular appendages or pits which may be single or multiple and commonly located in a line from the tragus to the corner of the mouth; middle ear anomaly with variable deafness; and hemivertebrae, hypoplastic or fused vertebrae with occipitalization of the atlas (Figs. 5.27 and 5.28).

The epibulbar dermoids or lipodermoids are quite common. They are usually located at the corneoscleral junction of the lateral portion of the eye and are bilateral in two-thirds of the patients [3]. Colobomas of the eyelid are also common and are unilateral (Fig. 5.27).

Occasional abnormalities include the following: mental deficiency, frontal bossing, ocular hypertelorism, microphthalmos, hypoplasia or colobomas of the iris, cataracts, a fibrous band from the corner of the mouth to the tragus area of the auricle, a bifid tongue, cleft lip, umbilical hernia, and scoliosis due to malformed vertebrae. In certain cases cardiac, pulmonary, intestinal, and renal anomalies may also be found at autopsy [5, 6].

Affected individuals do not always exhibit anomalies in all the characteristic anatomic areas such as the eyes, ears, and vertebrae. No single anomaly is a sine qua non for making the diagnosis. The various combinations and gradations of many of these anomalies, both unilateral and bilateral, suggest that a similar error in morphogenesis may be at the origin of a spectrum of presentations.

Inheritance. The great majority of cases are sporadic. However, familial cases have also been described [7, 8].

Treatment. The preauricular skin tags and the large dermoids require surgical excision. In the case of conductive deafness due to incompletely developed external auditory canals, hearing aids should be utilized from early infancy. Occasionally, an external canal can be created. Dental care for crowding of the teeth is necessary. After assessing the degree of spontaneous improvement in early childhood, reconstructive surgery in the zygomatic area and the mandible may be deemed necessary.

References

1. Von Arlt, F.: Klinischer Darstellung der Krankheiten des Auges, Vol. III, p. 376. Wien 1845; cited by Van Duyse, D.: Bride dermoïde oculopalpébrale et colobome partiel de la paupière avec remarques sur la génèse de ces anomalies. Ann. Oculist. (Paris) (Ser. 12) *88*, 101 (1882)
2. Goldenhar, M.: Associations malformatives de l'oeil et de l'oreille, en particulier le syndrome dermoïde épibulbaire-appendices auriculaires-fistula auris congenita et ses relations avec la dysostose mandibulo-faciale. J. Génét. hum. *1*, 243 (1952)
3. Gorlin, R.J., Jue, K.L., Jacobsen, U., Goldschmidt, E.: Oculoauriculo-vertebral dysplasia. J. Pediat. *63*, 991–999 (1963)
4. Pashayan, H., Pinsky, L., Fraser, F.C.: Hemifacial microsomia – oculoauriculo-vertebral dysplasia. A patient with overlapping features. J. med. Genet. 7, 185–188 (1970)
5. Smith, D.W.: Recognizable patterns of human malformation, 2nd ed., p. 136. Philadelphia: Saunders, W.B.Co. 1976
6. Opitz, J.M., Faith, G.C.: Visceral anomalies in an infant with the Goldenhar syndrome. In: The clinical delineation of birth defects. Bergsma, D. (ed.), Vol. V, No. 2, pt. II, pp. 104–105. Baltimore: Williams & Wilkins Co. 1969
7. Summitt, R.L.: Familial Goldenhar syndrome. In: The clinical delineation of birth defects. Bergsma, D. (ed.), Vol. V, No. 2, pt. II, pp. 106–109. Baltimore: Williams & Wilkins Co. 1969
8. McKusick, V.A.: Mendelian inheritance in man, 5th ed., p. 621. Baltimore: Johns Hopkins University Press 1978

Auriculo-Osteodysplasia

In 1967 Beals [1] described a syndrome with multiple osseous dysplasia, characteristic ear shape, and short stature. In 1972 possible linkage of auriculo-osteodysplasia to Rh and Duffy (i.e., to chromosome No. 1) was reported [2]. Inheritance is autosomal dominant.

References

1. Beals, R.K.: Auriculo-osteodysplasia. A syndrome of multiple osseous dysplasia, ear anomaly, and short stature. J. Bone Jt. Surg. *49*, 1541–1550 (1967)
2. Kimberling, W.: Computers and gene localization. In: Perspectives in cytology. Wright, S.W., Crandall, D.I., Boyer, P.D. (eds.), p. 131. Springfield: Charles C Thomas 1972

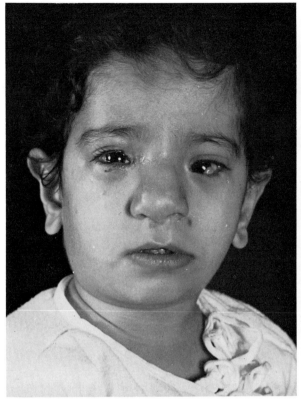

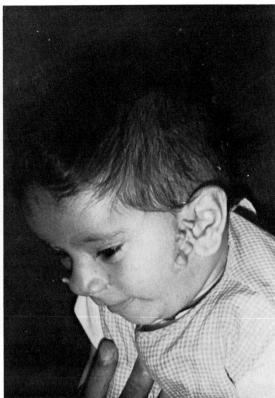

Fig. 5.27. Facioauriculovertebral anomalad. Note the epibulbar dermoid of the left eye, the coloboma of the right eyelid, and the left hemifacial atrophy

Fig. 5.28. Facioauriculovertebral anomalad. Note the preauricular appendages and the abnormal pinna

Syndactylies

Table 5.1. Classification of syndactylies[a]

Name	Inheritance	Clinical Presentation	Ref.
Syndactyly, type I (zygodactyly)	Autosomal dominant	Webbing between 3rd and 4th fingers (Fig. 5.29), occasionally with fusion of the distal phalanges In the feet, usually webbing between 2nd and 3rd toes, either complete or partial; sometimes only the hands are affected, sometimes only the feet	[2]
Syndactyly, type II (synpolydactyly)	Autosomal dominant	Syndactyly of 3rd and 4th fingers of the hand with polydactyly of all components or of part of 4th finger In the feet, polydactyly of the 5th toe in the web of syndactyly of the 4th and 5th toes	[3]
Syndactyly, type III (ring and little finger syndactyly)	Autosomal dominant	Syndactyly of 4th and 5th fingers, usually complete and bilateral; the 5th finger is short with absent or rudimentary middle phalanx The feet are not affected	[4]
Syndactyly, type IV (Haas type)	Autosomal dominant (probable)	Complete syndactyly in both hands with 6 metacarpals and 6 digits Flexion of fingers (cup-shaped hands)	[5]
Syndactyly, type V (metacarpal and metatarsal fusion)	Autosomal dominant	Most commonly fused metacarpals and metatarsals are the 4th and 5th or the 3rd and 4th Soft tissue syndactyly affects 3rd and 4th fingers and 2nd and 3rd toes	[6]
Synostoses (tarsal, carpal, and digital)	Autosomal dominant	Multiple carpal and tarsal synostoses, radial-head subluxation, aplasia or hypoplasia of the middle phalanges, metacarpophalangeal synostoses	[7]
Acrocephalosyndactyly, type I (typical Apert syndrome) (see also p. 107)	Autosomal dominant	Skull malformation (acrocephaly, brachysphenocephaly) Syndactyly of hands and feet (complete distal fusion)	[8]
Acrocephalosyndactyly, type II (Apert-Crouzon disease or Vogt cephalodactyly)	Autosomal dominant (probable)	Hand and foot malformations characteristic of Apert disease Facial characteristics of Crouzon disease due to an extremely hypoplastic maxilla Many doubt that this is a separate entity; they view it as Apert syndrome with unusually marked facial features	[9]

[a] After McKusick [1].

References

1. McKusick, V.A.: Mendelian inheritance in man, 5th ed. Baltimore: Johns Hopkins University Press 1978
2. Stern, C.: The problem of complete Y-linkage in man. Amer. J. hum. Genet. 9, 147–166 (1957)
3. Cross, H.E., Lerberg, D.B., McKusick, V.A.: Type II syndactyly. Amer. J. hum. Genet. 20, 368–380 (1968)
4. Johnston, O., Kirby, V.V.: Syndactyly of the ring and little finger. Amer. J. hum. Genet. 7, 80–82 (1955)
5. Haas, S.L.: Bilateral complete syndactylism of all fingers. Amer. J. Surg. 50, 363–366 (1940)
6. Kemp, T., Ravn, J.: Über erbliche Hand- und Fußdeformitäten in einem 140-köpfigen Geschlecht, nebst einigen Be-

merkungen über Poly- und Syndaktylie beim Menschen. Acta psychiat. neurol. 7, 275–296 (1932)
7. Pearlman, H.S., Edkin, R.E., Warren, R.F.: Familial tarsal and carpal synostosis with radial-head subluxation (Nievergelt's syndrome). J. Bone Jt. Surg. 46, 585–592 (1964)
8. Blank, C.E.: Apert's syndrome (a type of acrocephalosyndactyly). Observations on a British series of thirty-nine cases. Ann. hum. Genet. 24, 151–164 (1960)
9. Temtamy, S.A., McKusick, V.A.: The genetics of hand malformations. New York: National Foundation-March of Dimes 1975
10. Bartsocas, C.S., Weber, A.L., Crawford, J.D.: Acrocephalosyndactyly type III: Chotzen's syndrome. J. Pediat. 77, 267–272 (1970)

Table 5.1 (continued)

Name	Inheritance	Clinical Presentation	Ref.
Acrocephalosyndactyly, type III (Chotzen syndrome)	Autosomal dominant	Acrocephaly and asymmetry of the skull Partial soft tissue syndactyly of the 2nd and 3rd fingers and 3rd and 4th toes	[10]
Acrocephalosyndactyly, type V (Pfeiffer type)	Autosomal dominant	Broad, short thumbs and big toes Proximal phalanx of the thumb either triangular or trapezoid, thumb pointing outward	[11]
Acrocephalopolysyndactyly, type I (ACPS I, Noack syndrome)	Autosomal dominant (probable)	Acrocephaly Enlarged thumbs and great toes Duplication of great toes (preaxial polydactyly) Syndactyly Normal intelligence Pfeiffer thinks that this disorder is the same as acrocephalosyndactyly, type V	[12, 13]
Acrocephalopolysyndactyly, type II (ACPS II, Carpenter syndrome) (see also p. 109)	Autosomal recessive	Acrocephaly, peculiar facies Brachydactyly and syndactyly of hands Preaxial polydactyly and syndactyly of toes	[14, 15]
Polysyndactyly with peculiar skull shape (Greig cephalopolysyndactyly syndrome)	Autosomal dominant	Skull with high forehead and bregma; no evidence of precocious closure of cranial sutures Syndactyly or polysyndactyly	[16]
Mohr syndrome (Orofaciodigital syndrome II, OFD II)	Autosomal recessive	Syndactyly, polydactyly, brachydactyly Lobate tongue with papilliform protuberances (Figs. 5.30 and 5.31). High-arched palate and angular form of alveolar processes of mandible Episodic neuromuscular disturbance Conductive hearing loss	[17]
Roberts syndrome (see also p. 203)	Autosomal recessive	Tetraphocomelia, bilateral cleft lip and palate, ectrodactyly, syndactyly of the digits, hypertelorism with exophthalmos, congenital heart defect	[18]
Sclerosteosis	Autosomal recessive	Cortical hyperostosis with syndactyly	[19]
Orofaciodigital (OFD I) syndrome	X-linked dominant or autosomal dominant (lethal in male)	Same as in OFD II (see above) with prominent milia on pinnae and face	[1]

11. Martsolf, J.T., Cracco, J.B., Carpenter, G.G., O'Hara, A.E.: Pfeiffer syndrome. An unusual type of acrocephalosyndactyly with broad thumbs and great toes. Amer. J. Dis. Child 121, 257–262 (1971)

12. Noack, M.: Ein Beitrag zum Krankheitsbild der Akrozephalosyndaktylie (Apert). Arch. Kinderheilk. 160, 168–171 (1959)

13. Pfeiffer, R.A.: Associated deformities of the head and hands. In: The clinical delineation of birth defects. Bergsma, D. (ed.), Vol. V, No. 3, pt. III, pp. 18–34. Baltimore: Williams & Wilkins Co. 1969

14. Temtamy, S.A.: Carpenter's syndrome: acrocephalopolysyndactyly, an autosomal recessive syndrome. J. Pediat. 69, 111–120 (1966)

15. Der Kaloustian, V.M., Sinno, A.A., Nassar, S.I.: Acrocephalopolysyndactyly, type II (Carpenter syndrome). Amer. J. Dis. Child. 124, 716–718 (1972)

16. Hootnick, D., Holmes, L.B.: Familial polysyndactyly and craniofacial anomalies. Clin. Genet. 3, 128–134 (1972)

17. Rimoin, D.L., Edgerton, M.T.: Genetic and clinical heterogeneity in the oral-facial-digital syndromes. J. Pediat. 71, 94–102 (1967)

18. Zergollern, L., Hitrec, V.: Three siblings with Robert's syndrome. Clin. Genet. 9, 433–436 (1976)

19. Truswell, A.S.: Osteopetrosis with syndactyly. A morphologic variant of Albers-Schonberg's disease. J. Bone Jt.Surg. (Brit.) 40, 208–218 (1958)

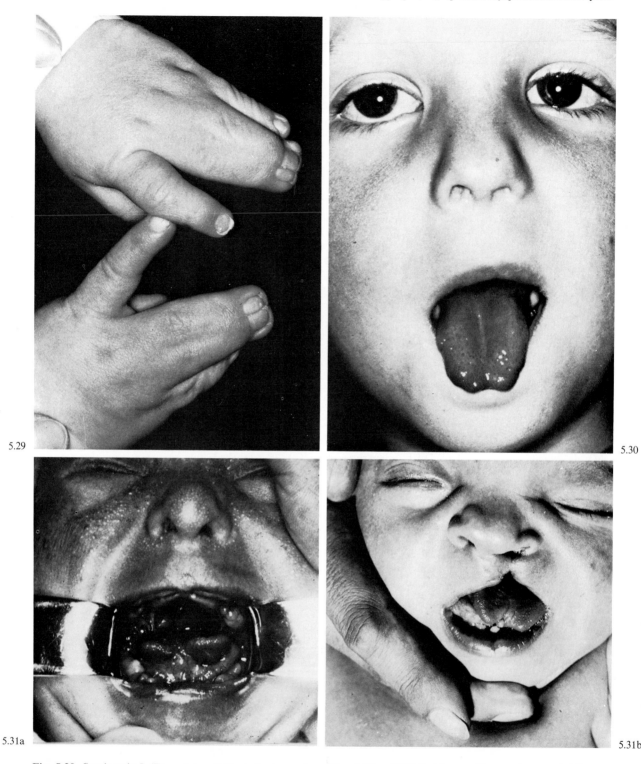

5.29

5.30

5.31a

5.31b

Fig. 5.29. Syndactyly I. (From Levy, E.P., et al.: Amer. J. Dis. Child. *128*, 531–533, 1974)

Fig. 5.30. OFD II (Mohr syndrome). Bilobate tongue. (Courtesy of Dr. F.C. Fraser)

Fig. 5.31a. OFD I. Note milia on face and bilobate tongue. (From Solomon, L.M., et al.: Arch. Derm. *102*, 598–602, 1970)

Fig. 5.31b. OFD II. Note bilobate tongue. (Courtesy of Dr. L. Vissian)

Acrocephalosyndactyly, Type I
(Apert Syndrome)

Gorlin and Pinborg [1] noted descriptions of this syndrome as early as 1842. However, eponymic credit is given to Apert [2] for his presentation in 1906. The syndrome is characterized by malformation of the skull and severe syndactyly of the hands and feet. Apert proposed the descriptive term *acrocephalosyndactyly* which has been widely accepted. Since other types of acrocephalosyndactyly (ACS) have also been described [3], Apert syndrome has been designated ACS type I.

Clinical Presentation. The acrocephaly is of the brachysphenocephalic type. The skull is towerlike because the growth is directed predominantly upward. The forehead is high and wide and the occiput is flat. The apex of the skull is at or near the bregma.

The face is flat. The eyes are protuberant and widely placed (Fig. 5.32). The palpebral fissures have a downward slant. The maxilla and the bridge of the nose are underdeveloped. A cleft palate and bifid uvula may be present.

Syndactyly of the hands and feet is of a special type, i.e., complete distal fusion with a tendency of the bony structures to fuse also. The hand, when all fingers are webbed, has been compared to a spoon or, when the thumb is free, to an obstetric hand. The nails of the second to fifth fingers are often fused (Figs. 5.33 and 5.34).

The patients are usually moderately to severely mentally retarded [3, 4].

All of those subjects who have passed puberty have moderate to severe acne vulgaris involving the face, chest, and back (Figs. 5.35 and 5.36). Comedones may be present on the upper and lower parts of the forearms. The acneiform eruption may extend to the buttocks and thighs [5]. The hair displays trichorrhexis nodosa [6].

In a review [4] of 54 patients, two clinical categories were distinguished: (a) "typical" acrocephalosyndactyly, to which Apert's name is applied; and (b) other forms lumped together as "atypical" acrocephalosyndactyly. The feature distinguishing the two types is a middigital handmass with a single nail common to digits II through IV, found in Apert syndrome and lacking in the others. However, it is generally thought that these two types are only phenotypic variations of the same disorder [7]. The incidence of this syndrome is said to be as low as 1 in 160,000 live births [4].

Pathology and Pathophysiology. The syndrome results from irregular bridging between early islands of the mesenchymal blastema destined to become bone. The organization of other tissues is also disturbed.

The craniofacial malformation is attributed to premature fusion of the coronal complex of sutures alone or together with the sagittal suture. This results in distorted growth of the neurocranium, producing a tall brachycephalic skull.

Of 24 patients studied cytogenetically, the total reported number of abnormal karyotypes in Apert syndrome is four. All of the anomalies involve chromosomes from group A, but with different structural rearrangements [8].

Inheritance. Most cases of Apert syndrome are sporadic. But several cases of parent-to-child transmission have been reported [9, 10]. The evidence strongly suggests dominant inheritance, presumably autosomal, in view of the equal sex ratio. Paternal age effect is suspected. Low frequency of consanguinity and failure to observe multiple affected sibs make recessive inheritance unlikely [3].

Treatment. It is recommended that the craniosynostosis be corrected in early infancy. Repair of the syndactyly should be performed in the first few years, if possible [11].

References

1. Gorlin, R.S., Pinborg, J.J.: Syndromes of the head and neck, p. 9. New York: McGraw-Hill Book Co. 1964
2. Apert, E.: De l'acrocéphalosyndactylie. Bull. Soc. Med. Hôp. (Paris) *23*, 1310–1330 (1906)
3. McKusick, V.A.: Mendelian inheritance in man. 5th. ed., p. 7. Baltimore: Johns Hopkins University Press 1978
4. Blank, C.E.: Apert's syndrome (a type of acrocephalosyndactyly) – observations on a British series of thirty-nine cases. Ann. hum. Genet. *24*, 151–164 (1960)
5. Solomon, L.M., Fretzin, D., Pruzansky, S.: Pilosebaceous abnormalities in Apert's syndrome. Arch. Derm. *102*, 381–385 (1970)
6. Moynahan, E.J.: Genetically determined diseases. In: Recent advances in dermatology. Rook, A. (ed.), No. 3, pp. 323–371. London: Churchill Livingstone 1973
7. Holmes, L.B., Moser, H.W., Halldórsson, S., Mack, C., Pant, S.S., Matzilevich, B.: Mental retardation. pp. 222–225. New York: Macmillan Co. 1972
8. Dodson, W.E., Museles, M., Kennedy, J.L., Jr., Al-Aish, M.: Acrocephalosyndactylia associated with a chromosomal translocation. 46, XX, t(2p− :Cq+). Amer. J. Dis. Child. *120*, 360–362 (1970)
9. Roberts, K.B., Hall, J.G.: Apert's acrocephalosyndactyly in mother and daughter: cleft palate in the mother. In: The clinical delineation of birth defects. Bergsma, D. (ed.), Vol. VII, No. 7, pt. XI, pp. 262–264, Baltimore: Williams & Wilkins Co. 1971
10. Weech, A.A.: Combined acrocephaly and syndactylism occurring in mother and daughter. A case report. Bull. Johns Hopk. Hosp. *40*, 73–76 (1927)
11. Hoover, G.H., Flatt, A.E., Weiss, M.W.: The hand and Apert's syndrome. J. Bone Jt. Surg. (Brit.) *52*, 878–895 (1970)

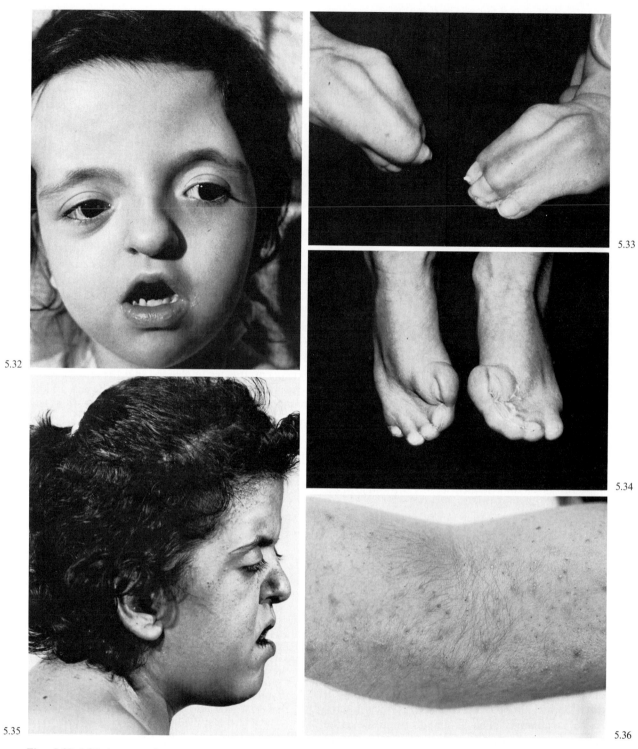

5.32

5.33

5.34

5.35

5.36

Figs. 5.32–5.36. Apert syndrome

Fig. 5.32. Note flat face and protuberant eyes. (Courtesy of Dr. F.C. Fraser)

Figs. 5.33 and 5.34. Hands and feet with severe syndactyly

Fig. 5.35. Adult with acneiform eruption. (Courtesy of Dr. L. M. Solomon)

Fig. 5.36. Acneiform eruption on upper limb. (Courtesy of Dr. L. M. Solomon)

Acrocephalopolysyndactyly, Type II (ACPS II, Carpenter Syndrome)

In 1901 Carpenter [1] described two sisters with acrocephaly, peculiar facies, brachydactyly and syndactyly of the hands, and preaxial polydactyly and syndactyly of the toes. In 1966 Temtamy [2] coined the eponym "Carpenter's syndrome." At least 18 cases of this disorder have been reported to date [3].

Clinical Presentation. Acrocephaly (Fig. 5.37), flat facial profile, flat nasal bridge, laterally displaced medial canthi, slight downward slant of the palpebral fissures, epicanthic folds, and micrognathia are the main features of this disease. The ears are usually low-set and malformed.

The most common hand anomalies are brachydactyly (brachymesophalangy) and partial syndactyly of the third and fourth fingers. Most patients also have ulnar deviation of the last two phalanges of the middle finger and radial deviation of the last two phalanges of the ring finger. All patients have polysyndactyly of the toes with medial deviation and duplication of either the first or second toe (Fig. 5.38). In older patients, obesity, mental subnormality, and hypogonadism have been noted.

Other less consistently observed features include congenital heart defects, duplication of the second phalanx of the thumb, metatarsus varus, flat acetabulum, flare of the pelvis, coxa valga, genu valgum, lateral displacement of patellae, pilonidal dimple, and abdominal hernias. Chromosome, amino acid, and mucopolysaccharide studies have been normal.

Pathology and Pathophysiology. Pathologic findings are inconsistent. They include congenital heart defects (patent ductus arteriosus, ventricular septal defect, pulmonic stenosis, transposition of the great vessels), unilateral hydroureter, small phallus and testes, biliary atresia, hypergyri of the cerebral cortex, and an accessory spleen [2].

Patients with premature fusion of all sutures have a small head. Those with premature closure of only the coronal and lambdoid sutures have a wide, flat brow and occiput and increased vertical diameter of the skull.

Inheritance. Autosomal recessive [2].

Treatment. Early surgical correction of the craniosynostosis and polysyndactyly is recommended (Fig. 5.39). Special shoes must be made or one toe must be surgically removed to allow the wearing of regular shoes.

References

1. Carpenter, G.: Two sisters showing malformations of the skull and other congenital abnormalities. Rep. Soc. Study Dis. Child (Lond.) *1*, 110–118 (1901)
2. Temtamy, S. A.: Carpenter's syndrome: acrocephalopolysyndactyly. An autosomal recessive syndrome. J. Pediat. *69*, 111–120 (1966)
3. Der Kaloustian, V.M., Sinno, A.A., Nassar, S.I.: Acrocephalopolysyndactyly type II (Carpenter syndrome). Amer. J. Dis. Child. *124*, 716–718 (1972)

Ectodermal Dysplasias

Anhidrotic Ectodermal Dysplasia (Christ-Siemens Syndrome)

Clinical Presentation. The characteristic features of this syndrome are absent or reduced skin appendages and defective dentition. Affected individuals have distinctive features: prominent frontal bosses, depressed central face, prominent chin, thick lips, and sparse hair [1, 2].

The skin is soft, dry, and finely wrinkled, especially around the eyes, giving the appearance of premature aging. The eccrine sweat glands are absent or greatly reduced (hypohidrotic ectodermal dysplasia [3]), resulting in poor heat tolerance. The ears may be small or large [1]. The nose is saddle-shaped with small conspicuous nostrils and recessed columella [2]. The eyebrows are often absent and the eyelashes delicate (Figs. 5.40 and 5.41). Periorbital pigmentation is present [2]. Milialike papules may appear on the face, due to hyperplastic sebaceous glands [4]. There may be injection of the conjunctiva. The scalp hair is characteristically sparse and fine. Occasionally there is total alopecia. Body hair is likewise sparse. Atopic dermatitis may be associated with this syndrome [2].

The temporary and permanent teeth may be absent or greatly reduced. When present, the teeth are defective: incisors, canines, and bicuspids are conical and curved, and molars have hooked cusps [2]. Pseudorhagades or furrows are frequently found [1]. The mouth and nose may be dry.

Other associated findings are mental deficiency [1], absent breasts [1], hypogonadism [1], and infections of the pharynx and respiratory tract.

Relatives of affected individuals and female carriers may show few of the features of the syndrome.

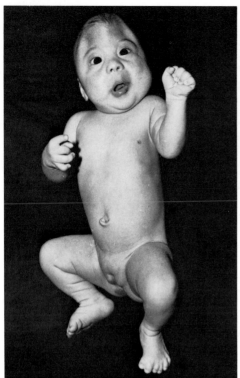

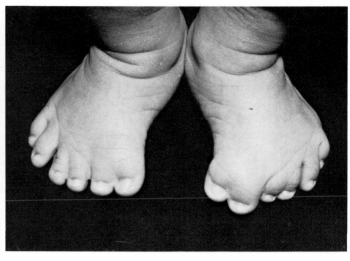

5.38

5.37

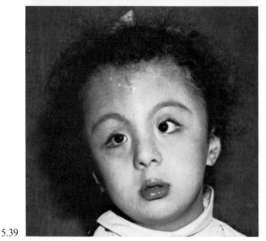

5.39

Figs. 5.37–5.39. Carpenter syndrome

Fig. 5.37. General view. Note towering skull, laterally displaced medial canthi, and downward slant of the palpebral fissures. (From Der Kaloustian, V.M., et al.: Amer. J. Dis. Child. *124*, 716–718, 1972)

Fig. 5.38. Polysyndactyly of the toes. (From Der Kaloustian, V.M., et al.: Amer. J. Dis. Child. *124*, 716–718, 1972)

Fig. 5.39. The same child at the age of 3 years. (Surgical correction of craniosynostosis was performed at the age of 5 months)

Some may show defective sweating and abnormal dermatoglyphics, whereas others may only show a few conical teeth [5].

A rare syndrome (Helweg-Larsen syndrome) [6] combines anhidrosis with neurolabyrinthitis developing in the fourth or fifth decade. There are no associated abnormalities of the hair or teeth. This syndrome is probably determined by a dominant gene.

A few families have been reported with anhidrosis, hypotrichosis, microdontia, nail dysplasia, cleft lip and palate, syndactyly, malformation in the genitourinary system, and mental retardation. Popliteal and perineal pterygia are present. The mode of inheritance is autosomal recessive [7]. These features are similar to those of the ectrodactyly-ectodermal dysplasia-cleft lip and palate (EEC) syndrome which is inherited as dominant [8, 9] (Fig. 5.42).

A kindred with anhidrotic ectodermal dysplasia and cleft lip and palate has been described with a probable autosomal dominant inheritance (Rapp-Hodgkin syndrome) [10].

Another variant is the Basan syndrome which is characterized by ectodermal dysplasia, absent dermatoglyphic pattern, nail changes, and simian

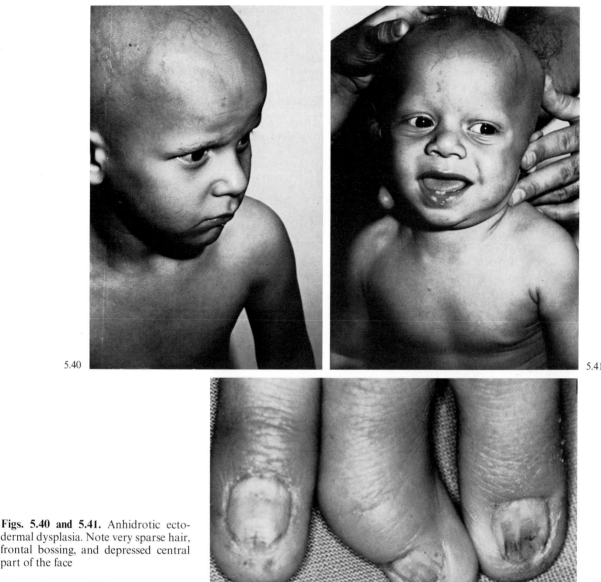

Figs. 5.40 and 5.41. Anhidrotic ecto-dermal dysplasia. Note very sparse hair, frontal bossing, and depressed central part of the face

Fig. 5.42. Note defective nails in a patient with the EEC syndrome. (Courtesy of Dr. F.C. Fraser)

crease [11, 12]. The inheritance in this syndrome is by an autosomal dominant gene.

Anhidrosis without any other abnormality characteristic of anhidrotic ectodermal dysplasia has been described in an Iranian sibship, with an autosomal recessive mode of inheritance [13].

One kindred of four sibs has been reported with facies resembling that of anhidrotic ectodermal dysplasia and reduced sweating [14]. This syndrome (Berlin) also includes infantilism, mental retardation, hypodontia, and hypotrichosis. Characteristic features of this syndrome are generalized mottled pigmentation, dry skin, and palmoplantar keratodermia. Inheritance is autosomal recessive.

A Brazilian family presents another syndrome with hypohidrotic ectodermal dysplasia [15, 16]. In this family, a brother and sister and two deceased brothers showed severe absence deformities of all four limbs, hypotrichosis, abnormal teeth, hypoplastic nipples and areolae, and deformed auricles. The consistent features included hypoplastic nails, hypogonadism, thyroid enlargement, incomplete cleft lip, mental retardation, and EKG and EEG abnormalities. Both living sibs showed an excess of tyrosine and/or tryptophane in the urine. The disorder is suspected to be inherited as an autosomal recessive.

Hypoplastic enamel, onycholysis, and hypohidrosis were described in members of a three generation kindred. The inheritance of this condition is autosomal dominant [17].

A newly described syndrome of ankyloblepharon, ectodermal defects, and cleft lip and palate (AEC syndrome) is probably inherited as autosomal dominant [18]. In this syndrome there is dry skin with reduced sweating, palmoplantar keratodermia, partial to total alopecia, severe nail dystrophy, and hypodontia. Associated features include supernumerary nipples, syndactyly, photophobia, lacrimal duct atresia, and deformed ears [18].

Pathology and Pathophysiology. The epidermis is usually atrophic and the eccrine sweat glands are absent or few and poorly developed. Other appendages may be few or normal.

In a group of patients with anhidrotic ectodermal dysplasia and atopic dermatitis, there appears to be some degree of cellular immune hypofunction. Such an abnormality may contribute to recurrent viral infections evidenced by bouts of fever [19].

Inheritance. Most pedigrees with only anhidrotic ectodermal dysplasia show an X-linked recessive type of inheritance. In inbred people of eastern Kentucky [20], and occasionally in females [21], an autosomal recessive mode of inheritance has been reported. The features in these pedigrees are phenotypically indistinguishable from those in males with the X-linked form. A few suggest autosomal recessivity [4].

Treatment. Management mainly entails avoidance of conditions that accentuate heat intolerance. Dental care is also important.

References

1. Upshaw, B.Y., Montgomery, H.: Hereditary anhidrotic ectodermal dysplasia. A clinical and pathological study. Arch. Derm. Syph. *60*, 1170–1183 (1949)
2. Reed, W.B., Lopez, D.A., Landing, B.: Clinical spectrum of anhidrotic ectodermal dysplasia. Arch. Derm. *102*, 134–143 (1970)
3. Katz, S.I., Penneys, N.S.: Sebaceous gland papules in anhidrotic ectodermal dysplasia. Arch. Derm. *103*, 507–509 (1971)
4. Crump, I.A., Danks, D.M.: Hypohidrotic ectodermal dysplasia. A study of sweat pores in the X-linked form and in a family with probable autosomal recessive inheritance. J. Pediat. *78*, 466–473 (1971)
5. Verbov, J.: Hypohidrotic (or anhidrotic) ectodermal dysplasia – an appraisal of diagnostic methods. Brit. J. Derm. *83*, 341–348 (1970)
6. Helweg-Larsen, H.F., Ludwigsen, K.: Congenital familial anhidrosis and neurolabyrinthitis. Acta derm.-venereol. (Stockh.) *26*, 489–505 (1946)
7. Rosselli, D., Gulienetti, R.: Ectodermal dysplasia. Brit. J. plast. Surg. *14*, 190–204 (1961)
8. Rüdiger, R.A., Haase, W., Passarge, E.: Association of ectrodactyly, ectodermal dysplasia, and cleft lip-palate. The EEC syndrome. Amer. J. Dis. Child. *120*, 160–163 (1970)
9. Bixler, D., Spivack, J., Bennett, J., Christian, J.C.: The ectrodactyly-ectodermal dysplasia-clefting (EEC) syndrome. Report of 2 cases and review of the literature. Clin. Genet. *3*, 43–51 (1972)
10. Rapp, R.S., Hodgkin, W.E.: Anhidrotic ectodermal dysplasia: autosomal dominant inheritance with palate and lip anomalies. J. med. Genet. *5*, 269–272 (1968)
11. Basan, M.: Ektodermale Dysplasie. Fehlendes Papillarmuster, Nagelveränderungen und Vierfingerfurche. Arch. klin. exp. Derm. *222*, 546–557 (1965)
12. Jorgenson, R.J.: Ectodermal dysplasia with hypotrichosis, hypohidrosis, defective teeth, and unusual dermatoglyphics (Basan syndrome?). In: The clinical delineation of birth defects. Bergsma, D. (ed.), Vol. X, No. 4, pt. XVI, pp. 323–325. Baltimore: Williams & Wilkins Co. 1974
13. Mahloudji, M., Livingston, K.E.: Familial and congenital simple anhidrosis. Amer. J. Dis. Child. *113*, 477–479 (1967)
14. Berlin, C.: Congenital generalized melanoleucoderma associated with hypodontia, hypotrichosis, stunted growth, and mental retardation occurring in two brothers and two sisters. Dermatologica (Basel) *123*, 227–243 (1961)
15. Freire-Maia, N.: A newly recognized genetic syndrome of tetramelic deficiencies, ectodermal dysplasia, deformed ears, and other abnormalities. Amer. J. hum. Genet. *22*, 370–377 (1970)
16. Cat, I., Costa, O., Freire-Maia, N.: Odontotrichomelic hypohidrotic dysplasia. A clinical reappraisal. Hum. Heredity (Basel) *22*, 91–95 (1972)
17. Witkop, C.J.,Jr., Brearley, L.J., Gentry, W.C.,Jr.: Hypoplastic enamel, onycholysis and hypohidrosis inherited as autosomal dominant trait: review of ectodermal dysplasia syndromes. Oral Surgery *39*, 71–86 (1975)
18. Hay, R.J., Wells, R.S.: The syndrome of ankyloblepharon, ectodermal defects, and cleft lip and palate: an autosomal dominant condition. Brit. J. Derm. *94*, 277–289 (1976)
19. Davis, J.R., Solomon, L.M.: Cellular immunodeficiency in anhidrotic ectodermal dysplasia. Acta derm.-venereol. (Stockh.) *56*, 115–120 (1976)
20. Passarge, E., Nuzum, C.T., Schubert, W.K.: Anhidrotic ectodermal dysplasia as autosomal recessive trait in an inbred kindred. Humangenetik *3*, 181–185 (1966)
21. Gorlin, R.J., Old, T., Anderson, V.E.: Hypohidrotic ectodermal dysplasia in females. A critical analysis and argument for genetic heterogeneity. Z. Kinderheilk. *108*, 1–11 (1970)

Fig. 5.43. Hidrotic ectodermal dysplasia. Dysplastic nails of child and parents. (Courtesy of Dr. F.C. Fraser)

Figs. 5.44 and 5.45. Hidrotic ectodermal dysplasia. Note sparse hair and absence of eyebrows. (Courtesy of Dr. F.C. Fraser)

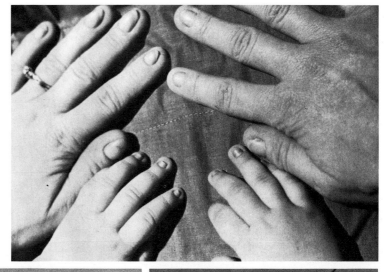

5.43

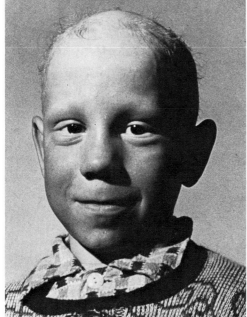

5.44

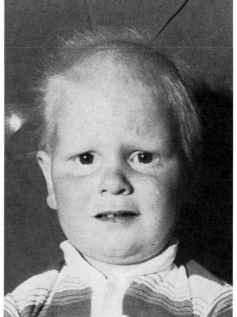

5.45

Hidrotic Ectodermal Dysplasia

Clouston, in 1929, was the first to draw attention to this abnormality [1].

Clinical Presentation. The main features are nail dystrophy, palmoplantar keratodermia, and defects of the hair [1, 2]. The nails are slow-growing and appear thick, striated, and discolored (Fig. 5.43). Paronychial infections are frequent. The palms and soles show diffuse thickening that may extend to the sides. The scalp hair, eyebrows, and eyelashes are sparse, thin, and fragile (Figs. 5.44 and 5.45). Body hair may be absent or sparse. Sweating is normal and the teeth are usually unaffected. Mental deficiency is rare.

Pathology and Pathophysiology. In the Clouston variety of hidrotic ectodermal dysplasia, the palms and soles show orthokeratotic hyperkeratosis. A study of the physical properties and chemical composition of the hair suggests that the structural gene of a matrix polypeptide is involved. Mutation of this gene causes deletion of a low sulfur segment of the polypeptide which results in the destabilization of intermolecular disulfide bonds [3]. The recent demonstration of proteins of abnormally low molecular weight in ectodermal dysplastic matrix has lent support to this hypothesis [4].

Onychodystrophy and neural deafness have been reported in a pedigree with probably recessive inheritance [5].

In another pedigree with hidrotic dysplasia, delayed primary and secondary dentition, syndactylism, and polydactylism, severe sensorineural deafness was an added feature. The inheritance in this pedigree is probably autosomal dominant [6].

Still another pedigree has been reported in which there is hidrotic ectodermal dysplasia, sensorineural hearing loss (due probably to a defect of the cells of the organ of Corti), and contracture of the fifth fingers [7]. The inheritance in this single pedigree is autosomal recessive.

Inheritance. Autosomal dominant [8].

Treatment. No specific treatment is available.

References

1. Clouston, H. R.: Hereditary ectodermal dystrophy. Can. med. Ass. J. *21*, 18–31 (1929)
2. Zlatkov, N.B., Konstantinova, B.: Genealogische und zyto-genetische Untersuchungen bei der hidrotischen Form der erblichen ektodermalen Dysplasie. Dermatologica (Berl.) *147*, 144–152 (1973)
3. Gold, R.J.M., Scriver, C.R.: Properties of hair keratin in an autosomal dominant form of ectodermal dysplasia. Amer. J. hum. Genet. *24*, 549–561 (1972)
4. Gold, R.J.M., Kachra, Z.: Molecular defect in hidrotic ectodermal dysplasia. In: The first human hair symposium. Brown, A.C. (ed.), pp. 250–276. New York: Medcom Press 1974
5. Feinmesser, M., Zelig, S.: Congenital deafness with onycho-dystrophy. Arch. Otolaryng. *74*, 507–508 (1961)
6. Robinson, G.C., Miller, J.R., Bensimon, J.R.: Familial ectodermal dysplasia with sensori-neural deafness and other anomalies. Pediatrics *30*, 797–802 (1962)
7. Mikaelian, D.O., Der Kaloustian, V.M., Shahin, N.A., Barsoumian, V.M.: Congenital ectodermal dysplasia with hearing loss. Arch. Otolaryng. *92*, 85–89 (1970)
8. Williams, M., Fraser, F.C.: Hidrotic ectodermal dysplasia – Clouston's family revisited. Can. med. Ass. J. *96*, 36–38 (1967)

Ellis-van Creveld Syndrome

Ellis and van Creveld described this syndrome in 1940 [1]. Since then, more than 100 patients have been reported in the literature [2–4]. The largest series is from an Amish kindred [3].

Clinical Presentation. The main manifestations of the syndrome consist of chondrodysplasia, ecto-dermal dysplasia, polydactyly, and congenital mor-bus cordis. The patients are dwarfed; they have short extremities, dystrophic nails and teeth (partial anodontia, small teeth, neonatal teeth), a shallow upper lip-gum groove, funnel chest, lumbar lor-dosis, genu valgum, and polydactyly of fingers and occasionally of toes (Figs. 5.46–5.48). The majority of cases also show some form of congenital heart disease from a mild to a severe one, most commonly a septal defect [2–4].

Occasionally the following abnormalities may oc-cur: mental retardation, scant or fine hair, cryptor-chidism, epispadias, and talipes equinovarus. The sweat mechanism is normal.

Roentgenography reveals generalized thickness and coarseness of bones; marked acceleration of second-ary centers of ossification in phalanges, metacar-pals, head of femur, and humerus; and retardation of primary centers of ossification in metacarpals and proximal and medial phalanges [5].

About half of the patients die in early infancy as a consequence of cardiorespiratory problems.

The very high frequency of this disorder in the Old Order Amish is considered a good illustration of the "founder effect" [4] (see Glossary).

Pathology and Pathophysiology. The basic patho-genesis of the syndrome is not known.

Inheritance. Autosomal recessive [4,6].

Treatment. There is no effective treatment.

References

1. Ellis, R.W.B., van Creveld, S.: A syndrome characterized by ectodermal dysplasia, polydactyly, chondrodysplasia, and congenital morbus cordis. Report of three cases. Arch. Dis. Child. *15*, 65–84 (1940)
2. Douglas, W.F., Schonholtz, G.J., Geppert, L.J.: Chondro-ectodermal dysplasia (Ellis-van Creveld syndrome). Amer. J. Dis. Child. *97*, 473–478 (1959)
3. McKusick, V.A., Egeland, J.A., Eldridge, R., Krusen, D.E.: Dwarfism in the Amish. I. The Ellis-Van Creveld syndrome. Bull. Johns Hopk. Hosp. *115*, 306–336 (1964)
4. Blackburn, M.G., Belliveau, R.E.: Ellis-Van Creveld syn-drome. A report of previously undescribed anomalies in two siblings. Amer. J. Dis. Child. *122*, 267–270 (1971)
5. Caffey, J.: Chondroectodermal dysplasia (Ellis-Van Creveld disease). Amer. J. Roentgenol. *68*, 875–886 (1952)
6. Metrakos, J.D., Fraser, F.C.: Evidence for a hereditary factor in chondroectodermal dysplasia (Ellis-Van Creveld syn-drome). Amer. J. hum. Genet. *6*, 250–269 (1954)

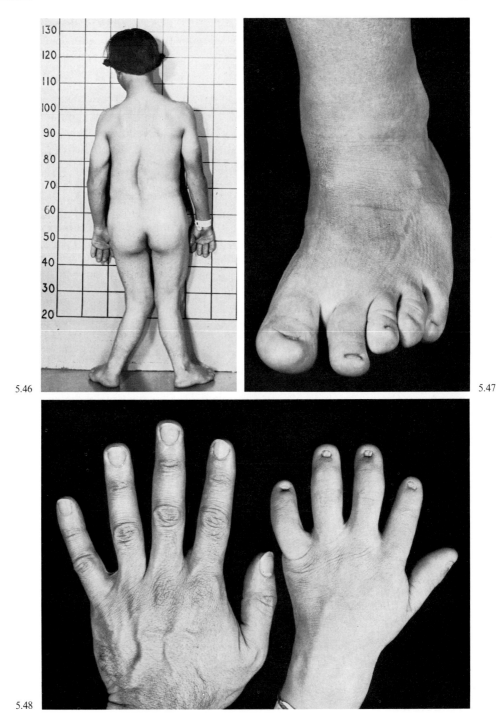

5.46

5.47

5.48

Fig. 5.46. Ellis-van Creveld syndrome. Note dwarfism. (Courtesy of Dr. V.A. McKusick)

Figs. 5.47 and 5.48. Ellis-van Creveld syndrome. Note dysplastic nails. (Courtesy of Dr. V.A. McKusick)

Congenital Ectodermal Dysplasia of the Face (Focal-Facial-Dermal Dysplasia and Facial Ectodermal Dysplasia)

Two syndromes which share several features are included under this title. Both syndromes are characterized by the appearance, at birth, of one to ten scarlike, symmetric, and usually hyperpigmented defects in the temporal region similar to "forceps marks" [1–3]. In both syndromes, the lateral thirds of the eyebrows are sparse. In focal-facial-dermal dysplasia, vertical linear depressions are present on the forehead [3, 4] as well as clefting of the chin [4]. Mental retardation and possibly abdominal cancer may be associated findings [4]. In the second syndrome, other abnormalities are present: low hairline, flat nasal bridge, fleshy nose, prominent epicanthic fold, absent eyelashes on the lower lids and distichiasis of the upper lid, arched eyebrows, and wrinkled chin [2, 3].

In focal-facial-dermal dysplasia, histologic studies show dermal atrophy with absence of connective and adipose tissues. Bundles of striated muscle are present in the dermis near the epidermis [4]. Focal-facial-dermal dysplasia is determined by an autosomal dominant gene [3, 4] and facial ectodermal dysplasia by a recessive gene [2].

References

1. Brauer, A.: Hereditärer symmetrischer systematisierter Naevus aplasticus bei 38 Personen. Derm. Wschr. *89*, 1163–1168 (1929)
2. Setleis, H., Kramer, B., Valcarcel, M., Einhorn, A.H.: Congenital ectodermal dysplasia of the face. Pediatrics *32*, 540–548 (1963)
3. Jensen, N.E.: Congenital ectodermal dysplasia of the face. Brit. J. Derm. *84*, 410–416 (1971)
4. McGeoch, A.H., Reed, W.B.: Familial focal facial dermal dysplasia. Arch. Derm. *107*, 591–595 (1973)

Syndromes with Premature Aging

Progeria (Hutchinson-Gilford Syndrome)

In 1886 Hutchinson [1] described this condition as "congenital absence of hair and mammary glands with atrophic condition of the skin and its appendages in a boy whose mother had been almost bald from alopecia areata from the age of six." Later, Gilford [2] termed the condition "progeria," meaning premature aging.

Clinical Presentation. The most striking feature is the alopecia with its onset between birth and 18 months. The skin is thin, taut, dry, wrinkled, and "sclerodermatous." Its surface is mottled and brownish orange in color. The superficial blood vessels are prominent (Figs. 5.49–5.52). Sweating is decreased. The nails are hypoplastic, brittle, curved, and yellowish. Right from infancy there is gradual loss of subcutaneous fat, ultimately involving the cheeks and pubic area. In most cases there is generalized hypotrichosis with absent eyebrows and eyelashes.

Deficient growth is evident between 6 and 18 months of age. At the age of 1–2 years, periarticular fibrosis develops, resulting in stiff or partially flexed prominent joints.

Skeletal hypoplasia is manifested by facial hypoplasia (resulting in craniofacial disproportion), frontal bossing, micrognathia, slim tubular bones, small thoracic cage, and thin calvarium. Coxa valga and a tendency toward ovoid vertebral bodies are evident. The teeth, both deciduous and permanent, have a delayed eruption and are crowded. The voice is high-pitched. Mental development is normal.

Patients usually die of coronary heart disease during the first or second decade of life.

Pathology and Pathophysiology. Since patients with classic progeria resemble aged individuals, an understanding of the pathophysiology of this disease may shed important light on the aging process.

The skin histopathology varies depending on the biopsy site and the age of the patient, but in general shows the following [3]: hyperkeratotic atrophic epidermis with heavy pigmentation in the basal cell layer; decreased numbers of sebaceous glands and hair follicles; normal to slightly decreased numbers of sweat glands; prominent arrectores pilorum muscles; decreased subcutaneous fat; disorganization, thickening, and "hyalinization" of collagen; normal or decreased elastic tissue; and normal to decreased numbers of blood vessels, frequently with thickened walls, but without obliteration of lumina.

Scanning electron microscopy of scalp hairs reveals abnormal longitudinal depressions with minor cuticular defects manifested by loose scales. Similar surface defects, however, may be seen in normal hairs following physical trauma [4].

In the cardiovascular system, varying degrees of generalized atherosclerosis, involving chiefly the larger arteries, are found. The development of atherosclerosis in these patients, however, is not accompanied by an obvious abnormality of lipid metabolism. Coronary occlusions with myocardial

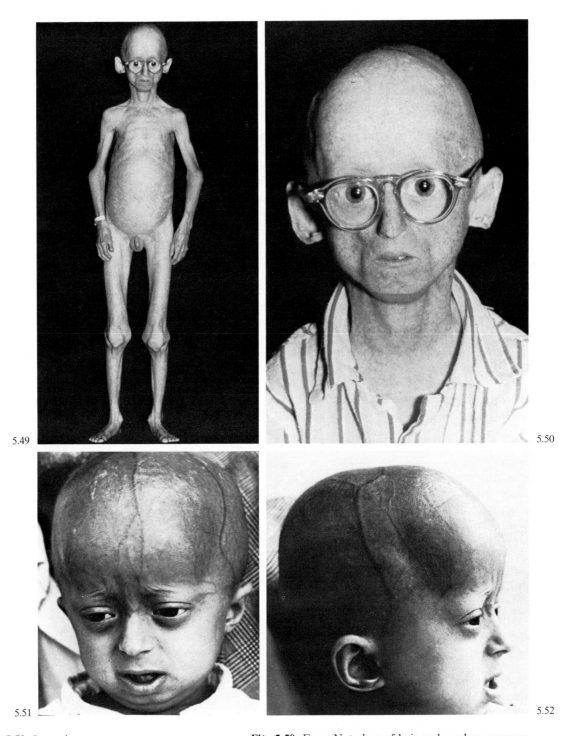

5.49

5.50

5.51

5.52

Figs. 5.49–5.52. Progeria

Fig. 5.49. General appearance. Note striking loss of subcutaneous fat and hypotrichosis. The patient is 15 years old. (Courtesy of Dr. F.C. Fraser)

Fig. 5.50. Face. Note loss of hair and aged appearance. (From Nora, J.J., Fraser, F.C.: Medical genetics, p. 177. Philadelphia: Lea & Febiger 1974)

Figs. 5.51 and 5.52. Note thin, taut skin and prominent blood vessels

infarctions are encountered more frequently than cerebral vascular lesions. In certain cases, however, the cardiac pathology consists of patchy and focal myocardial fibrosis and necrosis rather than typical myocardial infarction [5]. There may also be an accumulation of lipofuscin pigment in the myocardium [6].

Metabolic studies [7] suggest that progeria represents a form of mesenchymal dysplasia in which connective tissue cells are unresponsive to growth hormone influences. It is hypothesized that this failure to grow may account for the "older" collagen which may in turn produce structural abnormalities in vessel walls predisposing to atherosclerosis.

Skin fibroblast cultures have given conflicting results, either failure to grow [3] or a marked diminution in survival [8]. Other studies, however, have shown that cultured progeria fibroblasts have a lifespan within normal limits [9], but with a reduction in mitotic activity, DNA synthesis, and cloning efficiency [10].

An immune process may account for the extensive changes characteristic of progeria [11]. This observation is based on the presence of HL-A antigens on lymphocytes, but not on fibroblasts. Absorption studies on fibroblasts with two HL-A2 antisera reveal that HL-A antigens are either absent or have a drastically reduced expression on progeric fibroblasts.

In addition, it was shown [12] that at each passage progeria cells clearly contained a higher mean percentage of heat-labile G6PD and HGPRT than control strains. The most likely cause appears to be an aberration in protein synthesis or degradation, or both, although multiple somatic mutations cannot be ruled out.

Deficient DNA repair in human progeroid cells has also been reported [13].

Inheritance. The occurrence of the disease in siblings is suggestive of a genetic etiology; however, the pattern of inheritance is not definite. Cultures of cells from the parents of patients showed a somewhat reduced mitotic activity and DNA synthesis [10]. Although this favors the autosomal recessive pattern of inheritance, controversy still exists [14].

Treatment. No specific treatment is available except for protection against trauma. Short-term growth hormone therapy may decrease the discomfort in the joints [7]. Atherosclerosis develops in spite of a special dietary regimen. Assuming that a defect in vitamin E metabolism may be at the root of progeria, vitamin E has been recommended for its antioxidant effect [15].

References

1. Hutchinson, J.: Congenital absence of hair and mammary glands with atrophic condition of the skin and its appendages in a boy whose mother had been almost bald from alopecia areata from the age of six. Medico-Chirurgical Trans. roy. Med. Chir. Soc. Lond. *69*, 473–477 (1886)
2. Gilford, H.: Progeria: a form of senilism. Practitioner *73*, 188–217 (1904)
3. DeBusk, F.L.: The Hutchinson-Gilford progeria syndrome. Report of 4 cases and review of the literature. J. Pediat. *80*, 697–724 (1972)
4. Fleischmajer, R., Nedwich, A.: Progeria (Hutchinson-Gilford). Arch. Derm. *107*, 253–258 (1973)
5. Gabr, M., Hashem, N., Hashem, M., Fahmi, A., Safouh, M.: Progeria, a pathologic study. J. Pediat. *57*, 70–77 (1960)
6. Reichel, W., Garcia-Bunuel, R.: Pathologic findings in progeria: myocardial fibrosis and lipofuscin pigment. Amer. J. clin. Path. *53*, 243–253 (1970)
7. Villee, D.B., Nichols, G., Jr., Talbot, N.B.: Metabolic studies in two boys with classical progeria. Pediatrics *43*, 207–216 (1969)
8. Goldstein, S.: Lifespan of cultured cells in progeria. Lancet *1969 I*, 424
9. Martin, G.M., Sprague, C.A., Epstein, C.J.: Replicative lifespan of cultivated human cells. Effects of donor's age, tissue and genotype. Lab. Invest. *23*, 86–92 (1970)
10. Danes, B.S.: Progeria: a cell culture study on aging. J. clin. Invest. *50*, 2000–2003 (1971)
11. Singal, D.P., Goldstein, S.: Absence of detectable HL-A antigens on cultured fibroblasts in progeria. J. clin. Invest. *52*, 2259–2263 (1973)
12. Goldstein, S., Moermann, E.: Heat-labile enzymes in skin fibroblasts from subjects with progeria. New. Engl. J. Med. *292*, 1305–1309 (1975)
13. Epstein, J., Williams, J.R., Little, J.B.: Deficient DNA repair in human progeroid cells. Proc. nat. Acad. Sci. (Wash.) *70*, 977–981 (1973)
14. McKusick, V.A.: Mendelian inheritance in man, 5th ed., p. 645. Baltimore: Johns Hopkins University Press 1978
15. Ayres, S., Jr., Mihan, R.: Progeria: a possible therapeutic approach. J. Amer. med. Ass. *227*, 1381–1382 (1974)

Acrogeria

In 1940 Gottron described two siblings with premature aging of the skin confined to the extremities and present from birth [1].

Clinical Presentation. These patients have atrophy of the skin with telangiectasia and mottled hyperpigmentation on the extremities, especially the backs of the hands and feet. The nails are dystrophic or thickened. There are no leg ulcers. Micrognathia may be present. However, stature, scalp hair, and eyes are normal [2].

Pathology and Pathophysiology. The subcutaneous fat is reduced and may be almost absent in the most severely affected region. The dermis is atrophic with sparse, thin collagen bundles, but abundant elastic fibers which appear clumped.

Inheritance. Probably autosomal recessive [2].

Treatment. No special treatment is available.

References

1. Gottron, H.: Familiäre Akrogerie. Arch. Derm. Syph. (Berl.) *181*, 571–583 (1940)
2. Gilkes, J.J.H., Shavrill, D.E., Wells, R.S.: The premature ageing syndromes. Report of eight cases and description of a new entity named metageria. Brit. J. Derm. *91*, 243–262 (1974)

Metageria

In 1974 Gilkes et al. [1] described two patients who gave the appearance of premature aging. They called this new syndrome metageria.

Clinical Presentation. The patients have a tall, thin stature; birdlike, pinched face; and beaked nose. The skin is atrophied, especially on the limbs. There is mottled hyperpigmentation with telangiectasia. The scalp hair is fine and thin. The eyes are prominent, but there is no true exophthalmos. The nails are normal. The limbs have a generalized loss of subcutaneous fat. Ischemic leg ulcers may occur. Pubic hair is normal, but sparse.

There may be early onset of diabetes mellitus. The libido is normal. The genitalia are of normal size.

Pathology and Pathophysiology. Early atherosclerosis is present. There are no vascular calcifications. The skin is atrophic over the hands; there is hyperkeratosis over the plantar aspect of the heels and the balls of the feet.

Inheritance. Probably autosomal recessive.

Treatment. No special treatment is available.

Reference

1. Gilkes, J.J.H., Sharvill, D.E., Wells, R.S.: The premature ageing syndromes. Report of eight cases and description of a new entity named metageria. Brit. J. Derm. *91*, 243–262 (1974)

Werner Syndrome (Adult Progeria)

In 1904 Werner [1] first reported four sibs affected with this disorder. It was accepted as a separate syndrome after the paper by Oppenheimer and Kugel in 1934 [2] and the comprehensive study by Thannhauser in 1945 [3]. More than 200 cases of Werner syndrome have been reported.

Clinical Presentation. The principal characteristics of Werner syndrome are shortness of stature with a characteristic habitus, canities, premature baldness, scleropoikiloderma, trophic ulcers of the legs, juvenile cataracts, hypogonadism, tendency to diabetes, osteoporosis, metastatic calcifications, a high-pitched voice, and calcification of the blood vessels with coronary heart disease and infarction [3].
Atrophy of the skin results in shiny, smooth, taut skin. The principal areas of involvement are the face and distal extremities, especially the feet. There is also atrophy of the underlying connective tissue, muscle, and fat. The nose is thin and "pinched." There may be loss of circumorbital tissue and atrophy of the skin of the ears [4].
An early and prominent feature of the skin affection is hyperkeratosis over the bony prominences and the soles. The hyperkeratoses may be dislodged to form ulcers, especially over the heels, toes, malleoli, and Achilles tendons. Severe pain may ensue with difficulty in walking [4]. The nails are dystrophic. Patients with Werner syndrome have a high incidence of malignancy. The two principal causes of death, which occurs between 30 and 60 years of age, are malignancies and vascular accidents (myocardial, cerebrovascular) [4].

Pathology and Pathophysiology. There is atrophy of subcutaneous fat, skin appendages, and epidermis. The epidermis may be reduced to a thickness of two or three cell layers and the rete pegs are rarely conspicuous. There is frequently mild or diffuse hyperkeratosis. The basal layer of the epidermis is generally focally hypermelanotic. Dermal fibrosis is variable and ranges from mild subepidermal hyalinization to a striking sclerodermalike picture [4].
All patients reveal atherosclerosis of a severity not regularly encountered in this age group. The most striking of the cardiovascular lesions is the severe calcification of the aortic or mitral valve leaflets and rings. Male patients have testicular atrophy with hyalinized seminiferous tubules devoid of spermatogenic activity. Pathologic findings are noted also in the ovaries, kidneys, adrenals, thyroid, parathyroid, pituitary, liver, and brain.

Cultures of subcutaneous tissue grow more rapidly than those from the epidermis and dermis. After the rapid initial period of growth, mitotic activity ceases abruptly and mitotic figures can rarely be found after 6 weeks. Cultures can be passaged at most five times before entering the "degenerative" phase [4]. This may explain the short stature and the "progeria."

Chromosome karyotypes from leukocyte cultures reveal a significant number of aneuploid cells, but do not demonstrate any consistent chromosomal anomaly [4].

Many consider Werner syndrome as a form of premature aging or senescence (see also Progeria, p. 116, and Rothmund-Thomson Syndrome, p. 123). Relevant information derived from the study of Werner syndrome is valuable because of the importance of the aging process and the pathologic events associated with it [4]. However, certain features associated with aging occur to a much lesser degree. These include senile keratoses and other malignant lesions of the skin (basal and squamous cell carcinomas), senile elastosis (basophilic degeneration of dermal collagen), hyalinization of pancreatic islets, deposition of lipofuscin pigment (in hepatic cells, myocardial fibers, neurons), and the presence of corpora amylasea in the brain and spinal cord.

Inheritance. Autosomal recessive [4].

Treatment. Treatment is symptomatic.

References

1. Werner, O.: Über Katarakt in Verbindung mit Sklerodermie. Doctoral dissertation, Kiel University 1904
2. Oppenheimer, B.S., Kugel, V.H.: Werner's syndrome – a heredofamilial disorder with scleroderma, bilateral juvenile cataracts, precocious graying of the hair and endocrine stigmatization. Trans. Ass. Amer. Phycns. *49*, 358–370 (1934)
3. Thannhauser, S.J.: Werner's syndrome (progeria of the adult) and Rothmund's syndrome: two types of closely related heredofamilial atrophic dermatosis with juvenile cataracts and endocrine features; a critical study with five new cases. Ann. intern. Med. *23*, 559–626 (1945)
4. Epstein, C.J., Martin, G.M., Schultz, A.L., Motulsky, A.G.: Werner's syndrome. Review of its symptomatology, natural history, pathologic features, genetics and relationship to natural aging process. Med. (Baltimore) *45*, 177–221 (1966)

Cockayne Syndrome

In 1936 and again in 1946 Cockayne [1,2] described siblings with dwarfism, microcephaly, mental retardation, photosensitivity of the skin, retinal atrophy, and progressive neurologic deterioration. The disease is very rare; about 20 cases have been described [3–8].

Clinical Presentation. The appearance is normal at birth. Growth and development proceed at a normal rate in early infancy. The syndrome becomes evident around the age of 2–4 years. The main manifestations are microcephaly, mental deficiency (IQ < 50), growth retardation, peripheral neuropathy, characteristic facial features (loss of facial adipose tissue with slender nose, moderately sunken eyes, prominent maxilla), ophthalmologic abnormalities [3] (pigmentary retinal degeneration, optic atrophy, cataracts, loss of macular reflex, nystagmus), deafness, endocrinologic deficiencies, and skeletal abnormalities (disproportionately long limbs and large hands, restricted motion at the hip, knee, and ankle joints, relatively short trunk with biconvex flattening of the vertebrae, dorsal kyphosis) (Figs. 5.53–5.55). The endocrinologic deficiencies are manifested by poor breast development in females and cryptorchidism with a feminine pattern of pubic hair in males [2].

The skin reveals photosensitivity with a scaly erythematous dermatitis that develops over exposed areas such as the face, ears, hands, and legs. The dermatitis of the face may have a "butterfly" distribution. Older patients may have a thickened, wrinkled, freckled skin. Loss of subcutaneous fat gradually develops during childhood. The hair is sparse and may become prematurely gray.

By the age of 20 years, because of the neurologic involvement and the mental deficiency, these patients are unable to care for themselves and die in early adulthood from inanition and respiratory infections. Laboratory investigations may reveal increased CSF protein, diminished glomerular function, and hyperinsulinemia. Radiologically, there may be intracranial calcifications, especially in the region of the basal ganglia, a thickened calvarium, and anterior notching of the thoracic vertebrae.

Pathology and Pathophysiology. The skin changes are those of photosensitivity with premature aging. Atrophy of the cerebral cortex and cerebellum; marked symmetric calcification in the cortex, basal ganglia, and cerebellum [4]; and segmental demyelination in the peripheral nerves have been observed [5]. The kidneys may show glomerular and tubular abnormalities [9]. Cultured fibroblasts from patients have less than 30% of normal activity of the enzyme metabolizing phytanic acid, [10].

Inheritance. Autosomal recessive.

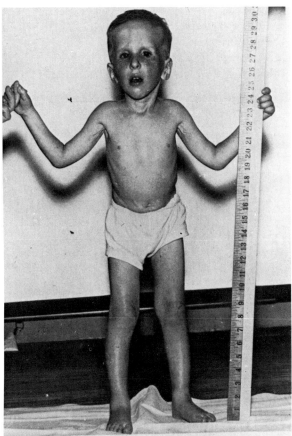

5.53

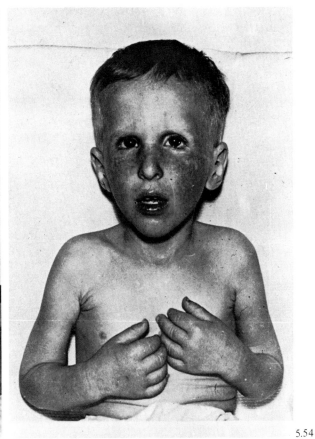

5.54

Figs. 5.53–5.55. Cockayne syndrome

Fig. 5.53. General appearance of affected child. Note long limbs. (From Windmiller, J., et al.: Amer. J. Dis. Child. *105*, 204–208, 1963)

Fig. 5.54. Photosensitive eruption of face and hands. (Courtesy of Dr. J. Windmiller)

Fig. 5.55. Face of affected adult. Note loss of adipose tissue, sunken eyes, and prominent maxilla. (From Coles, W.H.: Amer. J. Ophthal. *67*, 762–764, 1969)

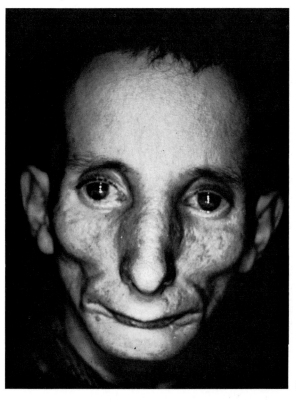

5.55

Treatment. Treatment is symptomatic and includes protection from sunlight and the use of sunscreens. Diet therapy may be tried, avoiding all foods containing chlorophyll, phytol, phytanic acid, or their precursors [10].

References

1. Cockayne, E.A.: Dwarfism with retinal atrophy and deafness. Arch. Dis. Child. *11*, 1–8 (1936)
2. Cockayne, E.A.: Case reports. Dwarfism with retinal atrophy and deafness. Arch. Dis. Child. *21*, 52–54 (1946)
3. Coles, W.H.: Ocular manifestations of Cockayne's syndrome. Amer. J. Ophthal. *67*, 762–764 (1969)
4. Moossy, J.: The neuropathology of Cockayne's syndrome. J. Neuropath. exp. Neurol. *26*, 654–660 (1967)
5. Moosa, A., Dubowitz, V.: Peripheral neuropathy in Cockayne's syndrome. Arch. Dis. Child. *45*, 674–677 (1970)
6. Fujimoto, W.Y., Greene, M.L., Seegmiller, J.E.: Cockayne's syndrome: report of a case with hyperlipoproteinemia, hyperinsulinemia, renal disease, and normal growth hormone. J. Pediat. *75*, 881–884 (1969)
7. Cotton, R.B., Keats, T.E., McKoy, E.E.: Abnormal blood glucose regulation in Cockayne's syndrome. Pediatrics *46*, 54–60 (1970)
8. Lanning, M., Similä, S.: Cockayne's syndrome. Report of a case with normal intelligence. Z. Kinderheilk. *109*, 70–75 (1970)
9. Ohno, T., Hirooka, M.: Renal lesions in Cockayne's syndrome. Tôhôku J. exp. Med. *89*, 151–166 (1966)
10. Lasser, A.E.: Cockayne's syndrome. Cutis *10*, 143–148 (1972)

Poikilodermas

Hereditary Sclerosing Poikiloderma

Weary et al. called attention to this syndrome in 1969 [1].

Clinical Presentation. There is extensive, mottled pigmentation appearing before the age of 4 years and gradually increasing in severity. The upper chest, face, and scalp are usually not involved. This mottled appearance is associated with skin atrophy and telangiectasia, especially over the knees, elbows, and interphalangeal joints. In the flexural regions of the axillae, antecubital fossae, and to a lesser extent the popliteal fossae, the mottling is associated with reticulated and linear hyperkeratotic and sclerotic bands. The palmar and plantar skin is sclerotic with irregular surfaces. Clubbing of the fingers and late-onset soft tissue calcification are other findings [1].

Pathology and Pathophysiology. There is homogenization of the collagen and decreased elastic tissue in addition to irregular distribution of melanin pigment [1]. The keratotic bands show focal hyperkeratosis.

Inheritance. Probably autosomal dominant.

Treatment. No definitive treatment is available.

Reference

1. Weary, P.E., Hsu, Y.T., Richardson, D.R., Caravati, C.M., Wood, B.T.: Hereditary sclerosing poikiloderma. Report of two families with an unusual and distinctive genodermatosis. Arch. Derm. *100*, 413–422 (1969)

Hereditary Acrokeratotic Poikiloderma

Weary et al., in 1971, described ten members of a family affected with this disorder [1].

Clinical Presentation. The usual age of onset is between 5 weeks and 6 months. The initial lesions are vesicles and/or vesicopustules over the hands and feet [1] and occasionally the trunk [2]. The lesions usually resolve in late childhood. In addition, there is a transient, widespread, eczematous dermatitis in flexural areas that resolves by the age of 5 years. Predominant in the flexural areas, but involving other areas with the exception of the face, scalp, and ears, is a gradually increasing diffuse poikiloderma with striate and reticulate atrophy. There is also development of keratotic lesions over the distal extremities, including the palms, soles, elbows, and knees. These lesions are firm lichenoid papules that persist throughout life.

Pathology and Pathophysiology. In the epidermis there is focal spongiosis and microvesicles with areas of hydropic degeneration of the basal cell layer. There are focal subepidermal, periappendageal, and perivascular inflammatory infiltrates. The histologic features of the nonvesicular lesions show epidermal atrophy, irregular pigmentation of the basal cell layer, incontinence of pigment, and mild perivascular inflammation. The acrokeratotic lesions show localized hyperkeratosis and irregular acanthosis [1].

There is a consistent elevation of IgG levels in affected individuals, and in some there is a positive test for rheumatoid factor. The significance of these abnormalities is not clear [1].

Inheritance. Probably autosomal dominant [1, 2].

Treatment. There is no specific treatment.

References

1. Weary, P.E., Manley, W.F., Jr., Graham, G.F.: Hereditary acrokeratotic poikiloderma. Arch. Derm. *103*, 409–422 (1971)
2. Aguadé, J.P., Herrero, C., Castello, C.A., Grimalt, F., Rueda Plata, L.A.: Congenital poikiloderma with vesiculobullous lesions: problems in classification of hereditary poikilodermas. Med. Cutanea *6*, 417–435 (1972)

Rothmund-Thomson Syndrome (Poikiloderma Congenitale)

In 1868 Rothmund [1] described several children with cataracts and a peculiar degeneration of the skin. In 1923 Thomson [2] described sisters who had poikiloderma congenitale, but no cataracts. Since the skin biopsy showed a type of hyperkeratosis similar to that described by Rothmund, the eponym of Rothmund-Thomson syndrome was coined. By 1966 more than 50 patients affected with this syndrome had been described [3].

Clinical Presentation. The most characteristic features are the abnormalities of the skin and eyes.
The skin lesions may be present at birth, but usually appear during the first 6 months of life. They start on the face, then spread to the ears, buttocks, and extremities, and finally to the whole body. The skin changes start with an erythema of the cheeks which later assumes a marmoreal appearance. The following lesions may be seen, sometimes in the same area: linear telangiectases, brown pigmentation, depigmentation, and punctate atrophy. Bullae may develop on exposure to sunlight [3, 4]. Occasionally, hyperkeratosis of the palms and soles may be present with verrucous lesions [5]. The skin lesions are progressive in the first years of life, but later remain stationary. In adults, carcinomatous changes of the skin may occur. The hair is sparse and prematurely gray. Some patients have total alopecia. In about one-fourth of the patients, the nails may be small, rough, ridged, and atrophic [4] (Figs. 5.56–5.60).
Zonular cataracts are the most frequent ophthalmic lesions [6]. They develop in half of the patients and are usually bilateral. Although these may appear as early as 4 months of age, they are usually noted by the age of 6 years. Degenerative, dystrophic changes of the cornea have also been described [4, 7] (Fig. 5.56).
Frequently, these patients have microdontia or malformations of the teeth with failure to erupt. They may also present with short stature, abnormalities of the limbs (asymmetry, syndactyly, ectrodactyly), cystic or sclerotic skeletal changes, scoli-

osis, microcephaly, and mental retardation [3, 4]. Hypogonadism with cryptorchidism may also be present in male patients. Females often suffer from amenorrhea [4].

Pathology and Pathophysiology. In the early stages, there is mild atrophy of the epidermis and hydropic degeneration of the basal cell layer with pigmentary incontinence. In the upper dermis, the capillaries are dilated and there is an infiltrate of chronic inflammatory cells and melanophages. Later, there is compact hyperkeratosis overlying an atrophic epidermis. The rete ridges are effaced. The dermal capillaries are dilated. Melanophages persist, but there is no inflammatory infiltrate. Elastic fibers are fragmented. Bowenoid dyskeratosis of the epidermis heralds carcinomatous changes [8, 9].

Inheritance. Autosomal recessive [4].

Treatment. Visual impairment due to the cataracts or degenerative changes of the cornea may be successfully treated surgically. Protection against sunlight and the use of sunscreens are essential. Surgical excision of carcinomas is indicated.

References

1. Rothmund, A.: Über Katarakt in Verbindung mit einer eigentümlichen Hautdegeneration. Albrecht v. Graefes Arch. Ophthal. *14*, 159–182 (1868)
2. Thomson, M.S.: An hitherto undescribed familial disease. Brit. J. Derm. *35*, 455–462 (1923)
3. Silver, H.K.: Rothmund-Thomson syndrome: an oculocutaneous disorder. Amer. J. Dis. Child. *111*, 182–190 (1966)
4. Taylor, W.B.: Rothmund's syndrome–Thomson's syndrome. Congenital poikiloderma with or without juvenile cataracts: a review of the literature, report of a case, and discussion of the relationship of the two syndromes. Arch. Derm. *75*, 236–244 (1957)
5. Kanitakis, C., Ktenides, M.A.: Lésions kératosiques et verruqueuses au cours du syndrome de Thomson. Ann. Derm. Syph. (Paris) *99*, 269–276 (1972)
6. François, J.: Syndromes with congenital cataract. Trans. Amer. Acad. Ophthal. Otolaryng. *64*, 433–471 (1960)
7. Wahl, J.W., Ellis, P.P.: Rothmund-Thomson syndrome. Amer. J. Ophthal. *60*, 722–726 (1965)
8. Rook, A., Davis, R., Stevanovic, D.: Poikiloderma congenitale; Rothmund-Thomson syndrome. Acta derm.-venereol. (Stockh.) *39*, 392–420 (1959)
9. Tritsch, H., Lischka, G.: Zur Histopathologie der kongenitalen Poikilodermie Thomson. Z. Haut- u. Geschl.-Kr. *43* (Suppl.), 155–166 (1968)

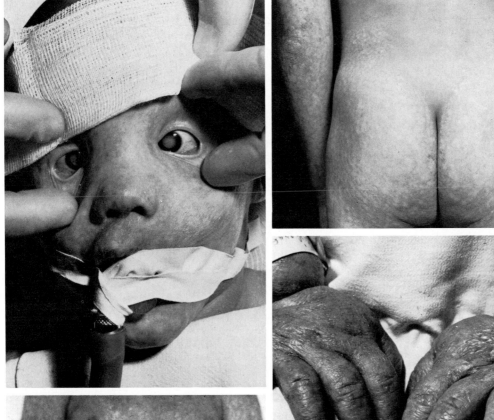

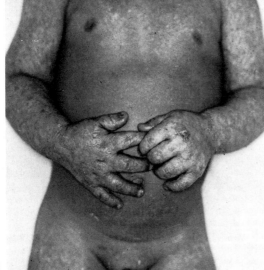

5.56

5.58

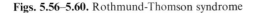

5.57

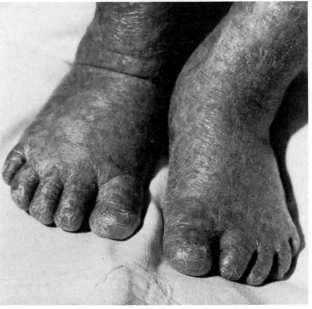

5.59

5.60

Figs. 5.56–5.60. Rothmund-Thomson syndrome

Fig. 5.56. Face. Note cataracts and erythema of the cheeks with cutis marmorata. (From Silver, H.K.: Amer. J. Dis. Child. *111*, 182–190, 1966)

Fig. 5.57. Poikilodermatous changes over the forearms and buttocks. (Courtesy of Dr. V.A. McKusick, from Nissim, J.E.: In: The clinical delineation of birth defects. Bergsma, D. (ed.), Vol. VII, No. 8, pt. XII, pp. 294–295. Baltimore: Williams & Wilkins Co., 1971)

Figs. 5.58–5.60. Note atrophic nails and the skin changes comprising hyper- and hypopigmentation with punctate atrophy. (From Silver, H.K.: Amer. J. Dis. Child. *111*, 182–190, 1966)

Cutis Verticis Gyrata

Cutis verticis gyrata is a descriptive term for hyperplasia and folding of the scalp. Such a morphologic picture is part of several inherited syndromes.

Pachydermoperiostosis

An inherited and an acquired form are known. The former manifests in the teens, the latter in later adulthood.

Clinical Presentation. The skin changes begin in the teens and consist of cutis verticis gyrata (with folding and furrowing of the forehead and cheeks as well), increased oiliness of the facial skin [1, 2], thickened skin over the hands and feet [1, 2], and palmoplantar hyperhidrosis [1] (Figs. 5.61–5.64). Other findings are columnar, thick extremities, clubbing of the fingers and toes, and arthropathy [2]. Periosteal thickening is demonstrable radiologically, but there is no increase in sellar size nor in endochondral bone growth [3].
The skin and skeletal changes progress until the third decade when they usually become stationary.

Pathology and Pathophysiology. The main features are hyperplasia of sebaceous and eccrine glands, thickening of the dermis, and, at the sites of the folds, a dense collection of fibrocytes with increased formation of collagen and acid mucopolysaccharides [2].

Inheritance. Probably autosomal dominant [1].

Treatment. Plastic surgery may be helpful for cosmetic purposes.

Acromegaloid Changes, Cutis Verticis Gyrata, and Corneal Leukoma

The syndrome consists of three components: corneal leukomas, acromegaloid features, and cutis verticis gyrata [4]. The corneal leukomas begin in childhood and may be uni- or bilateral. The entire cornea becomes involved, leading to blindness.
The acromegalic features include large hands and feet, tall stature, and prominent frontal bones.

The folds of the scalp in this syndrome characteristically have a longitudinal rather than transverse orientation [4]. The contiguous skin of the neck is not involved. Dermatoglyphic studies show splitting of many of the epidermal ridges in the midline of the ridges [4]. Inheritance is autosomal dominant.

Cutis Verticis Gyrata with Mental Deficiency

The extent of skin changes in cutis verticis gyrata varies from severe, in which 15 or more ridges are present, to mild, in which the folds are barely noticeable. In a Swedish study, these changes are reported to be associated with mental deficiency (IQ below 30–35) [5]. Other abnormalities are epilepsy, cerebral palsy, eye defects (strabismus, cataract, nystagmus, keratoconus), microcephaly, and short stature [5]. The chromosomal pattern is normal [6]. Inheritance is probably autosomal recessive.
In another Swedish study, five males in three sibships have thyroid aplasia as a common feature of cutis verticis gyrata and mental deficiency [7]. The inheritance seems to be X-linked [7].

References

1. Rimoin, D.L.: Pachydermoperiostosis (idiopathic clubbing and periostosis). Genetic and physiologic considerations. New Engl. J. Med. *272*, 923–931 (1965)
2. Hambrick, G.W., Jr., Carter, D.M.: Pachydermoperiostosis. Touraine-Solente-Golé syndrome. Arch. Derm. *94*, 594–608 (1966)
3. Harbison, J.B., Nice, C.M., Jr.: Familial pachydermoperiostosis presenting as an acromegaly-like syndrome. Amer. J. Roentgenol. *112*, 532–536 (1971)
4. Rosenthal, J.W., Kloepfer, H.W.: An acromegaloid, cutis verticis gyrata, corneal leukoma syndrome. A new medical entity. Arch. Ophthal. *68*, 722–726 (1962)
5. Åkesson, H.O.: Cutis verticis gyrata and mental deficiency in Sweden. I. Epidemiologic and clinical aspects. Acta med. scand. *175*, 115–127 (1964)
6. Åkesson, H.O.: Cutis verticis gyrata and mental deficiency in Sweden. II. Genetic aspects. Acta med. scand. *177*, 459–464 (1965)
7. Åkesson, H.O.: Cutis verticis gyrata, thyroaplasia and mental deficiency. Acta Genet. med. (Roma) *14*, 200–204 (1965)

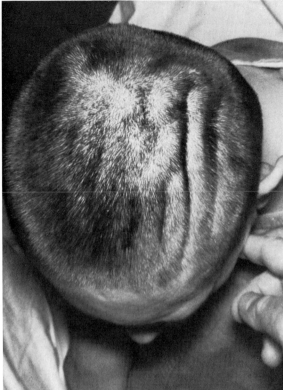

5.61

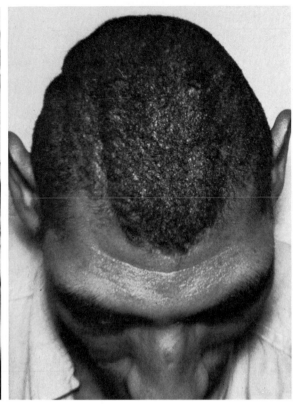

5.62

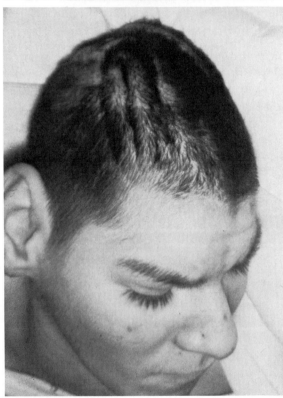

5.63

Figs. 5.61–5.63. Cutis verticis gyrata. (Courtesy of Dr. I. Zeligman)

Other Disorders

Acanthosis Nigricans

Curth [1, 2] has delineated the various types of acanthosis nigricans: the genetically determined "benign" type; benign acanthosis nigricans associated with a variety of syndromes; pseudoacanthosis nigricans associated with obesity or gigantism; and the malignant type which is constantly associated with malignant disease. This discussion is restricted to the inherited variety.

Clinical Presentation. The hallmark of the disease is a darkened, thickened skin with accentuated markings and a velvety feel. The usual sites of involvement are the neck, face, axillae, and groin (Figs. 5.65–5.68). Other intertriginous surfaces may also be involved. Soft papillomatous and verrucous papules and nodules may appear in the involved areas. Occasionally the mucous membranes, especially the buccal mucosa, may be affected (Fig. 5.68). Alopecia, palmoplantar hyperkeratosis, and striated brittle nails have been observed in some

Fig. 5.64. Hyperkeratotic lesions on the palms in pachydermoperiostosis. Cutis verticis gyrata may be an associated finding. See text, p. 125. (Courtesy of Dr. I. Zeligman)

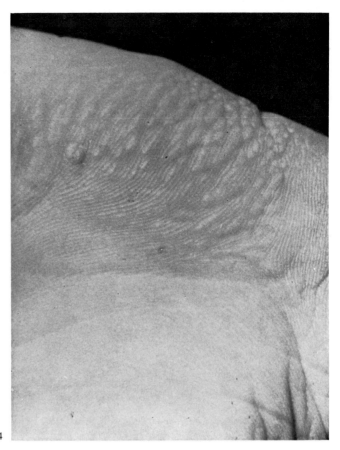

5.64

patients with acanthosis nigricans. Ocular involvement is manifested by loss of luster of the conjuctiva, which is hypertrophied and hyperpigmented [3].

The disorder usually becomes apparent during childhood and increases in severity until puberty. After puberty it may be stationary or show a gradual diminution.

Acanthosis nigricans may be a part of a number of inherited syndromes: Bloom syndrome (p. 140), Crouzon syndrome, Seip syndrome (p. 130), degenerative disorder of the pyramidal tracts, and phenylketonuria (p. 264) [1].

Pathology and Pathophysiology. The epidermis is hyperkeratotic and papillomatous with irregular acanthosis and atrophy.

Inheritance. Autosomal dominant.

Treatment. There is no treatment. Keratolytics may give some cosmetic improvement.

References

1. Curth, H.O.: The necessity of distinguishing four types of acanthosis nigricans. Proceedings of the XIIIth international congress of dermatology. Jadassohn, W., Schirren, C.G. (eds.), Vol. 1, pp. 557–558. Berlin, Heidelberg, New York: Springer 1968
2. Curth, H.O., Aschner, B.M.: Genetic studies on acanthosis nigricans. Arch. Derm. *79*, 55–56 (1959)
3. Lamba, P.A., Lal, S.: Ocular changes in benign acanthosis nigricans. Dermatologica (Basel) *140*, 356–361 (1970)

Congenital Localized Absence of Skin

Bart et al. first described this entity in 1966 in a kindred of 103 direct descendants of one affected person [1].

Clinical Presentation. The affected individual is born with a defect of the skin of the lower extremities, particularly the feet and medial surfaces of the lower legs and ankles [1, 2]. The affected areas are slightly depressed with a glistening moist base (Fig. 5.69). There is gradual healing by regrowth of epidermis from the border, leaving a fine scar [1, 2].

Blistering of the skin and mucous membranes appears in infancy and usually follows trauma [1, 2]. Bullae occur predominantly on the hands and feet. Healing is without scar formation. Many of the affected individuals have absent nails, lose their nails later on, or develop deformities in the form of "heaped up," yellowish gray discolorations or onychogryphosis [1, 2].

Pathology and Pathophysiology. In one patient with epidermolysis bullosa and congenital localized absence of the skin, the bulla was due to cleavage within the basal cell layer while the basement membrane was intact on the dermal side [3].

Inheritance. Autosomal dominant [2].

Treatment. No specific treatment is available.

References

1. Bart, B.J., Gorlin, R.J., Anderson, V.E., Lynch, F.W.: Congenital localized absence of skin and associated abnormalities resembling epidermolysis bullosa. A new syndrome. Arch. Derm. *93*, 296–304 (1966)
2. Bart, B.J.: Congenital localized absence of skin, blistering and nail abnormalities, a new syndrome. In: The clinical delineation of birth defects. Bergsma, D. (ed.), Vol. VII, No. 8, pt. XII, pp. 118–120. Baltimore: Williams & Wilkins Co. 1971
3. Bart, B.J.: Epidermolysis bullosa and congenital localized absence of skin. Arch. Derm. *101*, 78–81 (1970)

Acro-Osteolysis

In 1961 Lamy and Maroteaux [1] described a dominant form of this disease in a mother and son.

Clinical Presentation. Onset is around 6 years of age. Slowly progressive osteolysis of the phalanges in the hands and feet is associated with recurrent ulcers of the fingers and soles, elimination of bone sequestra, and healing with loss of toes or fingers. There is no basilar impression or other change in the skull or long bones to suggest the Cheney syndrome.

Pathology and Pathophysiology. The pathophysiology of the condition is not clear. There may be hypervascularization at the place where the osseous tissue has disappeared. This suggests a vascular origin for the disease. However, these vascular anomalies are considered to be secondary and other observations support a neurologic origin.

Inheritance. Autosomal dominant [1].

Treatment. No specific treatment is available.

Reference

1. Lamy, M., Maroteaux, P.: Acro-ostéolyse dominante. Arch. franç. Pediat. *18*, 693–702 (1961)

Sclero-Atrophic and Keratotic Dermatosis of the Limbs (Sclerotylosis)

In 1967 Mennecier [1] described this degenerative sclero-atrophic and keratodermic genodermatosis of the extremities. Later, Huriez et al. [2] presented two families with 42 affected members out of a total of 132.

Clinical Presentation. The skin lesions are symmetric and exclusively localized on the hands and feet. The entity consists of a triad [2]: (a) diffuse sclero-atrophy of the hands, varying from simple atrophic erythrocyanotic areas to frank sclerodactyly; (b) hypoplastic nail dystrophy, varying from koilonychia to plationychia to total aplasia; and (c) mild lamellar keratodermia, more accentuated in the palms than the soles and very well-circumscribed, sparing the wrist and the Achilles tendon.
There are no mucosal lesions or radiologic signs. The disease is identifiable at birth and remains stationary throughout adulthood. Squamous cell carcinoma is a serious complication and bowel cancer is a frequent cause of death [2].
The disease should be distinguished from scleroderma and palmoplantar keratodermia of the Thost-Unna type.

Pathology and Pathophysiology. The lesions are nonspecific with orthokeratosis, numerous congested capillaries, and sparse lymphocytic infiltrates. The degeneration is always of the spinocellular type, but greatly polymorphic.

Inheritance. Autosomal dominant, with complete penetrance. Linkage with the MNS blood group locus has been established [1, 2], the two genes probably being located on chromosome No. 2 [3].

Treatment. The treatment is symptomatic, aiming more specifically at the malignancies.

References

1. Mennecier, M.: Individualisation d'une nouvelle entité: la génodermatose scléro-atrophiante et kératodermique des extrémités, fréquemment dégénérative. Étude clinique et génétique (possibilité de linkage avec le système MNS). Thèse de doctorat, Université de Lille 1967

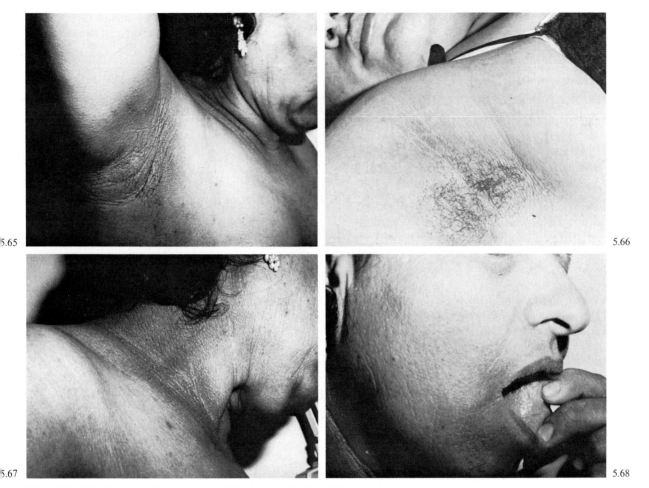

5.65

5.66

5.67

5.68

Figs. 5.65–5.68. Acanthosis nigricans. Axilla, neck, and sides of the mouth

Fig. 5.69. Congenital localized absence of skin. Depressed, well-defined, glistening area on the right leg

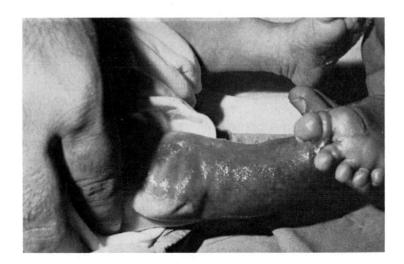

2. Huriez, C., Deminati, M., Agache, P., Delmas-Marsalet, Y., Mennecier, M.: Génodermatose scléro-atrophiante et kératodermique des extrémités. Ann. Derm. Syph. (Paris) 96, 135–146 (1969)
3. Lambert, D., Nivelon-Chevallier, A., Chapuis, J.-L.: Génodermatose scléro-atrophiante et kératodermique des extrémités. J. Génét. Hum. 26, 25–31 (1978)

Congenital Generalized Lipodystrophy (Berardinelli Syndrome, Seip Syndrome)

In 1946 Lawrence [1] reported a patient with total absence of subcutaneous fat. In 1954 Berardinelli [2] reported two additional cases of the syndrome. By 1975 about 50 patients affected with this syndrome had been reported [3].

Clinical Presentation. The most characteristic clinical findings are the following: paucity of subcutaneous fat noted early in infancy, hypertrichosis with curly scalp hair, general increase in pigmentation, acanthosis nigricans, prominent muscles, relatively large hands and feet, hepatomegaly, enlargement of penis or clitoris, and mental retardation (Figs. 5.70–5.73). Systemic cystic angiomatosis may accompany the syndrome [4].
X-rays reveal advanced skeletal maturation, epiphyseal hypertrophy, thickening of diaphyseal cortices, and mild metaphyseal sclerosis of the long bones [5]. Serum growth hormone, insulin, triglyceride, and free fatty acid levels are usually increased. Hyperglycemia is present in all affected adults, but occurs rarely in children [6–8].
Congenital generalized lipodystrophy is a progressive disease. Insulin resistance, glucose intolerance, elevation of plasma immunoreactive insulin, and abnormal human growth hormone homeostasis are absent in infancy but appear with age. Although the accelerated growth and bony maturation, the muscle hypertrophy, and the enlargement of the phallus are suggestive of androgen effect, the androgens and gonadotropins are not elevated. Fatty infiltration of the liver also increases with age. Cirrhosis with esophageal varices may be the cause of death.
There are two other types of lipodystrophy: the acquired generalized type and the partial or cephalothoracic type. The acquired generalized lipodystrophy differs from the congenital generalized type in the early onset of its manifestations, its greater severity, and its association with a more rapid, progressive insulin-resistant diabetes mellitus and cirrhosis. The partial lipodystrophy presents with loss of fat involving mainly the face and the trunk but sparing the hips, the buttocks, and the lower extremities. There is no evidence of a genetic etiology for either the acquired generalized or the partial type [9].

Pathology and Pathophysiology. The pathogenesis of congenital generalized lipodystrophy remains unknown. Rather than a primary abnormality of the adipose tissue, a diencephalic disturbance is suggested in most cases. [10].

Inheritance. Autosomal recessive [3].

Treatment. Management of the hyperglycemia and hyperlipemia is recommended. Both conditions improve with age.

References

1. Lawrence, R.D.: Lipodystrophy and hepatomegaly with diabetes, lipaemia, and other metabolic disturbances. A case throwing new light on the action of insulin. Lancet 1946I, 724–731
2. Berardinelli, W.: An undiagnosed endocrinometabolic syndrome: report of 2 cases. J. clin. Endocr. 14, 193–204 (1954)
3. Najjar, S.S., Salem, G.M., Idriss, Z.H.: Congenital generalized lipodystrophy. Acta paediat. scand. 64, 273–279 (1975)
4. Brunzell, J.D., Shankle, S.W., Bethune, J.E.: Congenital generalized lipodystrophy accompanied by cystic angiomatosis. Ann. intern. Med. 69, 501–516 (1968)
5. Wesenberg, R.L., Gwinn, J.L., Barnes, G.R., Jr.: The roentgenographic findings in total lipodystrophy. Amer. J. Roentgenol. 103, 154–164 (1968)
6. Seip, M., Trygstad, O.: Generalized lipodystrophy. Arch. Dis. Child. 38, 447–453 (1963)
7. Senior, B., Gellis, S.S.: The syndromes of total lipodystrophy and of partial lipodystrophy. Pediatrics 33, 593–612 (1964)
8. Senior, B., Loridan, L.: Fat cell function and insulin in a patient with generalized lipodystrophy. J. Pediat. 74, 972–975 (1967)
9. Salem, G.M., Najjar, S.S., Zeynoun, S.T., Farah, F.S.: Lipodystrophy. Lebanese med. J..26, 259–267 (1973)
10. Seip, M.: Generalized lipodystrophy. Ergebn. inn. Med. Kinderheilk. 31, 59–95 (1971)

Mandibulofacial Dysostosis (Treacher Collins Syndrome, Franceschetti-Zwahlen-Klein Syndrome)

In 1889 Berry [1] described two patients, a mother and daughter, with notched eyelids and a downward palpebral slant. In 1900 Treacher Collins [2] reported two patients with a similar appearance and emphasized the underdevelopment of the malar bones. In 1944 Franceschetti and Zwahlen [3] and in 1949 Franceschetti and Klein [4] described additional cases of the syndrome, with severe facial anomalies. Although the descriptive term of "man-

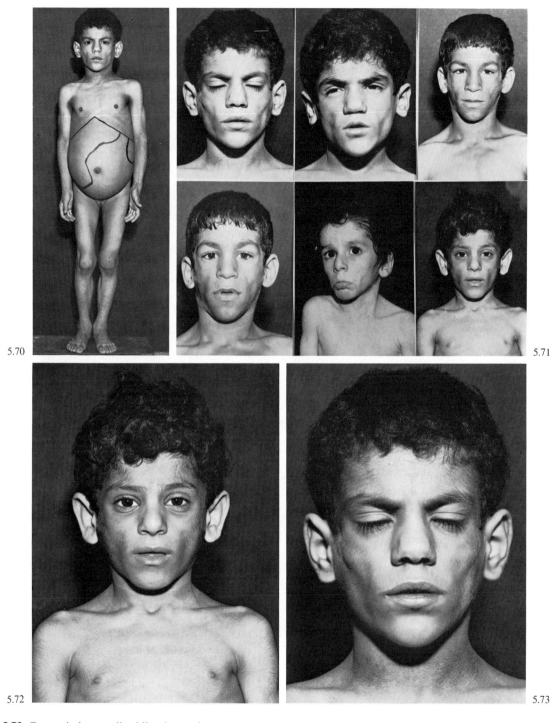

5.70

5.71

5.72

5.73

Figs. 5.70–5.73. Congenital generalized lipodystrophy

Fig. 5.70. General view. Note hepatosplenomegaly. (From Najjar, S.S., et al.: Acta paediat. scand. *64*, 273–279, 1975)

Fig. 5.71. Facial features of several unrelated patients. Note striking similarities and curly hair in most of them. (From Najjar, S.S., et al.: Acta paediat. scand. *64*, 273–279, 1975)

Fig. 5.72. Note hirsutism and curly hair. (From Najjar, S.S., et al.: Acta paediat. scand. *64*, 273–279, 1975)

Fig. 5.73. Note sunken cheeks and acanthosis nigricans of the neck. (From Najjar, S.S., et al.: Acta paediat. scand. *64*, 273–279, 1975)

dibulofacial dysostosis" was introduced, several eponyms are still used. The most common of these is Treacher Collins syndrome. More than 200 cases of the syndrome have been described [5, 6].

Clinical Presentation. The most characteristic anomalies involve the face, in general, and the eyes, in particular.

The most common abnormalities of the eyes are a downward palpebral slant, eyelid and iris colobomas, and microphthalmia.

The general facial anomalies are hypoplasia of the malar and zygoma areas and a small, retracted chin. About half of the patients have abnormalities of the external ear and atresia of the external auditory meatus. The patients with external ear anomalies may also have middle and inner ear defects (Figs. 5.74–5.77).

Consequent to the malar hypoplasia, the palate is narrow and high, and the teeth are crowded and malaligned. There may be abnormal hair patterns. The terminal hair may extend to the cheeks in a tongue-shaped process; in a few cases, circumscribed cicatricial alopecia may be present.

Most patients have a normal intelligence.

X-rays show poor development of the maxilla, malar bones, zygoma, mandible, middle ear ossicles, and paranasal sinuses.

Pathology and Pathophysiology. The hereditary defect involves structures derived from the first branchial area.

Inheritance. Autosomal dominant [7].

Treatment. Since the intelligence is normal, the deafness should be recognized early and corrected with hearing aids or surgery to ensure normal development. After childhood, cosmetic surgery for the facial appearance can be attempted, sometimes with striking improvement.

References.

1. Berry, G. A.: Note on a congenital defect (?coloboma) of the lower lid. R. Lond. Ophthalmic Hosp. Rep. *12*, 255–257 (1889)
2. Treacher Collins, E.: Case with symmetrical congenital notches in the outer part of each lower lid and defective development of the malar bones. Trans. ophthal. Soc. UK. *20*, 190–192 (1900)
3. Franceschetti, A., Zwahlen, P.: Un syndrome nouveau: la dysostose mandibulo-faciale. Bull. schweiz. Akad. med. Wiss. *1*, 60–66 (1944)
4. Franceschetti, A., Klein, D.: The mandibulo-facial dysostosis. A new hereditary syndrome. Acta ophthal. (Kbh.) *27*, 143–224 (1949)
5. Rogers, B.O.: Berry-Treacher Collins syndrome: a review of 200 cases (mandibulo-facial dysotosis; Franceschetti-Zwahlen-Klein syndrome). Brit. J. plast. Surg. *17*, 109–137 (1964)
6. Fernandez, A.O., Ronis, M.L.: The Treacher-Collins syndrome. Arch. Otolaryng. *80*, 505–520 (1964)
7. Fazen, L.E., Elmore, J., Nadler, H.L.: Mandibulo-facial dysostosis (Treacher-Collins syndrome). Amer. J. Dis. Child. *113*, 405–410 (1967)

Dyskeratosis Congenita (Zinsser-Cole-Engman Syndrome)

Although widely distributed, this is a rare disorder. It was first reported by Zinsser in 1906 [1] and affects predominantly males.

Clinical Presentation. The main manifestations are hyperpigmentation of the skin, nail dystrophy, and oral leukokeratosis. These appear around puberty and are well-developed during the second decade. The skin is gray-brown with a reticulate lacy pattern simulating poikiloderma, involving usually the face, neck, and trunk, but occasionally becoming more widespread. There may be generalized hyperpigmentation; deforming atrophic changes of the hands, elbows, knees, and feet with traumatic formation of bullae; and dystrophic nails, with longitudinal grooves or complete atrophy. There is palmoplantar hyperkeratosis and hyperhidrosis. The hair may be sparse.

The leukokeratosis of the oral mucosa, especially the buccal and lingual areas, appears as glazed white patches. Erosions and bullae may also appear. Similar mucosal involvement may be found in the anogenital areas and possibly the gastrointestinal tract. Other manifestations include epiphora due to obliteration of the lacrimal puncta; ectropion of the lower eyelids with loss of cilia; bullous conjunctivitis; transparent tympanic membranes; dysphagia; dental dystrophies (poorly aligned teeth, pyorrhea, gingivitis, caries); urogenital anomalies (hyperpigmentation of the penis, urethral bleeding, partial atresia of the meatus, small testes, atrophic bands on penis); frail skeletal structure; mental retardation; malnourished appearance; small sella turcica; heart block; enlargement of the left atrium; low blood pressure; splenomegaly; and premature graying of hair [2, 3]. Furthermore, there may be anemia and pancytopenia. Some patients develop Fanconi anemia.

Affected individuals have a poor prognosis because of the development of either a blood dyscrasia or carcinoma in the areas of leukoplakia.

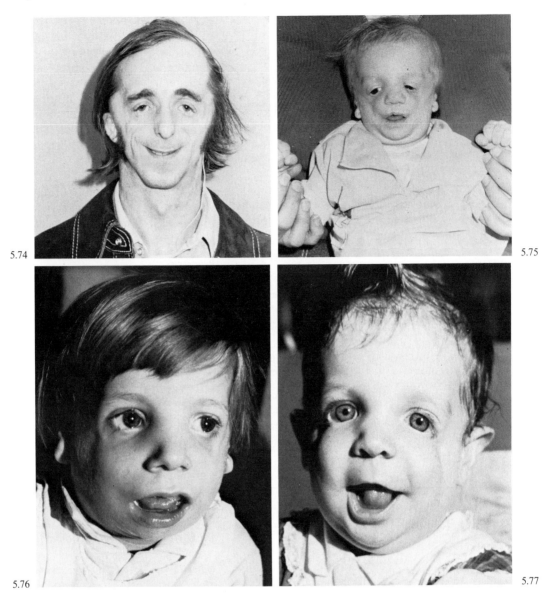

5.74

5.75

5.76

5.77

Figs. 5.74 and 5.75. Mandibulofacial dysostosis. Affected father and child. Note downward palpebral slant, striking hypoplasia of the malar and zygoma areas, and abnormal pinnae. The father has a hearing aid on the left side. (Courtesy of Dr. F.C. Fraser)

Figs. 5.76 and 5.77. Mandibulofacial dysostosis. Milder forms of the syndrome. (Courtesy of Dr. F.C. Fraser, from Nora, J.J., Fraser, F.C.: Medical genetics, p. 123. Philadelphia: Lea & Febiger 1974)

Pathology and Pathophysiology. The histologic appearance of the skin is not diagnostic. The changes include atrophy of the epidermis, hydropic degeneration of the basal cells, some homogenization of the collagen, and dilated capillaries in the upper dermis [3]. In the upper dermis there may be non-iron-bearing cells that are strongly dopa-positive [2]. The mucosal lesions exhibit slight parake-ratosis, marked focal acanthosis, and normally oriented epithelial cells [3].

Inheritance. X-linked recessive.

Treatment. There is no specific treatment. The patients should be kept under observation for early detection of malignant changes and institution of the appropriate treatment.

Dyskeratosis Congenita
(Scoggins Type)

One kindred has been described in which the main features of dyskeratosis congenita (Zinsser-Cole-Engman syndrome), skin hyperpigmentation, nail dystrophy, and oral leukokeratosis, are associated with hematologic, immunologic, and chromosomal changes very similar to those of Fanconi anemia (see p. 237) [4]. Other features encountered in this family are absent fingerprints, scanty hair, poor dentition, absent lacrimal puncta, and palmar hyperkeratosis. Inheritance in this syndrome is probably autosomal dominant.

References

1. Zinsser, F.: Atrophia cutis reticularis cum pigmentatione, dystrophia unguium et leukoplakia oris. Ikonogr. Derm. *219* (1906)
2. Costello, M.J., Buncke, C.M.: Dyskeratosis congenita. Arch. Derm. *73*, 123–132 (1956)
3. Sorrow, J.M., Jr., Hitch, J.M.: Dyskeratosis congenita. First report of its occurrence in a female and a review of the literature Arch. Derm. *88*, 340–347 (1963)
4. Scoggins, R.B., Prescott, K.J., Asher, G.H., Blaylock, W.K., Bright, R.W.: Dyskeratosis congenita with Fanconi-type anemia: investigations of immunologic and other defects. Clin. Res. *19*, 409 (1971)

Bird-Headed Dwarfism
(Montreal Type)

In 1970 Fitch et al. [1] described a form of bird-headed dwarfism clearly distinct from the Seckel type.

Clinical Presentation. The following features are characteristic of this syndrome: proportionate dwarfism, premature senility with premature graying and loss of scalp hair; increased number of minor palmar creases with redundant and wrinkled skin of the palms (Fig. 5.78); deficiency of subcutaneous tissue and profuse sweating; prominent beaked nose and micrognathia (birdlike face); low-set ears with abnormal pinnae; low posterior hairline; blepharoptosis; and cryptorchidism [1] (Fig. 5.79).
Radiograms reveal osteoporotic bones and coarse trabeculae. The epiphyses are closed and C-6 and C-7 vertebrae are fused. The vertebrae also have diminished anteroposterior diameter and accentuated height. The spine has a slight scoliosis. The karyotype is normal.

Pathology and Pathophysiology. Light microscopy of the skin reveals slight irregular atrophy of the epidermis with shortening of the rete pegs and thinning of the malpighian layers. The stratum corneum has a basket weave appearance. The basal layer shows focal vacuolization of the cells and disorganization of the cell layers. The epidermodermal junction is somewhat blurred in some areas. Elastotic degeneration of the collagen is noted in the dermis [1].

Inheritance. Probably autosomal recessive [2].

Treatment. No specific treatment is available.

References

1. Fitch, N., Pinsky, L., Lachance, R.C.: A form of bird-headed dwarfism with features of premature senility. Amer. J. Dis. Child. *120*, 260–264 (1970)
2. McKusick, V.A.: Mendelian inheritance in man, 5th ed., p. 436. Baltimore: Johns Hopkins University Press 1978

Pterygium Syndrome

Clinical Presentation. This syndrome comprises webbing of the neck and the antecubital and popliteal fossae, along with dystopia canthorum, sternal deformity, and male hypogonadism. Cutaneous depressions may be present on the back of the elbows and front of the knees [1, 2].

Pathology and Pathophysiology. Unknown.

Inheritance. Autosomal recessive. X-linked dominant inheritance is suggested in the report of a family [3].

Treatment. No specific treatment is available.

References

1. Norum, R.A., James, V.L., Mabry, C.C.: Pterygium syndrome in three children in a recessive pedigree pattern. In: The clinical delineation of birth defects. Bergsma, D. (ed.), Vol. V, No. 2, pt. II, pp. 233–235. Baltimore: Williams & Wilkins Co. 1969
2. Srivastana, R.N.: Arthrogryposis multiplex congenita. Case report of two siblings. Clin. Pediat. (Philadelphia) 7, 691–694 (1968)
3. Carnevale, A., Hernandez, A.L., De los Cobos, L.: Sindrome de pterygium familiar con probable transmission dominante ligada al cromosoma X. Rev. Invest. Clin. *25*, 237–244 (1973)

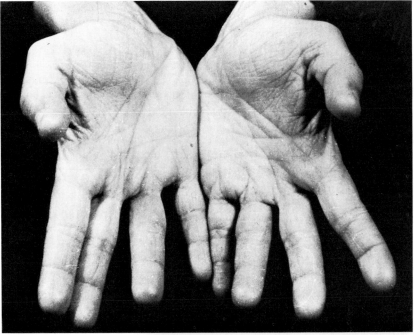

5.78

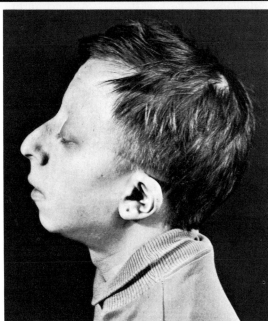

Fig. 5.78. Bird-headed dwarfism. Wrinkled palmar skin with increased creases. (From Fitch, N., et al.: Amer. J. Dis. Child. *120*, 260–264, 1970)

Fig. 5.79. Bird-headed dwarfism. Note prominent beaked nose, micrognathia, low-set ears with abnormal pinnae, low posterior hairline, and some loss of scalp hair. (From Fitch, N., et al.: Amer. J. Dis. Child. *120*, 260–264, 1970)

5.79

Congenital Absence of the Breasts and Nipples

Clinical Presentation. In 1965 Trier [1] reviewed the literature dealing with the absence of breasts and nipples. He collected 43 cases and divided them into 3 groups: (a) absence of breasts with ectodermal defects involving the skin, sweat glands, hair, and teeth; (b) unilateral absence of the corresponding pectoral muscles; and (c) bilateral absence of the breasts (Figs. 5.80 and 5.81) associated with congenital anomalies (atrophy of the pectoral muscles, anomalies of the limbs, sparse axillary and pubic hair, short stature, hypertelorism, high-arched or cleft palate). Even with pubertal changes, as evidenced by the cytology of the vaginal mucosa and the presence of follicle-stimulating hormone in the urine of female patients, breast tissue does not develop [2].

Pathology and Pathophysiology. Absence of breast tissue results from failure of the pectoral portions of the mammary ridges to develop [1].

Inheritance. Absence of breasts associated with anhidrotic ectodermal dysplasia follows the X-linked recessive pattern of inheritance. The inheritance of the other types is not clear. Pedigrees consistent with either dominant [3, 4] or recessive [5] inheritance have been reported.

Treatment. Treatment is surgical. When absence of breast tissue is not associated with other grossly deforming features, early reconstruction is desirable. Construction of nipples should be performed preferably before acute consciousness of the deformity causes distress for both child (boy or girl) and parents. For girls in the adolescent period, Silastic gel-filled breast prostheses may be implanted in cases of total absence of breast tissue [1].

References

1. Trier, W.C.: Complete breast absence. Case report and review of the literature. Plast. reconstr. Surg. *36*, 430–439 (1965)
2. Tawil, H.M., Najjar, S.S.: Congenital absence of the breasts. J. Pediat. *73*, 751–753 (1968)
3. Fraser, F.C.: Dominant inheritance of absent nipples and breasts. In: Novant' anni delle leggi mendeliane, pp. 360–362. Rome: Instituto Gregorio Mendel 1956
4. Goldenring, H., Cerlin, E.S.: Mother and daughter with bilateral congenital amastia. Yale J. Biol. Med. *33*, 466–467 (1961)
5. Kowlessar, M., Orti, E.: Complete breast absence in siblings. Amer. J. Dis. Child. *115*, 91–92 (1968)

Supernumerary Nipples

Polymastia (supernumerary breasts) and supernumerary nipples follow a pattern suggestive of autosomal dominant inheritance [1]. In females, the extra breasts enlarge in pregnancy and lactation.

Reference

1. Klinkerfuss, G.H.: Four generations of polymastia. J. Amer. med. Ass. *82*, 1247–1248 (1924)

Inverted Nipples

Inverted nipples (mammilla invertita) follow the autosomal dominant pattern of inheritance [1].

Reference

1. Romanus, T.: A pedigree showing the incidence of malformation of the nipples. Acta Genet. Statist. Med. *1*, 168–173 (1948)

Gardner Syndrome (Intestinal Polyposis III)

In 1953 Gardner and Richards [1] reported in one family the association of multiple polyposis of the colon with cystic lesions of the skin, fibrous tissue tumors, and osteomatosis. Although this was not the first report of such an association, it is Gardner's thorough evaluation and further reports that established this syndrome as a definite genetic entity [2].

Clinical Presentation. The most important feature of Gardner syndrome is multiple polyposis of the colon and rectum. Usually the polyps are relatively asymptomatic until malignancy develops, although melena, anemia, diarrhea, or vague abdominal pains may occur [3].

The disfiguring cutaneous lesions are either sebaceous or epidermal inclusion cysts and may be present from infancy (Fig. 5.82). In the majority of cases they arise on the scalp and face. In many they are observed on the trunk, scrotum, and extremities. The number and size of the cysts may increase slowly with time but then appear to level off. One of the most important features of the cystic lesions is their tendency to appear well in advance of the polyposis and thus suggest the presence of the disorder before malignancies develop [3].

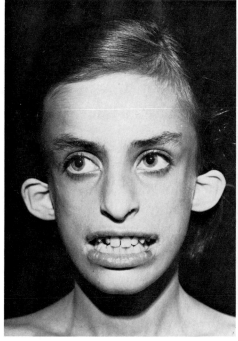
5.80

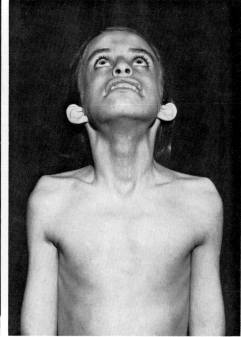
5.81

Figs. 5.80 and 5.81. Congenital absence of breasts. Note absence of nipples and associated low-set ears with abnormal pinnae. (From Tawil, H.M., Najjar, S.S.: J. Pediat. 73, 751–753, 1968)

Bony abnormalities, primarily osteomas, occur in slightly over 50% of cases. There is no report of their malignant alteration. Globoid osteomas of the mandible with overlying fibromas are characteristic [3]. Fibrous tissue tumors are reported in 45% of cases. The fibrous tissue abnormalities include fibromas, desmoid tumors, and fibrosarcomas [3]. Dental anomalies, such as cystic odontomas, supernumerary teeth, unerupted teeth, and follicular odontomas, may occur. Other miscellaneous lesions, such as leiomyomas, lipomas, trichoepitheliomas, and neurofibromas, may also occur [3]. A condition with perifollicular fibromatosis cutis and polyps of the colon was recently described [4]. This seems to be a distinct entity.

Pathology and Pathophysiology. The cystic lesions of the skin are more commonly epidermal inclusion cysts than sebaceous cysts. No case of malignancy arising in a cystic lesion has been noted [3]. Tetraploidy may be increased in skin fibroblast cultures from patients with Gardner syndrome [5].

Inheritance. Autosomal dominant [2].

Treatment. The treatment is aimed at the polyposis. A subtotal colectomy with ileoproctostomy or total colectomy with ileostomy are possible modes of treatment [6].

References

1. Gardner, E.J., Richards, R.C.: Multiple cutaneous and subcutaneous lesions occurring simultaneously with hereditary polyposis and osteomatosis. Amer. J. hum. Genet. 5, 139–147 (1953)
2. Gardner, E.J.: Follow-up study of a family group exhibiting dominant inheritance for a syndrome including intestinal polyps, osteomas, fibromas and epidermal cysts. Amer. J. hum. Genet. 14, 376–390 (1962)
3. Weary, P.E., Linthicum, A., Cawley, E.P., Coleman, C.C., Jr., Graham, G.F.: Gardner's syndrome. A family group study and review. Arch. Derm. 90, 20–30 (1964)
4. Hornstein, O.P., Knickenberg, M.: Perifollicular fibromatosis cutis with polyps of the colon: a cutaneointestinal syndrome Sui Generis. Arch. Derm. Res. 253, 161–175 (1975)
5. Danes, B.S.: The Gardner syndrome: increased tetraploidy in cultured skin fibroblasts. J. med. Genet. 13, 52–56 (1976)
6. MacDonald, J.M., Davis, W.C., Crago, H.R., Berk, A.D.: Gardner's syndrome and periampullary malignancy. Amer. J. Surg. 113, 425–430 (1967)

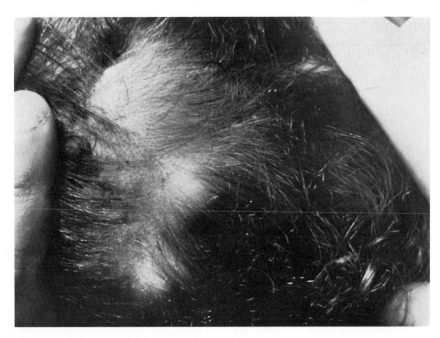

Fig. 5.82. Gardner syndrome. Epidermal inclusion cysts in the scalp. (Courtesy of Dr. W. Frain-Bell)

Familial Blepharophimosis

In 1889 Vignes [1] described this rare entity characterized predominantly by dysplasia of the eyelids. Recently, Sacrez et al. [2] made additions to the original report.

Clinical Presentation. The major manifestations involve the orbital structures and include bilateral blepharophimosis, blepharoptosis, and epicanthus inversus with telecanthus (Figs. 5.83 and 5.84). Deficiency of upper and lower eyelid tissue, elevation of the eyebrows, and absence of supraorbital rims and the ansoglabellar angle are also noted. Nystagmus and strabismus are occasionally found. Other findings include muscular hypotonia, hyperextensible joints, short stature, poor dentition, and high-arched palate. Occasionally, there are reports of skeletal findings, such as spina bifida and, rarely, congenital cardiomyopathy. The intelligence is usually normal.

Pathology and Pathophysiology. Almost invariably there is association with dystopia of the lower lacrimal puncta and frequently elongation of the lacrimal canaliculi, hypoplasia of the caruncle as plica semilunaris, and absence or poor development of the levator and superior rectus muscles causing limitation of the upward gaze. Other anomalies include slight lower-lid ectropion, doubling of the puncta, and stenosis of the lacrimal duct [3].

Inheritance. Autosomal dominant with high penetrance. There is a slight predominance of affected males.

Treatment. The treatment is surgical [4, 5]. For psychological reasons, it is preferable that surgery be performed before the patient goes to school. The epicanthus is first corrected, then the ptosis.

References

1. Vignes, N.I.: Epicanthus héréditaire. Rev. gén. Ophtal. (Paris) *8*, 438 (1889)
2. Sacrez, R., Francfort, J., Juif, J.G., de Grouchy, J.: Le blépharophimosis compliqué familial. Étude des membres de la famille Ble. Ann. Pediat. (Paris) *10*, 493–501 (1963)
3. Garden, J.W.: Blepharophimosis, ptosis, epicanthus inversus, and lacrimal stenosis. Amer. J. Ophthal. *67*, 153–154 (1969)
4. Lewis, S.R., Arons, M.S., Lynch, J.B., Blocker, T.G., Jr.: The congenital eyelid syndrome. Plast. reconstr. Surg. *39*, 271–277 (1967)
5. Johnson, C.C.: Surgical repair of the syndrome of epicanthus inversus, blepharophimosis and ptosis. Arch. Ophthal. *71*, 510–516 (1964)

Blepharochalasis (Dermatolysis Palpebrarum)

Several varieties of this disorder are recognized, one of which is hereditary [1].

Clinical Presentation. The disease is insidious in onset with progressive relaxation of the skin of the upper lids [2, 3]. By adulthood, the skin of the upper lids is discolored, erythematous, and hangs loosely over the eyes. Blepharochalasis may be associated with progressive enlargement of the upper lip (Ascher syndrome) [4]. The enlargement of

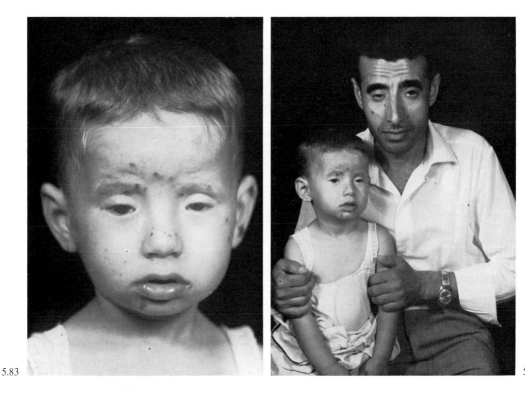

5.83   5.84

Figs. 5.83 and 5.84. Father and child with familial blepharophimosis syndrome

the lip starts in infancy or childhood, leading to a "double" lip (Fig. 5.85).

Pathology and Pathophysiology. There are telangiectases and a possible defect of elastic tissue of the eyelids [1]. The disorder may be considered as cutis laxa limited to the eyelids [5]. In Ascher syndrome, there is hypertrophy, inflammation, and fibrosis of the labial salivary glands [4].

Inheritance. Autosomal dominant [3].

Treatment. Plastic surgery may be of cosmetic help.

References

1. Klauder, J.V.: The interrelation of some cutaneous and ocular diseases. Particular discussion of blepharochalasis, sarcoid, erythema multiforme, ocular pemphigus, lupus erythematosus, melanosis of conjunctiva, length of cilia. Arch. Derm. *80*, 515–528 (1959)
2. Cockayne, E.A.: Inherited abnormalities of the skin and its appendages, p. 321. London: Oxford University Press 1933
3. Panneton, P.: La blépharo-chalazis. A propos de 51 cas dans une même famille. Arch. Ophtal. (Paris) *53*, 729–755 (1936)
4. Findlay, G.H.: Idiopathic enlargements of the lips: cheilitis granulomatosa, Ascher's syndrome and double lip. Brit. J. Derm. *66*, 129–138 (1954)
5. McKusick, V.A.: Heritable disorders of connective tissue, 4th ed., p. 378. Saint Louis: Mosby, C.V. Co. 1972

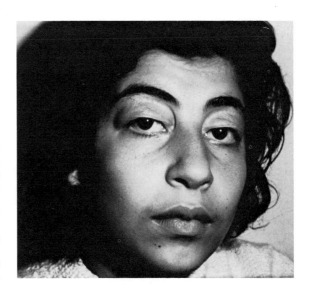

Fig. 5.85. Blepharochalasis. Note the ptotic and discolored upper lids

Chapter 6 Disorders with Photosensitivity

Contents

Bloom Syndrome

In 1954 Bloom [1] described this very rare syndrome with "three cardinal features" [2]: congenital facial telangiectatic erythema, sensitivity to sunlight, and stunted growth.

Clinical Presentation. The facial erythema may be present at birth or appear between the ages of 2 weeks and 3 years. The involved areas of the face are the cheeks and nose (the butterfly region), lips, forehead, ears, and margins of the eyelids. The dorsa of the hands and forearms may also be involved. The lesions consist of "erythematous telangiectatic spots," plaques, patches, or scattered, macular, slightly scaly areas (Figs. 6.1–6.3). In most cases the erythema is exacerbated upon first exposure to sunlight in the spring or summer. Thus, bullae may form on the lips, with bleeding, crusting, and exfoliation [2].

The birth weight is low for the gestational age and growth is slow. Sexual development is normal and the mental state is average. The dwarfism is of a special type with a slender build, narrow, fine-featured face, and dolichocephalic head [2]. Other defects associated with the syndrome are lichen pilaris, café-au-lait spots, ichthyotic skin, acanthosis nigricans, hypertrichosis, pilonidal cyst, fovea coccygea, syndactyly, polydactyly, clinodactyly, hypospadias, and cryptorchidism [2].

Leukemia or cancer occurs in many of these patients and may be responsible for their death. Moreover, many patients clearly have an increased susceptibility to infections. Serum immunoglobulin concentrations are abnormal with particularly low levels of IgA and IgM [3]. More than 50% of the patients are of Jewish ancestry of Eastern European origin [2].

Pathology and Pathophysiology. The epidermis is flattened with a variety of cellular changes. There is dilatation of the capillaries in the upper dermis. This may be associated with a mild perivascular infiltrate. Chromosomal anomalies in cultures of lymphocytes from venous blood [4] and skin fibroblasts [5] consist of isochromatid breaks, acentric fragments, transverse breakage at the centromere resulting in telocentric chromosomes, quadriradial configurations, triradials, and dicentrics.

As in ataxia telangiectasia and Fanconi anemia (see p. 237), the association of chromosomal changes and malignancy in Bloom syndrome suggests that the chromosomal anomalies, regardless of the underlying causes, may be of fundamental importance in the pathogenesis of neoplasia [5, 6].

The small size of the full-term newborn affected with Bloom syndrome is due to a smaller number of cells. This abnormally small number of cells in the term fetus is probably due to the high mortality, or inability to divide, of genetically unbalanced daughters of cells with chromosomal aberrations. This may also play a role in growth retardation after birth [6].

Using DNA fiber autoradiography, an estimation was made of the rate of DNA chain growth, one of the components of ongoing DNA replication. The rate in Bloom syndrome dermal fibroblasts in tissue culture was found to be significantly slower than that in normal control cells. Two possible explanations for the retarded chain growth may be

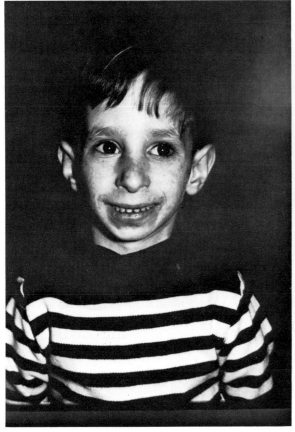

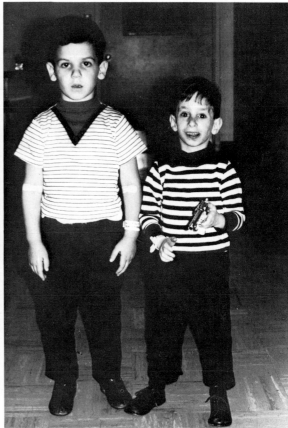

6.1

6.2

Figs. 6.1–6.3. Bloom syndrome

Fig. 6.1. Characteristic facial appearance with erythema and telangiectasias in areas of exposure to sunlight. (Courtesy of Dr. S. Harik)

Fig. 6.2. Note short stature of patient photographed with a child of the same age (6 years). (Courtesy of Dr. S. Harik)

Fig. 6.3. General view of the body showing telangiectasia on the face, dorsa of the hands, and lower extremities. (Courtesy of Dr. P. Dugois)

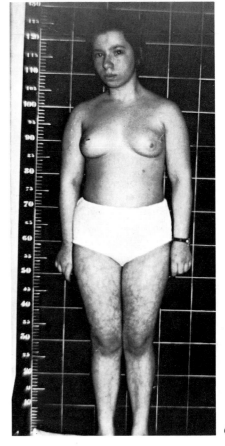

suggested. An enzyme (e.g., DNA polymerase) concerned directly with semiconservative DNA replication may be defective. Alternatively, an abnormal enzyme may affect replication indirectly by altering cellular metabolism [7].

Lymphocyte responses to pokeweed mitogen are reduced in Bloom syndrome [8].

Inheritance. Autosomal recessive [2].

Treatment. No satisfactory treatment for either the telangiectasia or the growth retardation has been found.

6.3

References

1. Bloom, D.: Congenital telangiectatic erythema resembling lupus erythematosus in dwarfs. Amer. J. Dis. Child. *88*, 754–758 (1954)
2. Bloom, D.: The syndrome of congenital telangiectatic erythema and stunted growth. J. Pediat. *68*, 103–113 (1966)
3. Bloom, D., German, J.: The syndrome of congenital telangiectatic erythema and stunted growth. Arch. Derm. *103*, 545–546 (1971)
4. German, J., Archibald, R., Bloom, D.: Chromosomal breakage in a rare and probably genetically determined syndrome of man. Science *148*, 506–507 (1965)
5. German, J., Crippa, L.P.: Chromosomal breakage in diploid cell lines from Bloom's syndrome and Fanconi's anemia. Ann. Génét. *9*, 143–154 (1966)
6. German, J.: Bloom's syndrome. I. Genetical and clinical observations in the first twenty-seven patients. Amer. J. hum. Genet. *21*, 196–227 (1969)
7. Hand, R., German, J.: A retarded rate of DNA chain growth in Bloom's syndrome. Proc. nat. Acad. Sci. (Wash.) *72*, 758–762 (1975)
8. Hütteroth, T.H., Litwin, S.D., German, J.: Abnormal immune responses of Bloom's syndrome lymphocytes in vitro. J. clin. Invest. *56*, 1–7 (1975)

Hartnup Disease

In 1956 Baron et al. [1] described this entity characterized by "hereditary pellagra-like skin rash with temporary cerebellar ataxia, constant renal amino-aciduria, and other bizarre biochemical features." The eponymic appellation for this disease, first found in the Hartnup family, is now generally accepted. The total number of patients described to date is less than 60 [2].

Clinical Presentation. The main clinical findings concern the skin and nervous system.
The onset is usually in childhood and occasionally in infancy. Commonly, the cutaneous eruption precedes the neurologic manifestations. The sites of skin involvement are those areas exposed to the sun, particularly the face, back of neck, and dorsa of hands. The eruption is variable from erythema and scaliness to vesiculation and exudation and is aggravated by exposure to sunlight. It resembles the rash seen in dietary pellagra [2].
A severe but fully reversible cerebellar ataxia may develop. This appears at times when the skin rash is most severe. Sometimes, instead of the ataxia, the patients may develop "collapsing" or fainting attacks. Nystagmus and double vision are also found. Psychiatric features range from mild emotional instability to complete delirium. Mental retardation may be present. The diagnosis can easily be made by two-dimensional paper or thin layer chromatography. Age brings a general improvement [2].

Pathology and Pathophysiology. There is a specific disturbance in the renal tubular reabsorption of the amino acids of the monoamino-monocarboxylic group, known to share a common system for renal membrane transport. All other tests of tubular function and renal clearance are normal. The same defect of amino acid absorption is most probably present in the small intestines as well. The cause of the symptomatology in Hartnup disease is primarily the absorption defect in the intestine. This defect allows the formation of decomposition products toxic to the central nervous system and diminishes the amount of nicotinamide synthesized from tryptophan, causing the "pellagra-like" condition [2]. The underlying enzymatic defect in this disease or the lesion at the molecular level is still unknown.

Inheritance. Autosomal recessive.

Treatment. The response to prolonged oral administration of nicotinamide is quite satisfactory [3]. Marked improvement in the dermatitis and neurologic picture usually follows.

References

1. Baron, D.N., Dent, C.E., Harris, H., Hart, E.W., Jepson, J.B.: Hereditary pellagra-like skin rash with temporary cerebellar ataxia, constant renal amino-aciduria, and other bizarre biochemical features. Lancet *1956 II*, 421–428
2. Jepson, J.B.: Hartnup disease. In: The metabolic basis of inherited disease. Stanbury, J.B., Wynngaarden, J.B., Fredrickson, D.S. (eds.), 4th ed., pp. 1563–1577. New York: McGraw-Hill Book Co. 1978
3. Wong, P.W.K., Lambert, A.M., Pillai, P.M., Jones, P.M.: Observations on nicotinic acid therapy in Hartnup disease. Arch. Dis. Child. *42*, 642–646 (1967)

Hereditary Polymorphic Light Eruption

Clinical Presentation. The condition seems to affect predominantly individuals of American Indian descent. Both sexes are affected although females have a higher incidence [1]. The age of onset is below 5 years in 35% of cases and below 10 years in 70% [1].
In young children, the eruption appears on the face as diffuse erythema, with small papules, exudation, and crusting. The involved areas are those exposed to sunlight. Often there is an acute exudative and crusted cheilitis, especially of the lower lip, which at

times may be the only manifestation [1]. On the exposed areas of the upper extremities and legs, prurigolike papules, usually with small crusts, appear [1, 2]. No vesiculo-bullae appear and there is no scarring (Figs. 6.4 and 6.5).

The lesions become less marked as the children approach puberty and this pattern continues into adulthood. Rarely, adults may have thickened erythematous plaques on the exposed parts of the face [1, 2] (Figs. 6.6 and 6.7). All of these lesions are pruritic but there is no burning sensation.

The lesions appear in the spring and tend to recur every year. Few lesions persist throughout the winter.

Pathology and Pathophysiology. The main histologic features are areas of hyperkeratosis alternating with parakeratosis, follicular plugging, acanthosis, subepidermal edema, and perivascular infiltrate [2]. In addition, the eczematous lesions show extravasation of erythrocytes and epidermal edema [2]. There is no evidence of an abnormal porphyrin metabolism [1].

Inheritance. Probably autosomal dominant [1].

Treatment. Trisoralen (5–10 mg daily), if started in February and continued throughout summer, gives substantial improvement [1].

References

1. Birt, A.R., Davis, R.A.: Hereditary polymorphic light eruption of American Indians. Int. J. Derm. *14*, 105–111 (1975)
2. Everett, M.A., Crockett, W., Lamb, J.H., Minor, D.: Light-sensitive eruptions in American Indians. Arch. Derm. *83*, 243–248 (1961)

Porphyrias

The porphyrias are disorders of the biosynthesis of protoheme, the ferrous iron complex of protoporphyrin IX. They are characterized by specific patterns of porphyrin and porphyrin precursor overproduction, accumulation, and excretion [1].

The two main clinical features of porphyria are the sensitivity of the skin to sunlight and neurologic lesions which characteristically cause severe abdominal pain, peripheral neuropathy, and often mental disturbance, frequently precipitated by drugs [1].

The first case of porphyria recorded in the literature was reported by Schultz [2] and Baumstark [3] in 1874 under the diagnosis of "pemphigus leprosus."

Since then, many forms have been reported. The modern classification of porphyrias, based on the site of origin of the porphyrins, is as follows [1].

Erythropoietic – congenital erythropoietic porphyria (Günther disease)
Erythrohepatic – erythrohepatic protoporphyria
Hepatic porphyrias
    Hepatic porphyrias inherited as autosomal dominant
        Acute intermittent porphyria
        Variegate porphyria
        Hereditary coproporphyria
    Symptomatic cutaneous hepatic porphyria (porphyria cutanea tarda)
    Cutaneous porphyria due to hepatic tumors

Congenital Erythropoietic Porphyria (Günther Disease)

Congenital erythropoietic porphyria (Günther disease) is very rare. Less than 100 cases have been reported to date.

Clinical Presentation. The first sign is usually the excretion of red urine noted at birth or during infancy. The red color may show considerable daily or seasonal fluctuation, increasing during periods of active photodermatitis and varying from a faint pink to a Burgundy red or a reddish brown color [4]. Photosensitivity becomes apparent during the first years of life with increased exposure to sunlight. It produces a severe "burning" sensation. A vesicular eruption appears on the exposed parts of the body, particularly the face and the back of the hands. The serous fluid of the vesicles reveals a red fluorescence. The lesions become crusted, often impetiginized, heal slowly, and leave depressed pigmented scars (Figs. 6.8 and 6.9). Repeated attacks over the years may lead to severe contractions of the face and mutilation of the digits and the ears. Hypertrichosis is frequently present, with blond lanugolike hair covering the face and the extremities [4]. There may be patchy baldness due to scarring of the scalp, as well as damage to terminal phalanges and nails. The nasal and aural cartilages are usually eroded.

The teeth, both deciduous and permanent, may show a red or brownish discoloration (erythrodontia) and a red fluorescence under UV light (Wood's) (Fig. 6.10). Splenomegaly and a hemolytic anemia are present in almost all patients. Uroporphyrin and coproporphyrin in the urine are increased and reveal the characteristic red fluorescence under UV light. The feces contain large amounts of coproporphyrin [4, 5].

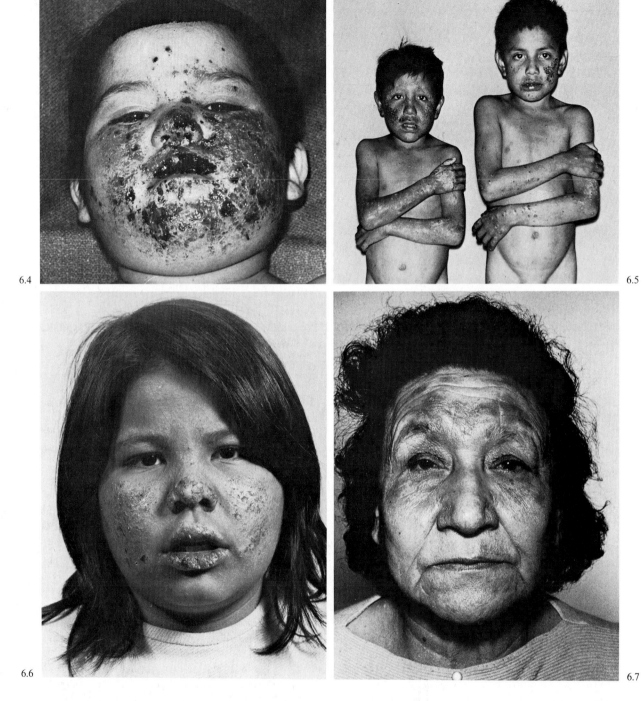

6.4

6.5

6.6

6.7

Figs. 6.4–6.7. Hereditary polymorphic light eruption

Fig. 6.4. Involvement of the face with erythema, exudation, and crusting. (From Birt, A.R., Davis, R.A.: Int. J. Derm. *14*, 105–111, 1975)

Fig. 6.5. Prurigolike papules on the exposed areas of the upper extremities. (From Birt, A.R., Davis, R.A.: Int. J. Derm. *14*, 105–111, 1975)

Figs. 6.6 and 6.7. Note that with increasing age the lesions become less exudative and appear as thickened plaques on the face. (From Birt, A.R., Davis, R.A.: Int. J. Derm. *14*, 105–111, 1975)

Fig. 6.8. Erythropoietic porphyria–Günther disease. Note the crusted lesions on the face and dorsa of the hands

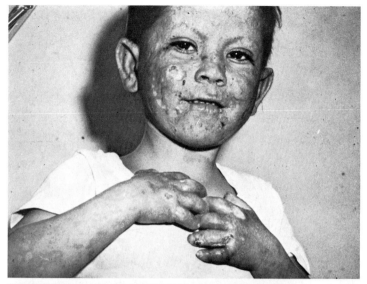

Fig. 6.9. Erythropoietic porphyria. Involvement of the dorsa of the hands with impetiginization

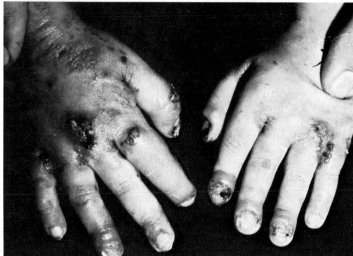

Fig. 6.10. Erythropoietic porphyria. Erythrodontia

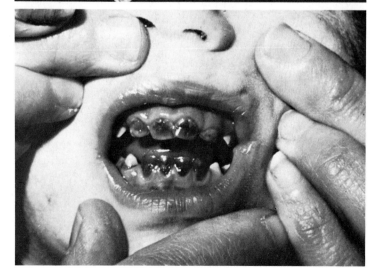

Pathology and Pathophysiology. "Photosensitizers" are molecules which absorb radiation and transfer it to other molecules, thereby making them reactive. The photochemical reaction in porphyria has the following components [6]: (a) a photosensitizing substance (a porphyrin); (b) radiation of an appropriate wavelength (400 nm and to a lesser extent 500–600 nm) that can pass through window glass; (c) molecular oxygen, which is available by normal circulation of arterial blood; and (d) a substrate.

The nature of the possible course of events after the initial photochemical reactions leading to the cutaneous lesions is not clear. Some investigators [7, 8] suggest that light causes lysosome rupture in the skin and release of the lysosomal hydrolytic enzymes, thereby initiating the release of chemical mediators of the skin lesion, such as histamine or histaminelike compounds.

Among the natural lesions occurring in porphyria due to photosensitivity, the most common is erythema. There is no evidence as to what the chemical mediator could be, but bradykinin is a good possibility.

Other types of lesions that are due to photosensitivity include a delayed edema reaction, petechiae, and bullae. Their pathophysiology has not yet been explained.

There is a marked decrease in uroporphyrinogen III cosynthetase activity in the erythrocytes and cultured skin fibroblasts from patients with erythropoietic porphyria [9, 10]. Asymptomatic heterozygotes can be detected because of the reduced enzymatic activity in circulating erythrocytes [11]. The mechanism responsible for the hemolytic process is not understood. At autopsy, under Wood's light, all the viscera, particularly the liver, kidneys, and intestines, and the bones show orange-red fluorescence [12].

Inheritance. Autosomal recessive.

Treatment. Patients should be protected by avoiding sunlight, wearing proper clothing, and using sunfilter preparations. Splenectomy has been advocated. Oral β-carotene may be helpful. Secondary infections should be controlled [4].

Erythrohepatic Protoporphyria

In 1961 Magnus and his co-workers [13] described this disease which differs from the classic erythropoietic porphyria. In recent years it has become apparent that in this type of porphyria the porphyrins are produced in excess in both erythropoietic and hepatic cells. Thus, the appellation of erythrohepatic protoporphyria was suggested instead of erythropoietic protoporphyria [14].

Clinical Presentation. In most cases of protoporphyria, the cutaneous manifestations are first noted in childhood or adolescence and persist throughout life. There is a very characteristic subjective "burning" sensation. The skin lesions appear in the form of solar urticaria or solar eczema. Exposure to sunlight for a few minutes results in pruritus, erythema, edema, and, rarely, blisters. This condition subsides in 12–24 h, without leaving scars, atrophy, or pigmentation. Some skin lesions may progress to a chronic eczematous phase lasting several weeks and leaving scars [4] (Figs. 6.11–6.14).

The disease may be associated with cholelithiasis, the gallstones consisting of precipitated protoporphyrin [15].

The concentration of free protoporphyrin in circulating erythrocytes is increased 5- to 30-fold. Up to half of the erythrocytes in the blood and bone marrow exhibit intense fluorescence. Large amounts of protoporphyrin are excreted in the stools [4]. However, the urinary excretion of porphyrins and their precursors is normal.

Some points of differentiation from the classic erythropoietic porphyria are the absence of erythrodontia, hirsutism, and hyperpigmentation, and normal urinary porphyrin excretion. In protoporphyria, the exposed parts of the skin show neither the abnormal mechanical fragility nor the chronic bullous eruptions of the other photosensitive porphyrias.

Pathology and Pathophysiology. The microscopic anatomy of the cutaneous changes in porphyria cutanea tarda, erythrohepatic porphyria, variegate porphyria, and coproporphyria is characteristic and similar, differing only in quantity rather than quality. On light microscopy, the primary alterations consist of a homogeneous thickening of the upper dermal blood vessel walls which contain a PAS-positive, diastase-resistant mucopolysaccharide. Fluorescent microscopic studies reveal the deposition of immunoglobulins, primarily IgG, in a similar perivascular distribution and at times at the epidermodermal junction. Electron microscopy reveals that the upper dermal blood vessels are also most prominently involved. These findings consist of reduplication of the vascular basal lamina and the deposition of a fine fibrillar material. The changes are most severe in the exposed erythrohepatic protoporphyria skin at all microscopic levels.

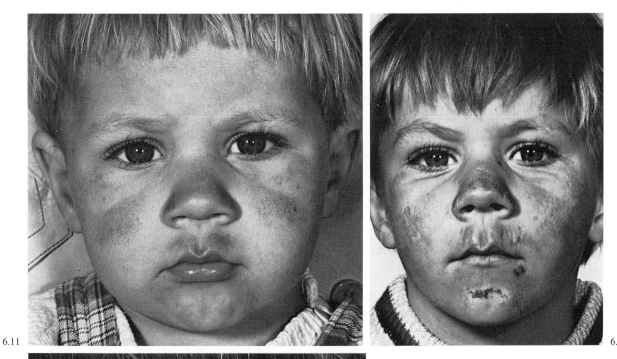

6.11

6.12

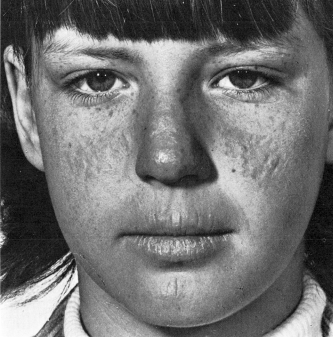

6.13

Fig. 6.11. Erythrohepatic protoporphyria. Note the initial erythema and edema on exposure to sunlight. There are no vesicles. (Courtesy of Dr. K. Thomsen, from Schmidt, H., et al.: Arch. Derm. *110*, 58–64, 1974)

Fig. 6.12. Erythrohepatic protoporphyria. Eczematous lesions with early scarring. (Courtesy of Dr. K. Thomsen, from Schmidt, H., et al.: Arch. Derm. *110*, 58–64, 1974)

Fig. 6.13. Erythrohepatic protoporphyria. Pitted scars over the cheeks. (Courtesy of Dr. K. Thomsen, from Schmidt, H., et al.: Arch. Derm. *110*, 58–64, 1974)

These results suggest that the primary injury occurs in the upper dermal blood vessels due to the presence of porphyrin molecules and sunlight energy. Additional damage is present in porphyria cutanea tarda and variegate porphyria at the epidermodermal zone, which may be responsible for the unique fragility of the sun-exposed skin in these conditions [16].

In protoporphyria, the pigment in circulating erythrocytes has the structure of isomer type IX protoporphyrin. There is increased δ-aminolevulinic acid (ALA) synthetase activity in both erythroid and hepatic tissues [17]. However, the fundamental defect in this disease appears to be a deficiency of the mitochondrial ferrochelatase enzyme, which converts protoporphyrin IX to heme [18].

Inheritance. Autosomal dominant.

Treatment. These patients respond poorly to antihistaminics, antimalarials, and topically applied sunscreens. Recently, β-carotene (100–200 mg orally per day) has been shown to be effective in suppressing the photosensitivity of these patients [19, 20].

Hepatic Porphyrias

Hepatic Porphyrias Inherited as Autosomal Dominant

Acute Intermittent Porphyria

This condition follows the autosomal dominant pattern of inheritance. The main manifestations are abdominal and neurologic. The only dermatologic finding is a pigmentation of the skin which is not diagnostic. The disease is presumably due to decreased activity of hepatic uroporphyrinogen I synthetase [21].

Variegate Porphyria

Since 1951 a large group of porphyric individuals has been reported in the white population of South Africa where the incidence of the disease in Afrikaners is 3 per 1000 [22, 23]. This high frequency is an important example of the founder effect (see p. Glossary).

Clinical Presentation. The main features are increased sensitivity of the exposed skin to minor mechanical trauma and light, transient episodes of acute abdominal and neurologic manifestations precipitated by the ingestion of drugs, and continuous excretion of increased amounts of protoporphyrin and coproporphyrin in the feces.

The skin lesions may be the only manifestations of variegate porphyria in half of the patients and are usually noted during the third decade. They are chronic and are limited to the parts of the body exposed to sunlight, especially the face and the back of the hands. Mechanical trauma leads to abrasions, erosions, and formation of bullae which heal with scarring. Direct sensitivity of the skin to light is less conspicuous than increased mechanical fragility. Hyperpigmentation of the exposed parts is observed. Hypertrichosis of the face is common in women [4].

Acute attacks of abdominal pain and neuropathy may accompany the skin lesions in half of the cases. They usually follow the onset of chronic cutaneous involvement by many years. The neurologic manifestations are variable and may involve the peripheral nerves, autonomic nervous system, brain stem, cranial nerves, or cerebral function [4].

The acute attacks may be precipitated by the ingestion of barbiturates or sulfonamides or by the administration of other hepatotoxic agents, such as general anesthetics, ethanol, or chloroquine. During an acute episode the mortality rate is around 25%. Otherwise the acute attacks resolve completely; however, neuropathic changes persist long after the end of the acute episode [4].

The characteristic chemical finding is the continuous excretion of large amounts of protoporphyrin and coproporphyrin in the feces and porphobilinogen in the urine.

Pathology and Pathophysiology. For the skin changes, see under Erythrohepatic Protoporphyria. Major anatomic abnormalities or histologic and laboratory evidence of major hepatic dysfunction are lacking.

The primary metabolic defect in porphyrin metabolism most probably results in an exaggerated responsiveness of hepatic δ-aminolevulinic acid (ALA) synthetase [4].

Inheritance. Autosomal dominant.

Treatment. A high carbohydrate diet may be helpful [24].

Fig. 6.14. Erythrohepatic protoporphyria. Dorsa of hands of a 6-year-old boy, showing coarse lichenified plaques. (Courtesy of Dr. K. Thomsen, from Schmidt, H., et al.: Arch. Derm. *110*, 58–64, 1974)

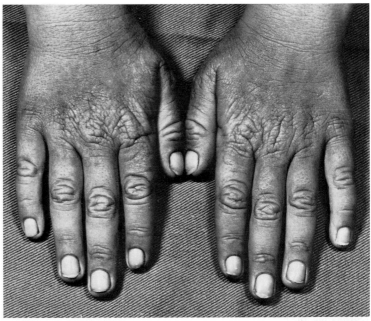

Fig. 6.15. Porphyria cutanea tarda. Bullae and ulcerations on dorsa of the hands. (Courtesy of Dr. I. Zeligman)

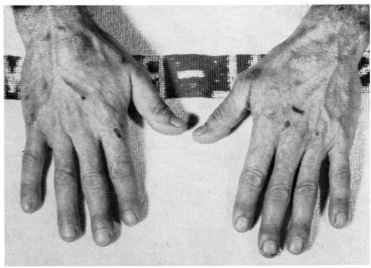

Hereditary Coproporphyria

Clinically, hereditary coproporphyria resembles a milder form of variegate porphyria. However, it has a unique pattern of porphyrin excretion, consisting of an unremitting excretion of large amounts of coproporphyrin III in the feces. Coproporphyrin excretion is also frequently increased in the urine, particularly during acute attacks. Porphobilinogen and ALA excretion is normal except during an acute attack. A fragment of liver tissue obtained from a patient showed an intense red fluorescence. Activity of coproporphyrinogen oxidase (CPG oxidase) is lower in fibroblasts from patients with hereditary coproporphyria than in cells from controls or patients with other types of porphyria [25]. The inheritance is autosomal dominant. There

is no specific treatment. β-Carotene administration may be tried.

Symptomatic Cutaneous Hepatic Porphyria (Porphyria Cutanea Tarda)

The major clinical manifestations are limited to the skin with frequent association of hepatic dysfunction. Although the disease has been reported in many parts of the world, its highest incidence occurs in the Bantu population of South Africa. Bullae, pigmentation, hypertrichosis, and sclerodermoid changes are the cardinal features, occurring on exposed areas of the skin (Fig. 6.15). Linear, atrophic, radiating scars around the mouth may simulate rhagades.

Hemochromatosis is one of the complications. Hepatic involvement is always present and overt cirrhosis may develop. The disease occurs particularly in alcoholics.

A genetically determined idiosyncrasy is suspected [26]. The disease apparently results from the combination of an inherited defect in uroporphyrinogen decarboxylase and an acquired factor, usually siderosis associated with alcoholic liver disease [27]. The decreased enzyme activity appears to be inherited as an autosomal dominant trait. Phlebotomy may be symptomatically and biochemically beneficial [28]. Small doses of chloroquine (250 mg twice weekly) may be helpful.

Toxic acquired porphyria has occurred in thousands of individuals exposed to hexachlorobenzene or other toxic chemicals.

Cutaneous Porphyria
Due to Hepatic Tumors

The purely cutaneous form of porphyria may be due to overproduction of porphyrin by a tumor (benign hepatic adenoma or malignant primary hepatoma) surrounded by normal liver tissue. The condition is not hereditary [29, 30].

References

1. Elder, G.H., Gray, C.H., Nicholson, D.C.: The porphyrias: a review. J. clin. Path. 25, 1013–1033 (1972)
2. Schultz, J.H.: Ein Fall von Pemphigus Leprosus, kompliziert durch Lepra visceralis. Ph. D. thesis, Greifswald 1874
3. Baumstark, F.: Zwei pathologische Harnfarbstoffe. Pflüger's Arch. ges. Physiol. 9, 568–584 (1874)
4. Meyer, V.A., Schmid, R.: The porphyrias. In: The metabolic basis of inherited disease. Stanbury, J.B., Wyngaarden, J.B., Fredrickson, D.S. (eds.), 4th ed., pp. 1166–1220. New York: McGraw-Hill Book Co. 1978
5. Idriss, Z.H., Najjar, S.S., Der Kaloustian, V.M., Shamaa, A.R.: Congenital erythropoietic porphyria. Amer. J. Dis. Child. 129, 701–702 (1975)
6. Magnus, I.A.: The cutaneous porphyrias. Semin. Hemat. 5, 380–408 (1968)
7. Slater, T.F., Riley, P.A.: Photosensitization and lysosomal damage. Nature (Lond.) 209, 151–154 (1966)
8. Allison, A.C., Magnus, I.A., Young, M.R.: Role of lysosomes and of cell membranes in photosensitization. Nature (Lond.) 209, 874–878 (1966)
9. Romeo, G., Levin, E.Y.: Uroporphyrinogen III cosynthetase in human congenital erythropoietic porphyria. Proc. nat. Acad. Sci. (Wash.) 63, 856–863 (1969)
10. Romeo, G., Kaback, M.M., Levin, E.Y.: Uroporphyrinogen III cosynthetase activity in fibroblasts from patients with congenital erythropoietic porphyria. Biochem. Genet. 4, 659–664 (1970)
11. Romeo, G., Glenn, B.L., Levin, E.Y.: Uroporphyrinogen III cosynthetase in asymptomatic carriers of congenital erythropoietic porphyria. Biochem. Genet. 4, 719–726 (1970)

12. Bhutani, L.K., Sood, S.K., Das, P.K., Deshpande, S.G., Mulay, D.N., Kandhari, K.C.: Congenital erythropoietic porphyria. An autopsy report. Arch. Derm. 110, 427–431 (1974)
13. Magnus, I.A., Jarrett, A., Prankerd, T.A.J., Rimington, C.: Erythropoietic protoporphyria. A new porphyria syndrome with solar urticaria due to protoporphyrinaemia. Lancet 1961 II, 448–451
14. Scholnick, P., Marver, H.S., Schmid, R.: Erythropoietic protoporphyria: evidence for multiple sites of excess porphyrin protoporphyrin formation. J. clin. Invest. 50, 203–207 (1971)
15. Cripps, D.J., Scheuer, P.J.: Hepatobiliary changes in erythropoietic protoporphyria. Arch. Path. 80, 500–508 (1965)
16. Epstein, J.H., Tufanelli, D.L., Epstein, W.L.: Cutaneous changes in the porphyrias. A microscopic study. Arch. Derm. 107, 689–698 (1973)
17. Miyagi, K.: The liver aminolaevulinic acid synthetase activity in erythropoietic protoporphyria by means of the new micro method. J. Kyushu Haemat. Soc. 17, 397–412 (1967)
18. Bottomley, S.S., Tanaka, M., Everett, M.A.: Diminished erythroid ferrochelatase activity in protoporphyria. J. lab. clin. Med. 86, 126–131 (1975)
19. Mathews-Roth, M.M., Pathak, M.A., Fitzpatrick, T.B.: Beta-carotene as a photoprotective agent in erythropoietic protoporphyria. New Engl. J. Med. 282, 1231–1234 (1970)
20. Baart de la Faille, H., Suurmond, D., Went, L.N., van Steveninck, J., Schothorst, A.A.: β-Carotene as a treatment for photohypersensitivity due to erythropoietic protoporphyria. Dermatologica (Basel) 145, 389–394 (1972)
21. Sassa, S., Solish, G., Levere, R.D., Kappas, A.: Studies in porphyria. IV. Expression of gene defect of acute intermittent porphyria in cultured skin fibroblasts and amniotic cells: prenatal diagnosis of the porphyria trait. J. exp. Med. 142, 722–731 (1975)
22. Dean, G., Barnes, H.D.: The inheritance of porphyria. Brit. med. J. 1955 II, 89–94
23. Dean, G.: The porphyrias. A story of inheritance and environment, 2nd ed., pp. 4–13. London: Pitman Medical 1971
24. Perlroth, M.G., Tschudy, D.P., Ratner, A., Spaur, W., Redeker, A.: The effect of diet in variegate (South African genetic) porphyria. Metabolism 17, 571–581 (1968)
25. Elder, G.H., Evans, J.O., Thomas, N., Cox, R., Brodie, M.J., Moore, M.R., Goldberg, A., Nicholson, D.C.: Primary enzyme defect in hereditary coproporphyria. Lancet 1976 II, 1217–1219
26. McKusick, V.A.: Mendelian inheritance in man, 5th ed., p. 328. Baltimore: Johns Hopkins University Press 1978
27. Kushner, J.P., Barbuto, A.J., Lee, G.R.: An inherited enzymatic defect in porphyria cutanea tarda: decreased uroporphyrinogen decarboxylase activity. J. clin. Invest. 58, 1089–1097 (1976)
28. Epstein, J.H., Redeker, A.G.: Porphyria cutanea tarda. A study of the effect of phlebotomy. New Engl. J. Med. 279, 1301–1304 (1968)
29. Tio, T.H., Leijnse, B., Jarrett, A., Rimington, C.: Acquired porphyria from a liver tumour. Clin. Sci. 16, 517–527 (1957)
30. Thompson, R.P.H., Nicholson, D.C., Farnan, T., Whitmore, D.N., Williams, R.: Cutaneous porphyria due to a malignant primary hepatoma. Gastroenterology 59, 779–783 (1970)

Xeroderma Pigmentosum

In 1874 Hebra and Kaposi [1] described this syndrome characterized by sun sensitivity, freckles, and skin cancers. The association of these features with microcephaly, hypogonadism, and subnormal intelligence was reported by de Sanctis and Cacchione [2] in 1932.

Clinical Presentation. The disease usually appears in the first or second year of life, the first sign being freckling of the skin in areas exposed to sunlight. The lesions are scattered over the face, ears, neck, hands, and forearms. As the disease progresses, the lesions are no longer limited to the exposed parts of the skin, but occur on the trunk and lower extremities. Interspersed among the pigmented lesions are white, parchmentlike, atrophic areas, sometimes covered with fine scales. Later, keratotic patches, waxy elevations, and pedunculated and malignant growths develop [3] (Figs. 6.16–6.18).

Photophobia, conjunctivitis, and excess lacrimation occur early in the disease, along with blepharitis, symblepharon, ectropion, and keratitis [3].

Some patients have microcephaly, hypogonadism, and mental retardation (de Sanctis-Cacchione syndrome) with the dermatologic anomalies (Fig. 6.19).

The course of xeroderma pigmentosum is chronic and usually fatal before adulthood, as a result of malignancies. However, mild forms of the disease are seen in adults [4].

Pathology and Pathophysiology. Histologic examination of the skin reveals relative and absolute hyperkeratosis; a varying degree of atrophy of the prickle cell layer, especially over the papillae; irregular proliferation and prolongation of the rete pegs; intracellular epidermal edema with pyknosis or karyorrhexis; edema of the pars papillaris and upper parts of the dermis with narrowing of the rete pegs; some dilatation of the superficial vessels and perivascular cellular infiltration; and spotty melanin pigmentation of the epidermis with pigment-laden melanophages in the upper dermis. Recently, muscle pathology consisting of massive accumulations of glycogen and subsarcolemmal mitochondrial aggregates has also been described [5]. The neoplasms encountered include those of epithelial as well as mesenchymal origin.

The defect in xeroderma pigmentosum is increased susceptibility to UV light with a wavelength of 280–310 nm. The effect of UV at the molecular level is the production of cyclobutyl pyrimidine dimers in the DNA. In normal individuals, these "lesions" are repaired in the dark by excision of the dimers and repair replication and rejoining of the DNA strand. Studies on fibroblasts from most patients with xeroderma pigmentosum reveal that the repair replication occurs at a reduced rate or not at all [6].

Cells from obligate heterozygotes have also shown in one study reduced DNA repair when they were subjected to high doses of UV which presumably exceed the threshold for repair capacity of heterozygotes [7].

Experiments of complementation with somatic cell hybridization have demonstrated that the defect is genetically heterogeneous [3, 8, 9] (see also p. 12). The non-neurologic forms comprise three groups: C, E, and a "variant." The neurologic forms also consist of three groups: A, B, and D. Groups A, B, C, D, and E are all defective in varying degrees at an early stage in excision repair involving the removal of damaged sites from DNA [4].

Endonuclease activity (see p. 1) upon depurinated DNA is slightly reduced in cell lines from certain complementation groups. But cell lines from one complementation group (D) have only one-sixth of the normal activity [10].

Xeroderma pigmentosum variants have been described with the clinical manifestations of the disease, but with cells that exhibit normal sensitivity to UV and normal DNA repair [7, 11]. The tumor cells of such patients resemble the other cells in DNA repair capacity and do not represent a minor cell population with defective DNA repair as reflected in reduced UV-induced thymidine incorporation [12].

Variants whose cells are completely normal in the excision repair process have an abnormality in the manner in which DNA is synthesized after UV irradiation. The time taken to convert initially low-molecular-weight DNA synthesized in UV-irradiated cells into high-molecular-weight DNA similar in size to that in untreated cells is much greater in these variants than in normal cells [13].

In normal cells, UV-induced cyclobutyl pyrimidine dimers in DNA are monomerized in normal light by an enzyme which restores biological activity to the DNA [14]. This is the photoreactivating enzyme. Fibroblasts of certain cell lines from patients with XP contain low levels of this enzyme as compared to normal cells.

Finally, XP cells deficient in excision of UV-induced pyrimidine dimers may have a diminished post-UV irradiation colony-forming ability (CFA) [15].

The multiplicity of complementation groups coupled with the wide range of phenotypes and repair

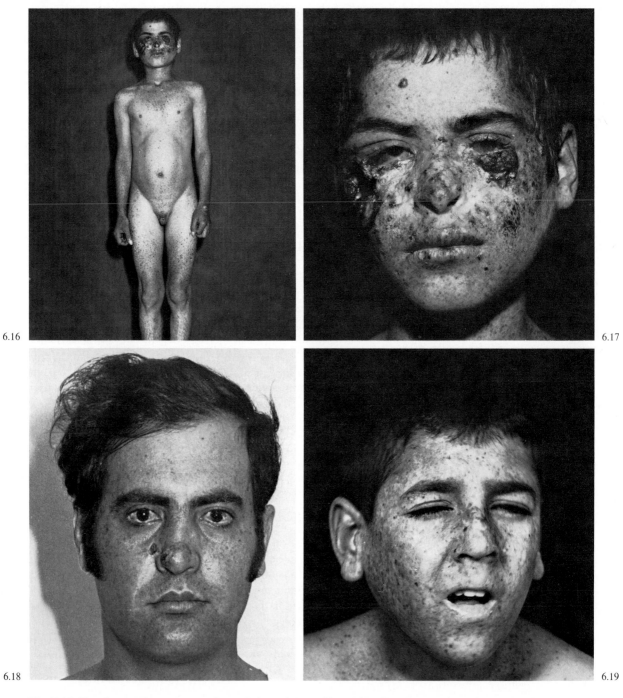

6.16

6.17

6.18

6.19

Fig. 6.16. Xeroderma pigmentosum. General view of the body. Note the involvement of the areas exposed to sun

Fig. 6.17. Xeroderma pigmentosum. Note hypo- and hyperpigmentation, whitish atrophic scars, and a variety of skin tumors

Fig. 6.18. Xeroderma pigmentosum. Mild form in an adult. Note the paranasal neoplastic ulcer

Fig. 6.19. de Sanctis-Cacchione syndrome

deficiencies of the cultured cell lines suggests that the XP groups have multiple repair defects [10].

Since XP patients may have abnormalities not only of the skin but also of the nervous, endocrine, and immune systems, it is possible that the effectiveness of DNA repair in humans may play a role in the normal and pathologic aging of various organ systems [15].

Inheritance. Autosomal recessive [3].

Treatment. Avoidance of sunlight, the use of sunscreens and topical 5-fluorouracil, and dermabrasion are the mainstays of treatment. Once tumors appear, they should be treated by surgery or electrosurgery.

A rapid, sensitive method for prenatal diagnosis is available [16]. In the matter of precise diagnosis in utero, interpretations of laboratory findings in homozygotes versus heterozygotes are still not clear-cut.

References

1. Hebra, F., Kaposi, M.: On diseases of the skin, Vol. 3, p. 252. London: New Sydenham Society 1874
2. de Sanctis, C., Cacchione, A.: L'idiozia xerodermica. Riv. sper. Freniat. *56*, 269–292 (1932)
3. Robbins, J.H., Kraemer, K.H., Lutzer, M.A., Festoff, B.W., Conn, H.G.: Xeroderma pigmentosum. An inherited disease with sun sensitivity, multiple cutaneous neoplasms, and abnormal DNA repair. Ann. intern. Med. *80*, 221–248 (1974)
4. Cleaver, J.E.: Xeroderma pigmentosum. In: The metabolic basis of inherited disease. Stanbury, J.B., Wyngaarden, J.B., Fredrickson, D.S. (eds.), 4th ed., pp. 1072–1095. New York: McGraw-Hill Book Co. 1978
5. Afifi, A.K., Der Kaloustian, V.M., Mire, J.J.: Muscular abnormality in xeroderma pigmentosum. High resolution light-microscopy and electron-microscopic observations. J. neurol. Sci. *17*, 435–442 (1972)
6. Cleaver, J.E.: Xeroderma pigmentosum: a human disease in which an initial stage of DNA repair is defective. Proc. nat. Acad. Sci. (Wash.) *63*, 428–435 (1969)
7. Cleaver, J.E.: Xeroderma pigmentosum: variants with normal DNA repair and normal sensitivity to ultraviolet light. J. invest. Derm. *58*, 124–128 (1972)
8. de Weerd-Kastelein, E.A., Keijzer, W., Bootsma, D.: Genetic heterogeneity of xeroderma pigmentosum demonstrated by somatic cell hybridization. Nature (Lond.) New Biol. *238*, 80–83 (1972)
9. Der Kaloustian, V.M., de Weerd-Kastelein, E.A., Kleijer, W.J., Keijzer, W., Bootsma, D.: The genetic defect in the de Sanctis-Cacchione syndrome. J. invest. Derm. *63*, 392–396 (1974)
10. Kuhnlein, U., Penhoet, E.E., Linn, S.: An altered apurinic DNA endonuclease activity in group A and D xeroderma pigmentosum fibroblasts. Proc. nat. Acad. Sci. (Wash.) *73*, 1169–1173 (1976)
11. Robbins, J.H., Levis, W.R., Miller, A.E.: Xeroderma pigmentosum epidermal cells with normal UV-induced thymidine incorporation. J. invest. Derm. *59*, 402–408 (1972)
12. Robbins, J.H., Kraemer, K.H., Flaxman, B.A.: DNA repair in tumor cells from the variant form of xeroderma pigmentosum. J. invest. Derm. *64*, 150–155 (1975)
13. Lehmann, A.R., Kirk-Bell, S., Arlett, C.F., Paterson, M.C., Lohman, P.H.M., de Weerd-Kastelein, E.A., Bootsma, D.: Xeroderma pigmentosum cells with normal levels of excision repair have a defect in DNA synthesis after UV-irradiation. Proc. nat. Acad. Sci. (Wash.) *72*, 219–223 (1975)
14. Sutherland, B.M., Rice, M., Wagner, E.K.: Xeroderma pigmentosum cells contain low levels of photoreactivating enzyme. Proc. nat. Acad. Sci. (Wash.) *72*, 103–107 (1975)
15. Andrews, A.D., Barrett, S.F., Robbins, J.H.: Relation of D.N.A. repair processes to pathological ageing of the nervous system in xeroderma pigmentosum. Lancet *1976I*, 1318–1320
16. Regan, J.D., Setlow, R.B., Kaback, M.M., Howell, R.R., Klein, E., Burgess, G.: Xeroderma pigmentosum: a rapid sensitive method for prenatal diagnosis. Science *174*, 147–150 (1971)

Chapter 7   Inherited Disorders with Immune Deficiency

Contents

Along with advances in genetics, the last two decades have witnessed a very significant upswing in the field of immunology in general and the study of inherited diseases with immune deficiency in particular.

For the sake of completeness, we included in this chapter most of the inherited diseases that may have some form of immune deficiency with dermatologic findings. We elected to present them in table form for practical, quick reference and also to save space. However, some of them (e.g., Aldrich syndrome, ataxia telangiectasia) are also presented separately, and at greater length, to cover their important clinical and basic aspects.

Since we do not review here the basic principles of modern immunology, we suggest the excellent reference of Stiehm and Fulginiti (Stiehm, E.R., Fulginiti, V.A.: Immunologic disorders in infants and children. Philadelphia: Saunders, W.B. Co. 1973).

Table 7.1. Antibody deficiency diseases

Disorder	Mode of inheritance	Clinical and immunologic abnormalities	Cutaneous manifestations	Ref.
Infantile agamma-globulinemia	X-linked recessive	Marked depression of all immunoglobulins Plasma cells absent from bone marrow, nodes, spleen, and gastrointestinal tract Intact cell-mediated immunity Normal thymus Normal numbers of circulating lymphocytes (T cells) Normal resistance to some gram-negative organisms and to viral and fungal infections Increased incidence of allergic disorders and autoimmune connective tissue disease	Severe furunculoses, pyoderma Warts	[1]
Immune deficiency with raised IgM	X-linked recessive	Lack of follicles in lymphoid structures Abundance of "plasmacytoid" cells containing IgM Virtual absence of IgG and IgA; very high IgM Recurrent cyclic or persistent neutropenia, hemolytic anemia, and thrombocytopenia	Widespread development of warts Indolent oral ulcerations	[2]

Table 7.2. Immunodeficiencies with thymic hypoplasia or dysplasia

Disorder	Mode of inheritance	Clinical and immunologic abnormalities	Cutaneous manifestations	Ref.
Severe combined immunodeficiency	Autosomal recessive and X-linked recessive	Susceptibility to viral, fungal, and bacterial infections Vestigial thymus and absence of thymus-dependent or immunoglobulin-producing systems Decreased circulating lymphocytes in many Extremely low levels of all 3 major immunoglobulins No benefit from γ-globulin administration No delayed hypersensitivity Chronic diarrhea and recurrent pulmonary infections Death at age 1–2 years from overwhelming infections	Massive candidiasis Vaccinia	[1, 3]
Immune defect with deficiency of adenosine deaminase	Probably autosomal recessive	Probably heterogeneous Respiratory infections and lymphopenia Impaired cellular and humoral immunity Absent red cell adenosine deaminase (ADA) Absence of lymphoid elements	Candidiasis	[4]
Immunodeficiency with lymphopenia (Nèzelof syndrome)	Autosomal recessive	Fever, diarrhea Persistent candidal broncho-pulmonary infection Death at an early age Aplasia of thymus Lymphopenia or alymphocytosis Lymphoid hypoplasia Normoglobulinemia	Erythematosquamous dermatosis Recurrent pyoderma	[5]
Reticular dysgenesis (congenital aleukia)	?	Complete absence of leukocytes Sepsis and death in first 10 days of life Thymic alymphoplasia Presence of megakaryocytes, hematocytoblasts, normoblasts, and monocytes	Staphylococcal infections of the mouth and conjunctiva	[6, 7]

Table 7.3. Other cellular immunodeficiencies

Disorder	Mode of inheritance	Clinical and immunologic abnormalities	Cutaneous manifestations	Ref.
Ataxia telangiectasia (see also p. 244)	Autosomal recessive	Progressive cerebellar degeneration Frequent sinopulmonary infections Absent or hypoplastic thymus Decreased cellular immune responses Complete lack of or marked decrease in IgA in 70% IgE deficiency	Ocular and cutaneous telangiectases	[8]
Aldrich syndrome (see also p. 161)	X-linked recessive	Thrombocytopenia, bloody diarrhea Susceptibility to fungal, viral, and bacterial infections Death usually before age of 10 years Cellular and humoral immune deficiency Hypercatabolism of IgG, IgA, and IgM	Thrombocytopenic purpura Eczema Multiple subcutaneous abscesses	[9, 10]
Familial chronic mucocutaneous candidiasis (FCMC)	Autosomal recessive	Candidal pharyngitis and laryngitis in severe cases Chest infections Hypoadrenocorticism or hypoparathyroidism in some Abnormalities of lymphocyte function Lymphocytes unable to produce migratory inhibitory factor	Candidal involvement of oral mucous membranes, scalp, face, hands, and groin (Figs. 7.1–7.4) Bilateral, symmetric, angular cheilitis Chronic candidal paronychia and onychomycosis (Fig. 7.3).	[11–14]
Immunodeficiency with short-limb dwarfism (achondroplasia and Swiss-type agammaglobulinemia)	Autosomal recessive	Lymphopenia, agammaglobulinemia, ectodermal dysplasia Thymic hypoplasia Metaphyseal chondrodysplasia	Skin forms redundant folds around the neck and extremities	[15]
Cartilage-hair hypoplasia (metaphyseal chondrodysplasia, McKusick type) (see also p. 182)	Autosomal recessive	Short-limb dwarfism Neutropenia and abnormal cellular immunity	Fine, sparse, and light-colored hair Thinner and weaker hair	[16, 17]
Episodic lymphopenia with lymphocytotoxin (immunologic amnesia)	Autosomal recessive	Recurrent bacterial and viral infections Recurrent otitis, pneumonia, meningitis Episodes of lymphopenia Dysgammaglobulinemia Impaired cellular immunity Absent immunologic memory Presence of complement-dependent lymphocytotoxic factor	Herpes simplex stomatitis Eczema Cellulitis	[18]

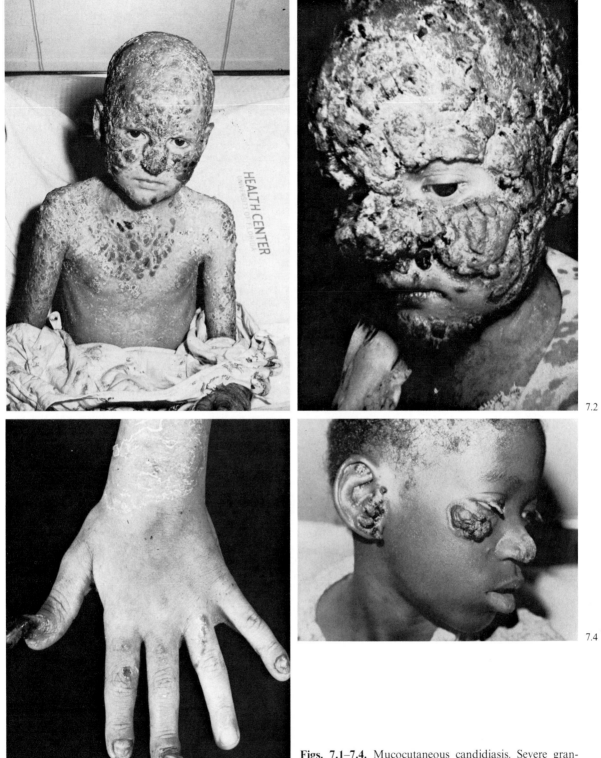

7.1

7.2

7.3

7.4

Figs. 7.1–7.4. Mucocutaneous candidiasis. Severe granulomatous lesions involving extensive areas of the skin and nails. (Courtesy of Dr. E. M. Ayoub)

Table 7.4. Disorders of the phagocytic system

Disorder	Mode of inheritance	Clinical and immunologic abnormalities	Cutaneous manifestations	Ref.
Chronic granulomatous disease due to leukocyte malfunction	X-linked recessive and autosomal recessive	Recurrent suppurative lymphadenitis Chronic pulmonary disease Hepatosplenomegaly Normal or elevated serum γ-globulins Leukocytes defective in postphagocytic metabolic burst Leukocytes phagocytize, but cannot kill catalase-positive organisms	Chronic dermatitis Skin rash: scaly, seborrheic, eczematoid, dry or weeping, frequently becoming red and pustular Development of skin hypersensitivity Organisms associated with chronic infection include staphylococci, aerobacter, salmonella, klebsiella, and serratia species	[19–23]
Myeloperoxidase deficiency	Autosomal recessive	No frequent or unusual bacterial infections Absence of activity of the lysosomal enzyme myeloperoxidase (MPO) in neutrophils and monocytes	Disseminated candidiasis	[24]
Chédiak-Higashi syndrome (see also p. 65)	Autosomal recessive	Photophobia and nystagmus Peculiar malignant lymphoma Increased susceptibility to infections Neutropenia Peroxidase-positive inclusion bodies in myeloblasts and promyelocytes	Decreased pigmentation of hair and eyes	[25]
Job syndrome	Autosomal recessive	Defect in local resistance to staphylococcal infection Most patients have red hair and fair skin Profound defect in neutrophil granulocyte chemotaxis and very high serum IgE levels found in 4 females Neutrophil random migration, phagocytosis, and bactericidal activity are normal	Indolent "cold" staphylococcal abscesses	[26, 27]
Defective neutrophil chemotaxis (see also p. 32)	Probably autosomal dominant	Abnormality of neutrophil movement with chemotaxis Normal number, morphology, phagocytic, and bactericidal activities of neutrophils	Congenital ichthyosis *Trichophyton rubrum* infection	[28]

Table 7.4 (continued)

Disorder	Mode of inheritance	Clinical and immunologic abnormalities	Cutaneous manifestations	Ref.
Defective monocyte chemotaxis	Probably autosomal recessive	Unresponsiveness of mono-cytes to lymphokine	Chronic mucocutaneous candidiasis and cutaneous anergy	[29, 30]
Chronic familial neutropenia	Autosomal dominant	Chronic neutropenia Hyperglobulinemia Clubbing of fingers No severe infections	Hyperplastic gingivitis Recurrent furuncles in many	[31]
Cyclic neutropenia	Probably autosomal dominant	Periodic neutropenia with infection (every 15–35 days) Fever, arthralgia, and vomiting Neutropenia may be accompanied by mono-cytosis, anemia, eosino-philia, and thrombo-cytopenia	Oral ulcerations Skin infections and recurrent furunculoses	[32, 33]
Infantile agranulocytosis of Kostmann	Autosomal recessive	Lower respiratory tract infections Otitis and mastoiditis Complete agranulocytosis Pronounced maturation arrest in myelopoiesis Cell-poor bone marrow containing mainly erythro-cyte precursors	Stubborn pyogenic skin infections very early in life	[34]
Fanconi anemia (see also p. 237)	Autosomal recessive	Malformations of heart, kidneys, and extremities Leukemia is a fatal complication Anemia, leukopenia, and thrombocytopenia	Pigmentary changes in skin	[35]
Familial C5 dysfunction	Unclear	Failure to thrive Diarrhea Recurrent sepsis due primarily to staphylococci and gram-negative enteric bacilli Leukocytosis and hyper-globulinemia Treatment with frequent infusions of fresh normal plasma and purified human C5	Severe seborrheic dermatitis	[36]

Table 7.5. Metabolic and other disorders

Disorder	Mode of inheritance	Clinical and immunologic abnormalities	Cutaneous manifestations	Ref.
Glycinemia (hyper-glycinemia with keto-acidosis and leukopenia)	Autosomal recessive	Episodic vomiting, lethargy, and ketosis Neutropenia (persistent) Periodic thrombocytopenia Hypogammaglobulinemia Developmental retardation Intolerance to protein Hyperglycinemia and hyper-glycinuria	Characteristic facies with puffy cheeks Exaggerated Cupid's bow of the upper lip Periodic purpura	[37, 38]
Tuftsin deficiency	Probably autosomal dominant	Deficiency of *tuftsin* Repeated severe infections	Multiple skin abscesses	[39, 40]
Vulnerability to leprosy	? Monogenic	Leprosy	Leprosy	[41]

References

1. Good, R.A.: Progress toward a cellular engineering. J. Amer. med. Ass. *214*, 1289–1300 (1970)
2. Rosen, F.S., Craig, J.M., Vawter, G., Janeway, C.A.: The dysgammaglobulinemias and X-linked thymic hypoplasia. In: Immunologic deficiency diseases in man. Bergsma, D. (ed.), Vol. IV, No. 1, pp. 67–70. New York: National Foundation 1968
3. Hoyer, J.R., Cooper, M.D., Gabrielsen, A.H., Good, R.A.: Lymphopenic forms of congenital immunologic deficiency: clinical and pathologic patterns. In: Immunologic deficiency diseases in man. Bergsma, D. (ed.), Vol. IV, No. 1, pp. 91–103. New York: National Foundation 1968
4. Yount, J., Nichols, P., Ochs, H.D., Hammar, S.P., Scott, C.R., Chen, S.-H., Giblett, E.R., Wedgwood, R.J.: Absence of erythrocyte adenosine deaminase associated with severe combined immunodeficiency. J. Pediat. *84*, 173–177 (1974)
5. Nèzelof, C., Jammet, M.-L., Lortholary, P., Labrune, B., Lamy, M.: L'hypoplasie héréditaire du thymus: sa place et sa responsabilité dans une observation d'aplasie lympho-cytaire, normoplasmocytaire et normoglobulinémique du nourrisson. Arch. franç. Pédiat. *21*, 897–920 (1964)
6. de Vaal, O.M., Seynhave, V.: Reticular dysgenesis. Lancet *1959II*, 1123–1125
7. Gitlin, D., Vawter, G., Craig, J.M.: Thymic alymphoplasia and congenital aleukocytosis. Pediatrics *33*, 184–192 (1964)
8. Peterson, R.D.A., Good, R.A.: Ataxia-telangiectasia. In: Immunologic deficiency diseases in man. Bergsma, D. (ed.), Vol. IV, No. 1, pp. 370–377. New York: National Foundation 1968
9. Cooper, M.D., Chase, H.P., Lowman, J.T., Krivit, W., Good, R.A.: Wiskott-Aldrich syndrome. An immunologic deficiency disease involving the afferent limb of immunity. Amer. J. Med. *44*, 499–513 (1968)
10. Blaese, R.M., Strober, W., Levy, A.L., Waldmann, T.A.: Hypercatabolism of IgG, IgA, IgM, and albumin in the Wiskott-Aldrich syndrome. A unique disorder of serum protein metabolism. J. clin. Invest. *50*, 2331–2338 (1971)
11. Wells, R.S., Higgs, J.M., McDonald, A., Valdimarsson, H., Holt, P.J.L.: Familial chronic muco-cutaneous candidiasis. J. med. Genet. *9*, 302–310 (1972)
12. Valdimarsson, H., Moss, P.D., Holt, P.J.L., Hobbs, J.R.: Treatment of chronic mucocutaneous candidiasis with leukocytes from HL-A compatible sibling. Lancet *1972I*, 469–472
13. Spinner, M.W., Blizzard, R.M., Childs, B.: Clinical and genetic heterogeneity in idiopathic Addison's disease and hypoparathyroidism. J. clin. Endocr. *28*, 795–804 (1968)

14. Öckerman, P.A.: Mannosidosis. In: Lysosomes and storage diseases. Hers, H.G., Van Hoof, F. (eds.), pp. 291–304. New York: Academic Press 1973
15. Gatti, R.A., Platt, N., Pomerance, H.H., Hong, R., Langer, L.O., Kay, H.E.M., Good, R.A.: Hereditary lymphopenic agammaglobulinemia associated with a distinctive form of short-limbed dwarfism and ectodermal dysplasia. J. Pediat. *75*, 675–684 (1969)
16. Coupe, R.L., Lowry, R.B.: Abnormality of the hair in the cartilage-hair hypoplasia. Dermatologica (Basel) *141*, 329–334 (1970)
17. Lux, S.E., Johnston, R.B., Jr., August, C.S., Say, B., Penchaszadeh, V.B., Rosen, F.S., McKusick, V.A.: Chronic neutropenia and abnormal cellular immunity in cartilage-hair hypoplasia. New Engl. J. Med. *282*, 231–236 (1970)
18. Kretschmer, R., August, C.S., Rosen, F.S., Janeway, C.A.: Recurrent infections, episodic lymphopenia and impaired cellular immunity. Further observations on "immunologic amnesia" in two siblings. New Engl. J. Med. *281*, 285–290 (1969)
19. Carson, M.J., Chadwick, D.L., Brubaker, C.A., Cleland, R.S., Landing, B.H.: Thirteen boys with progressive septic granulomatosis. Pediatrics *35*, 405–412 (1965)
20. Baehner, R.L., Karnovsky, M.L.: Deficiency of reduced nicotinamideadenine dinucleotide oxidase in chronic granulomatous disease. Science *162*, 1277–1279 (1968)
21. Baehner, R.L., Nathan, D.G.: Quantitative nitroblue tetrazolium test in chronic granulomatous disease. New Engl. J. Med. *278*, 971–976 (1968)
22. Holmes, B., Park, B.H., Malawista, S.E., Quie, P.G., Nelson, D.L., Good, R.A.: Chronic granulomatous disease in females. A deficiency of leukocyte glutathione peroxidase. New Engl. J. Med. *283*, 217–221 (1970)
23. Curnutte, J.T., Whitten, D.M., Babior, B.M.: Defective superoxide production by granulocytes from patients with chronic granulomatous disease. New Engl. J. Med. *290*, 593–597 (1974)
24. Lehrer, R.I., Cline, M.J.: Leukocyte myeloperoxidase deficiency and disseminated candidiasis; the role of myeloperoxidase in resistance to *Candida* infection. J. clin. Invest. *48*, 1478–1488 (1969)
25. Blume, R.S., Wolff, S.M.: The Chédiak-Higashi syndrome: studies in four patients and a review of the literature. Med. (Baltimore) *51*, 247–280 (1972)
26. Davis, S.D., Schaller, J., Wedgwood, R.J.: Job's syndrome. Recurrent, "cold", staphylococcal abscesses. Lancet *1966I*, 1013–1015

27. Hill, H.R., Ochs, H.D., Quie, P.G., Clark, R.A., Pabst, H.F., Klebanoff, S.J., Wedgwood, R.J.: Defect in neutrophil granulocyte chemotaxis in Job's syndrome of recurrent "cold" staphylococcal abscesses. Lancet 1974II, 617–619

28. Miller, M.E., Norman, M.E., Koblenzer, P.J., Schonauer, T.: A new familial defect of neutrophil movement. J. Lab. clin. Med. 82, 1–8 (1973)

29. Snyderman, E.P., Anderson, J.L., Chen, S.-H., Teng, Y.-S., Cohen, F.: Uridine monophosphate kinase: a new genetic polymorphism with possible clinical implications. Amer. J. hum. Genet. 26, 627–635 (1974)

30. Lehner, T., Wilton, J.M.A., Ivanyi, L.: Immunodeficiencies in chronic muco-cutaneous candidosis. Immunology 22, 775–787 (1972)

31. Cutting, H.O., Lang, J.E.: Familial benign chronic neutropenia. Ann. intern. Med. 61, 876–887 (1964)

32. Hahneman, B.M., Alt, H.L.: Cyclic neutropenia in a father and daughter. J. Amer. med. Ass. 168, 270–272 (1958)

33. Morley, A.A., Carew, J.P., Baikie, A.G.: Familial cyclical neutropenia. Brit. J. Haemat. 13, 719–738 (1967)

34. Kostmann, R.: Infantile genetic agranulocytosis (agranulocytosis infantilis hereditaria). A new recessive lethal disease in man. Acta paediat. scand. 105 (Suppl.), 1–78 (1956)

35. Fanconi, G.: Familial constitutional panmyelocytopathy, Fanconi's anemia (F.A.). I. Clinical aspects. Sem. Hemat. 4, 233–240 (1967)

36. Miller, M.E., Nilsson, U.R.: A familial deficiency of the phagocytosis-enhancing activity of serum related to a dysfunction of the fifth component of complement (C5). New Engl. J. Med. 282, 354–358 (1970)

37. Childs, B., Nyhan, W.L., Borden, M., Bard, L., Cooke, R.E.: Idiopathic hyperglycinemia and hyperglycinuria: a new disorder of amino acid metabolism. I. Pediatrics 27, 522–538 (1961)

38. Ando, T., Rasmussen, K., Nyhan, W.L., Donnell, G.N., Barnes, N.D.: Propionic acidemia in patients with ketotic hyperglycinemia. J. Pediat. 78, 827–832 (1971)

39. Constantopoulos, A., Najjar, V.A., Smith, J.W.: Tuftsin deficiency: a new syndrome with defective phagocytosis. J. Pediat. 80, 564–572 (1972)

40. Constantopoulos, A., Najjar, V.A.: Tuftsin deficiency syndrome. A report of two new cases. Acta paediat. scand. 62, 645–648 (1973)

41. Beiguelman, B.: Some remarks on the genetics of leprosy resistance. Acta Genet. med. (Roma) 17, 584–594 (1968)

Wiskott-Aldrich Syndrome
(Aldrich Syndrome)

In 1937 Wiskott [1] described three brothers with eczema, thrombocytopenia, and frequent infections. In 1954 Aldrich et al. [2] recognized the X-linked mode of inheritance of this condition.

Clinical Presentation. The disease is characterized by eczema, thrombocytopenia, and immunologic deficiency. The eczema is evident mostly during infancy. It mimics that of atopic dermatitis. The thrombocytopenia is present from early infancy, causing gastrointestinal bleeding and purpura. The immunologic deficiency results in recurrent in-

fections of the skin, middle ear, sinuses, and lungs. Lymphopenia, low IgM, high IgA, and low isoagglutinins are also noted (see also p. 156).

Occasional abnormalities include joint effusions, anemia, eosinophilia, and leukocytosis with myeloid hyperplasia.

Malignancies such as reticulum cell sarcoma, malignant lymphoma, myelogenous leukemia, or astrocytoma may develop.

Most patients die in infancy or childhood from bleeding, infection, or malignant neoplasia. The oldest survivor was 14 years old [3].

Pathology and Pathophysiology. The thymus is usually hypoplastic. The megakaryocytes are diminished. There may be eosinophilia and leukocytosis with myeloid hyperplasia [3].

In 1968 the immunologic defect was considered to be in the processing or recognition of antigens [4]. Later, evidence was presented that the defect involves the afferent limb of immunity [5].

Inheritance. X-linked recessive.

Treatment. Splenectomy and treatment with hydrocortisone analogues or γ-globulin have not been appreciably successful. Therapy with transfer factor has been attempted [6]. Bone marrow transplantation has been very successful [7].

References

1. Wiskott, A.: Familiärer angeborener Morbus Werlhofii? Mschr. Kinderheilk. 68, 212 (1937)

2. Aldrich, R.A., Steinberg, A.G., Campbell, D.C.: Pedigree demonstrating a sex-linked recessive condition characterized by draining ears, eczematoid dermatitis and bloody diarrhea. Pediatrics 13, 133–139 (1954)

3. Wolff, J.A.: Wiskott-Aldrich syndrome. Clinical, immunologic, and pathologic observations. J. Pediat. 70, 221-232 (1967)

4. Blaese, R.M., Strober, W., Brown, R.A., Waldmann, T.A.: The Wiskott-Aldrich syndrome. A disorder with a possible defect in antigen processing or recognition. Lancet 1968I, 1056–1060

5. Cooper, M.D., Chase, H.P., Lowman, J.T., Krivit, W., Good, R.A.: Wiskott-Aldrich syndrome. An immunologic deficiency disease involving the afferent limb of immunity. Amer. J. Med. 44, 499–513 (1968)

6. Levin, A.S., Spitler, L.E., Stiles, D.P., Fundenberg, H.H.: Wiskott-Aldrich syndrome, a genetically determined cellular immunologic deficiency: clinical and laboratory responses to therapy with transfer factor. Proc. nat. Acad. Sci. (Wash.) 67, 821–828 (1970)

7. Parkman, R., Rappeport, J., Geha, R., Belli, J., Cassady, R., Levey, R., Nathan, D.G., Rosen, F.S.: Complete correction of the Wiskott-Aldrich syndrome by allogeneic bone-marrow transplantation. New Engl. J. Med. 298, 921–927 (1978)

Chapter 8   Connective Tissue Disorders

Contents

Cutis Laxa (Chalazodermia, Dermatolysis, Dermatochalasis)

There are several varieties, genetic as well as acquired.

Clinical Presentation. The characteristic changes are present at birth or appear shortly afterwards [1] and progress to the stage in which the skin hangs in loose folds (Figs. 8.1 and 8.2). The facial appearance is of premature senility with the sagging jowls of the "bloodhound" facies (Figs. 8.3 and 8.4). The general skin surface is involved. The skin is extensible but not elastic or easily bruised. The face also shows a long upper lip, a tendency toward hook nose, shortening of the columella, and long earlobes [2]. Affected children have normal growth. The disease affects internal organs, especially the lungs (with emphysema and its sequelae). Other defects are hernias; rectal prolapse, gastrointestinal and urinary bladder diverticulae, large arteries, and excess of tissue around the vocal cords which gives a husky voice. Males with cutis laxa are impotent.

There is probably a distinct syndrome in which cutis laxa is associated with clouding of the cornea and mental retardation [2]. The corneal clouding is due to degeneration in the Bowman membrane. Congenital athetosis is also present.

Another syndrome is the association of cutis laxa with bone dystrophy [3]. The latter includes open and persistent fontanels, oxycephaly, hip dislocation, pigeon breast, and static scoliosis.

Pathology and Pathophysiology. The characteristic changes in the skin and other affected organs are reduction, fragmentation, and granular disruption of elastic fibers [1]. There is also an increase in acid mucopolysaccharides, while the collagen is normal [1].

Inheritance. Both autosomal dominant and autosomal recessive forms exist [4]. The dominant form is apparently free of pulmonary and other internal complications. The syndrome of cutis laxa, corneal clouding, and mental retardation is probably inherited as autosomal dominant, whereas that of cutis laxa and bone dystrophy is probably autosomal recessive.

Treatment. Plastic surgery gives good cosmetic results. Affection of each organ has to be managed as it arises.

References

1. Goltz, R.W., Hult, A.-M., Goldfarb, M., Gorlin, R.J.: Cutis laxa – a manifestation of generalized elastolysis. Arch. Derm. *92*, 373–387 (1965)
2. De Barsy, A.M., Moens, E., Dierckx, L.: Dwarfism, oligophrenia, and degeneration of the elastic tissue in skin and cornea. A new syndrome? Helv. paediat. Acta *23*, 305–313 (1968)
3. Fittke, H.: Über eine ungewöhnliche Form "multipler Erbabartung" (Chalodermie und Dysostose). Z. Kinderheilk. *63*, 510–523 (1942)
4. McKusick, V.A.: Heritable disorders of connective tissue, 4th ed., pp. 372–389. Saint Louis: Mosby, C.V. Co 1972

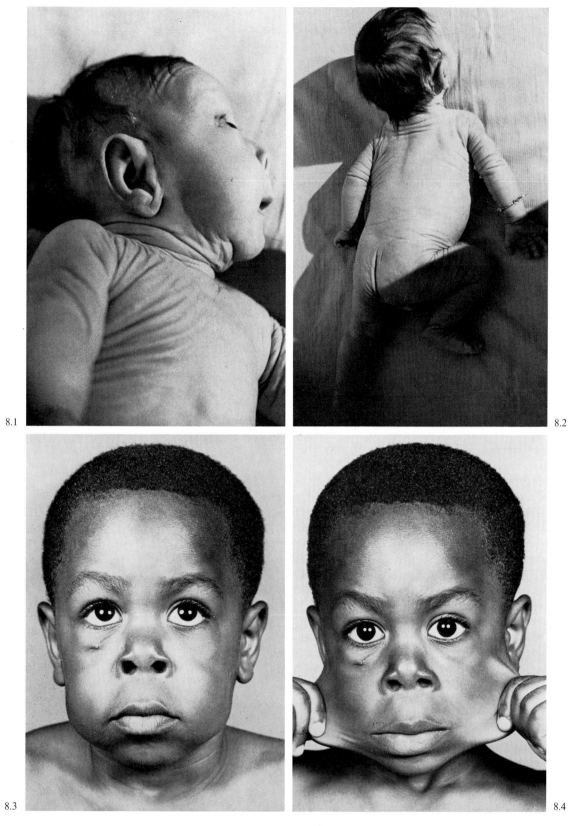

8.1

8.2

8.3

8.4

Figs. 8.1 and 8.2. Cutis laxa. Note loose folds of the skin. (Courtesy of Dr. F. C. Fraser)

Figs. 8.3 and 8.4. Cutis laxa. Lax skin of the cheeks giving the appearance of "bloodhound." The skin is extensible, but not elastic. Note long philtrum and short columella. (Courtesy of Dr. V. A. McKusick)

Ehlers-Danlos Syndrome
(Cutis Hyperelastica)

In 1682 van Meekeren described and illustrated the first definitive case [1]. The eponym refers to Ehlers [2] who described the loose-jointedness and subcutaneous hemorrhages and Danlos [3] who emphasized the pseudotumors.

Clinical Presentation. The syndrome is characterized by hyperelasticity of the skin, fragility of the tissues and blood vessels, and hyperextensibility of the joints.

The skin is velvety, chamoislike, and hyperextensible, but immediately returns to its original position when released (Figs. 8.5 and 8.6). Later in life it becomes lax and hangs in folds, especially around the elbows. It is fragile and easily bruised. Minor trauma results in gaping wounds. Healing is slow with formation of thin scars through which "molluscoid pseudotumors" develop, especially at pressure points (Figs. 8.7 and 8.8), and small pea-sized "spherules" of fat-containing cysts appear [4, 5]. The latter are frequently calcified.

Over the palms and soles the skin may be redundant [4]. Striae atrophicans are not formed. Acrocyanosis may frequently be encountered and Miescher elastoma may occur.

Hyperextensibility of the joints is characteristic, but of variable intensity (Figs. 8.9 and 8.10). "India-rubber men" and contortionists are persons with such skin and joint abnormalities. The ears project from the head, and there is ease in touching the tip of the nose with the tongue. Other skeletal abnormalities include joint effusions, kyphoscoliosis, spina bifida occulta, spondylolisthesis, ectopic bone formation, and short stature [4].

The eye changes include redundant folds around the eyes, epicanthic folds, hypertelorism, and strabismus [4]. Blue sclerae, corneal abnormalities, angioid streaks, and ectopic lenses occasionally occur. There may be gastrointestinal diverticula and bleeding, spontaneous rupture of the bowel, pneumothorax, dissecting aortal aneurysm, and rupture of large vessels. Affected fetuses are born prematurely because of early rupture of the membranes. The disease has been classified into the following seven types because of the heterogeneity of the syndrome [5]:

Type I or gravis type. The hyperelasticity, fragility, and bruisability of the skin and the hypermobility of the joints are severe.

Type II or mitis type. The manifestations are mild.
Type III or benign hypermobile type. The joint affection is severe while the skin changes are minimal.

Type IV or ecchymotic, arterial, or sack type. The main features are thin skin and prominent venous network. Bruisability is marked.

Type V or X-linked form with lysyl oxidase deficiency. The skin hyperelasticity is pronounced.

Type VI or protocollagen lysyl hydroxylase-deficient (or ocular) type. The skin and joint changes are associated with ocular complications [6].

Type VII or procollagen protease-deficient (arthrochalasis multiplex congenita) type. There is severe loose-jointedness and mild stretchability and bruisability of the skin [7].

Pathology and Pathophysiology. There do not seem to be any consistent histologic abnormalities in the collagen or elastic fibers. Foreign body giant cells may be seen in the pseudotumors. Calcification may be present there too. The evidence, in one syndrome type, of a deficiency of lysyl hydroxylase leading to paucity of hydroxylysyl residues in collagen [6] and, in another type, of a deficiency of procollagen protease which cleaves off the N-terminal end of collagen after it has been secreted from fibroblasts [7] lends support to the concept of a primary defect in the collagen fibers. This is further supported by the recent observation that fibroblasts from the skin of patients with type IV synthesize only type I collagen [8]. The absence of type III collagen in Ehlers-Danlos syndrome IV patients may lead to the fragility in their skin, blood vessels, and intestines.

Inheritance. Type V is inherited as X-linked, types VI and VII as autosomal recessive, and the others, which constitute the majority of cases, as autosomal dominant [4].

Treatment. The skin and joints should be protected from trauma. Pressure dressings and adhesive closures are recommended for wounds.

With asorbic acid supplementation, one patient affected with type VI or lysyl hydroxylase-deficient type was able to increase his urinary hydroxylysine excretion to near normal. His muscle strength and wound healing ability improved dramatically [9].

References

1. van Meekeren, J. A.: De dilatabilitate extraordinaria cutis. In: Observations medicochirugicae, Chap. 32. Amsterdam 1682
2. Ehlers, E.: Cutis laxa. Neigung zur Haemorrhagien in der Haut, Lockerung mehrerer Artikulationen. Derm. Z. *8*, 173–174 (1901)

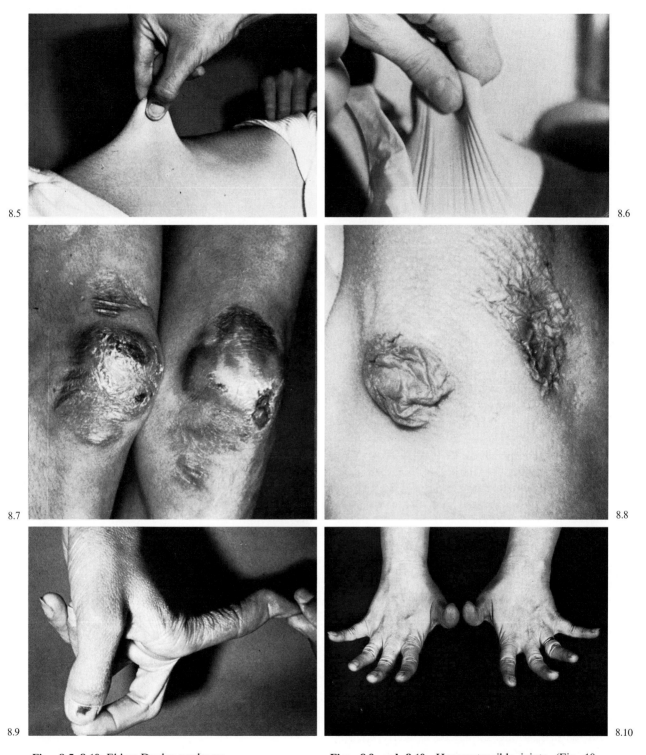

8.5

8.6

8.7

8.8

8.9

8.10

Figs. 8.5–8.10. Ehlers-Danlos syndrome

Figs. 8.5 and 8.6. Velvety, hyperextensible skin. (Fig. 6 – courtesy of Dr. F. C. Fraser)

Figs. 8.7 and 8.8. Thin scars and molluscoid pseudotumors at areas of pressure. (Courtesy of Dr. B. Moroz)

Figs. 8.9 and 8.10. Hyperextensible joints. (Fig. 10 – courtesy of Dr. V.A. McKusick, from Char, F.: In: The clinical delineation of birth defects. Bergsma, D. (ed.), Vol. VII, No. 8, pt. XII, pp. 300–301. Baltimore: Williams & Wilkins Co. 1971)

3. Danlos, M.: Un cas de cutis laxa avec tumeurs par contusion chronique des coudes et des genoux (xanthome juvénile pseudo-diabétique de M. M. Hallopeau et Macé de Lépinay). Bull. Soc. franç. Derm. Syph. *19*, 70–72 (1908)
4. McKusick, V.A.: Heritable disorders of connective tissue, 4th ed., pp. 292–371. Saint Louis: Mosby, C.V. Co. 1972
5. Beighton, P.: The Ehlers-Danlos syndrome. London: Heinemann 1970
6. Pinnell, S.R., Krane, S.M., Kenzora, J.E., Glimcher, M.J.: A heritable disorder of connective tissue. Hydroxylysine-deficient collagen disease. New Engl. J. Med. *286*, 1013–1020 (1972)
7. Lichtenstein, J.R., Martin, G.R., Kohn, L.D., Byers, P.H., McKusick, V.A.: Defect in conversion of procollagen to collagen in a form of Ehlers-Danlos syndrome. Science *182*, 298–300 (1973)
8. Pope, F.M., Martin, G.R., Lichtenstein, J.R., Penttinen, R., Gerson, B., Rowe, D.W., McKusick, V.A.: Patients with Ehlers-Danlos syndrome type IV lack type III collagen. Proc. nat. Acad. Sci. (Wash.) *72*, 1314–1316 (1975)
9. Elsas, L.J., Hollins, B., Pinnell, S.R.: Hydroxylysine-deficient collagen disease: effect of ascorbic acid. Amer. J. hum. Genet. *26*, 28A (1974)

Pseudoxanthoma Elasticum (Gronblad-Strandberg Syndrome)

Rigal first described this disorder in 1881 as an atypical xanthoma [1]. Darier, in 1896, identified it as a separate nonxanthomatous entity [2].

Clinical Presentation. The manifestations are mainly in the skin, eyes, and cardiovascular system.

The onset of the skin lesions is in early life. The classic lesions are yellowish papules or rhomboidal plaques bounded by skin lines [3]. The early lesions appear as accentuated skin lines, whereas the more advanced stages show redundant folds of lax skin [3] (Fig. 8.11). The neck and axillae are predominantly involved (Figs. 8.12–8.14). The inguinal folds, antecubital and popliteal areas, abdominal wall, cheeks, forehead, and penis may also be involved. Occasionally, elastosis perforans serpiginosa (Miescher elastoma) may be present.

The mucosal surface of the lips, palate, and vagina and the buccal mucosa may be similarly involved [3].

Angioid streaks of the fundus are the characteristic eye changes and appear in about 85% of cases [3]. Retinal pigmentation is frequently present and chorioretinal scarring with visual disturbances may result [3]. The severity of the eye changes does not parallel those of the skin.

The arterial involvement is manifested by weak pulse, arterial insufficiency in the extremities, coronary insufficiency, radiologic evidence of premature medial calcification of peripheral arteries, hemorrhage in several areas, and hypertension [4]. The most serious of these is gastrointestinal bleeding [3]. Psychiatric disorders may be encountered in these patients [4].

Pathology and Pathophysiology. The earliest abnormality seems to be calcification of elastic fibers, whereas the well-developed changes consist of masses of elastic-staining material in the middermis [3]. Similar changes occur in the elastic tissue of the Bruch membrane of the eye, the endocardium, and blood vessels. Ultrastructurally, the elastic fibers have unusual shapes, granular appearance, and calcium deposition [5]. There are no abnormalities in collagen biosynthesis but there may be increased degradation of connective tissue components [6]. The elastic modulus is higher in certain types of pseudoxanthoma elasticum (recessive type I) and lower in others (dominant types I and II) than in controls [7].

The present concept is that the primary defect is in the elastic fibers [4].

Inheritance. There is genetic heterogeneity in this disease. There seem to be four types of pseudoxanthoma elasticum: two autosomal recessives (recessive I and recessive II) and two autosomal dominants (dominant I and dominant II). In the dominant I and recessive I, the involvement is typically in the flexural areas with vascular disease and retinopathy. In dominant II and recessive II, the skin involvement is more generalized, but the systemic involvement is minimal [8, 9].

Pseudoxanthoma elasticum has been reported in association with Paget disease of bone, tumoral calcinosis with hyperphosphatemia, oculocutaneous albinism, hyperphosphatasia, and partial trisomy 14⁻ [10].

Treatment. There is no specific treatment. Vitamin E has been used. Plastic surgery may be of cosmetic help. The complications should be managed as they appear.

References

1. Rigal, D.: Observation pour servir à l'histoire de la chéloide diffuse xanthélasmique. Ann. Derm. Syph. (Paris) *2*, 491–493 (1881)
2. Darier, J.: Pseudoxanthoma elasticum. Mschr. Prakt. Derm. *23*, 609–611 (1896)
3. Goodman, R.M., Smith, E.W., Paton, D., Bergman, R.A., Siegel, C.L., Ottesen, O.E., Shelley, W.M., Pusch, A.L., McKusick, V.A.: Pseudoxanthoma elasticum: a clinical and histopathological study. Med. (Baltimore) *42*, 297–334 (1963)

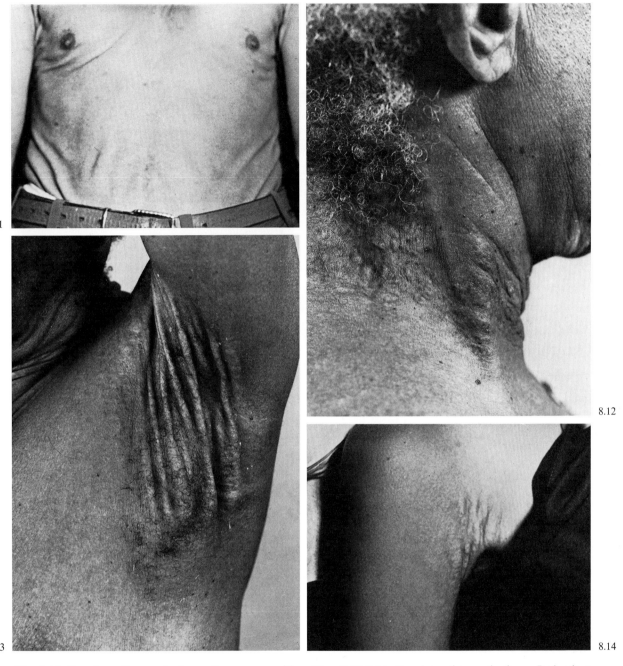

8.11

8.12

8.13

8.14

Fig. 8.11. Pseudoxanthoma elasticum. Severe case with generalized involvement of the skin

Figs. 8.12–8.14. Pseudoxanthoma elasticum. Redundant folds yellowish plaques in axillae and neck. (Figs. 12 and 13 – courtesy of Dr. V. A. McKusick, from Heard, M.G.: The clinical delineation of birth defects. Bergsma, D. (ed.), Vol. VII, No. 8, pt. XII, pp. 298–299. Baltimore: Williams & Wilkins Co. 1971)

4. McKusick, V.A.: Heritable disorders of connective tissue, 4th ed., pp. 475–520. Saint Louis: Mosby, C.V. Co. 1972
5. Piérard, J., Kint, A.: Le pseudoxanthome élastique. Sa structure en microscopie électronique. Ann. Derm. Syph. (Paris) 97, 481–492 (1970)
6. Uitto, J., Lindy, S., Turto, H., Danielsen, L.L.: Biochemical characterization of pseudoxanthoma elasticum: collagen biosynthesis in the skin. J. invest. Derm. 57, 44–48 (1971)
7. Harvey, W., Pope, F.M., Grahame, R.: Cutaneous extensibility in pseudo-xanthoma elasticum. Brit. J. Derm. 92, 679–683 (1975)
8. Pope, F.M.: Two types of autosomal recessive pseudoxanthoma elasticum. Arch. Derm. 110, 209–212 (1974)
9. Pope, F.M.: Autosomal dominant pseudoxanthoma elasticum. J. med. Genet. 11, 152–157 (1974)
10. Pinnel, S.R.: Disorders of collagen. In: The metabolic basis of inherited disease. Stanbury, J.B., Wyngaarden, J.B., Fredrickson, D.S. (eds.), 4th ed., pp. 1366–1394. New York: McGraw-Hill Book Co. 1978

Marfan Syndrome (Arachnodactyly, Dolichostenomelia)

In 1896 Marfan first described the syndrome which now bears his name [1].

Clinical Presentation. The syndrome consists of defects in the skeletal, ocular, and cardiovascular systems. There is excessive elongation of the limbs, loose-jointedness, scoliosis, anterior chest deformity, ectopic lenses, myopia, retinal detachment, and a defect in the tunica media of the ascending aorta leading to diffuse and/or dissecting aneurysm and mitral regurgitation [2] (Figs. 8.15–8.17). Other abnormalities include malformations of the cardiovascular system, lungs, eyes, kidneys, and stomach [1].
The skin involvement is rare. Elastoma perforans (Miescher) [3] and striae of the skin in the pectoral and deltoid areas may occur [4].
Kindreds with combinations of some features of Marfan syndrome and Ehlers-Danlos syndrome have been reported [5, 6]. In general, affected individuals have a marfanoid habitus, heart lesions, joint hypermobility, and skin stretchability. These features may constitute a separate syndrome, "marfanoid hypermobility syndrome," which is probably inherited as autosomal dominant.

Pathology and Pathophysiology. In the affected aorta, there is degeneration of the elastic lamellae [2]. Histologic studies of other organs including the skin are inconsistent. The basic defect may be in the elastic fibers or, more likely, in collagen.

Inheritance. Autosomal dominant with variable penetrance. New mutations are responsible for around 15% of the patients and are often associated with increased parental age [7].

Treatment. Treatment is along four lines: inhibition of growth by hormonal induction of puberty, use of anabolic steroids, use of β-blockers to reduce stress on the aorta, and surgical intervention for complications [2].

References

1. Marfan, A.B.: Un cas de déformation congénitale des quatre membres plus prononcée aux extrémités charactérisée par l'allongement des os avec un certain degré d'amincissement, Bull. Mem. Soc. med. Hôp. Paris 13, 220 (1896)
2. McKusick, V.A.: Heritable disorders of connective tissue, 4th ed., pp. 61–223. Saint Louis: Mosby, C.V. Co. 1972
3. Haber, H.: Miescher's elastoma (elastoma intrapapillare perforans verruciforme) Brit. J. Derm. 71, 85–96 (1959)
4. Loveman, A.B., Gordon, A.M., Fliegelman, M.T.: Marfan's syndrome. Some cutaneous aspects. Arch. Derm. 87, 428–435 (1963)
5. Goodman, R.M., Wooley, C.F., Frazier, R.L., Covault, L.: Ehlers-Danlos syndrome occurring together with the Marfan syndrome. Report of a case with other family members affected. New Engl. J. Med. 273, 514–519 (1965)
6. Walker, B.A., Beighton, P.H., Murdoch, J.L.: The Marfanoid hypermobility syndrome. Ann. intern. Med. 71, 349–352 (1969)
7. Murdoch, J.L., Walker, B.A., McKusick, V.A.: Parental age effects on the occurrence of new mutations for the Marfan syndrome. Ann. hum. Genet., 35, 331–336 (1972)

Osteogenesis Imperfecta

Clinical Presentation. The main features of this disease are "brittle bones," deafness, and blue sclerae. The joints are loose and hernias frequently occur. The fractures may be present at birth (osteogenesis imperfecta congenita) or occur later in life (osteogenesis imperfecta tarda).
The skin is thin and translucent, resembling the skin of the aged. Healing of wounds results in wide scars. Capillary fragility is increased [1]. Macular atrophy of the skin has been described [2].

Pathology and Pathophysiology. The defect is in the maturation of collagen or in the synthesis of a different species of collagen [3]. The collagen content per unit area is decreased [4]. Cells cultured from the skin of certain patients with osteogenesis imperfecta synthesize a higher proportion of type III collagen than cells from normal skin [5].

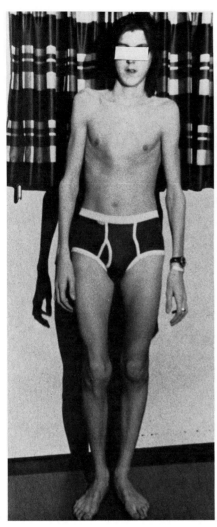

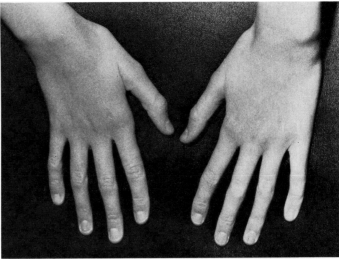

8.16

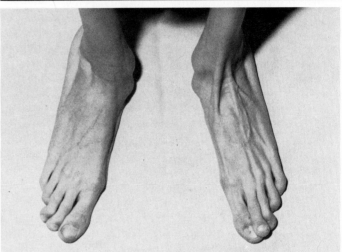

8.15   8.17

Figs. 8.15–8.17. Marfan syndrome

Fig. 8.15. General view showing long limbs, long face, and pectus carinatum. (Courtesy of Dr. F. C. Fraser)

Fig. 8.16. Arachnodactyly. (Courtesy of Dr. F. C. Fraser)

Fig. 8.17. Long feet. (Courtesy of Dr. F. C. Fraser)

Inheritance. Osteogenesis imperfecta is very heterogeneous [6]. The inheritance is usually autosomal dominant, although a rare form is inherited as autosomal recessive [3, 6]. The congenita and tarda forms may coexist in the same family.

Treatment. Surgical correction of leg deformities may be helpful. Several treatments have been recommended including fluoride, androgens, magnesium oxide, and calcitonin. This last treatment shows the most promise of being effective [7].

References

1. Siegel, B.M., Friedman, I.A., Schwartz, S.O.: Hemorrhagic disease in osteogenesis imperfecta. Study of platelet functional defect. Amer. J. Med. *22*, 315–321 (1957)
2. Blegvad, O., Haxthausen, H.: Blue sclerotics and brittle bones, with macular atrophy of the skin and zonular cataract. Brit. med. J. *1921II*, 1071–1072
3. McKusick, V.A.: Heritable disorders of connective tissue, 4th ed., pp. 390–454. Saint Louis: Mosby, C.V. Co. 1972
4. Stevenson, C.J., Bottoms, E., Shuster, S.: Skin collagen in osteogenesis imperfecta. Lancet *1970I*, 860–861
5. Penttinen, R.P., Lichtenstein, J.R., Martin, G.R., McKusick, V.A.: Abnormal collagen metabolism in cultured cells in osteogenesis imperfecta. Proc. nat. Acad. Sci. (Wash.) *72*, 586–589 (1975)
6. Beighton, P.: Inherited disorders of the skeleton, pp. 87–96. Edinburgh: Churchill Livingstone 1978
7. Pinnel, S.R.: Disorders of collagen. In: The metabolic basis of inherited disease. Stanbury, J.B., Wyngaarden, J.B., Fredrickson, D.S. (eds.), 4th ed., pp. 1366–1399. New York: McGraw-Hill Book Co. 1978

Puretic Syndrome

This syndrome is characterized by the appearance around the age of 3 months of painful contractures of the shoulders, elbows, hips, and knees; deformities of face and skull; stunted growth; osteolysis of terminal phalanges; multiple, large subcutaneous nodes, some calcified; sclerodermoid and atrophic changes in the skin; and repeated suppurative infections of the skin, eyes, and ears [1].

The nodes are formed as a result of changes in the connective tissue of the lower dermis: PAS-positive, diastase-resistant, homogeneous amorphous masses, with very fine fibrils and granules and absent elastic fibers [1]. The skin has a low fat content and a high protein content, with an unusually low hydroxyproline and high hexosamine [1]. Inheritance is autosomal recessive. Treatment is aimed primarily at combating secondary infection. The affected joints are helped by corticosteroids and physiotherapy.

Reference

1. Puretić, S., Puretić, B., Fiser-Herman, M., Adamćić, M.: A unique form of mesenchymal dysplasia. Brit. J. Derm. *74*, 8–19 (1962)

Elastosis Perforans Serpiginosa (Miescher Elastoma, Elastoma Intrapapillare Perforans Verruciforme)

First described by Lutz in 1953 [1], this disease was further delineated by Miescher in 1955 [2].

Clinical Presentation. The majority of patients are young adults. Both sexes are affected. The eruption has a predilection for the sides of the neck and upper extremities and occurs less frequently on the face, trunk, and lower extremities [3]. The primary lesion is a keratotic, conical papule, 2–5 mm in diameter, discrete or clustered to form an annular, serpiginous, or arcuate arrangement [3, 4] (Fig. 8.18). When the plug is forcibly removed, a bleeding crater remains. On healing, the skin is erythematous, hypopigmented, or atrophic [4]. The eruption is usually asymptomatic. Keloid formation is frequent.

The disease is associated with inherited disorders of connective tissue in more than one-third of the cases. The usual associated disorders are Down syndrome (mongolism), Ehlers-Danlos syndrome, osteogenesis imperfecta, Marfan syndrome, pseudoxanthoma elasticum, Rothmund-Thomson syndrome, and acrogeria [3, 4]. One family (a sister and two brothers) has been reported with elastosis perforans serpiginosa as an isolated trait [5].

Pathology and Pathophysiology. Characteristically, there are transepidermal, parafollicular, or transfollicular channels of perforation filled with elastic fibers, cellular debris, and keratin [3, 4]. The epidermis is hyperkeratotic and acanthotic. The dermis around the channel shows an inflammatory reaction with foreign body giant cells [3, 4] and thick elastic fibers [3]. It is postulated that the basic defect is in the connective tissue which incites a transepithelial elimination [3, 4].

Inheritance. Probably autosomal dominant.

Treatment. Most therapeutic measures have been unsatisfactory. Cryotherapy or occlusion with cellophane tape may be helpful [3]. Electrosurgery often results in keloids and is not recommended.

References

1. Lutz, W.: Keratosis follicularis serpiginosa. Dermatologica (Basel) *106*, 318–320 (1953)
2. Miescher, G.: Elastoma intrapapillare perforans verruciforme. Dermatologica (Basel) *110*, 254–266 (1955)
3. Mehregan, A.H.: Elastosis perforans serpiginosa. A review of the literature and report of 11 cases. Arch. Derm. *97*, 381–393 (1968)
4. Smith, E.W., Malak, J.A., Goodman, R.M., McKusick, V.A.: Reactive perforating elastosis: a feature of certain genetic disorders. Bull. Johns Hopkins Hosp. *111*, 235–251 (1962)
5. Woerdeman, M.J., Bour, D.J.H., Bijlsma, J.B.: Elastosis perforans serpiginosa. Report of a family with a chromosomal investigation. Arch. Derm. *92*, 559–560 (1965)

Familial Reactive Collagenosis

In 1967 Mehregan et al. drew attention to this entity [1]. Since then, several reports of familial occurrence have appeared [2–5].

Clinical Presentation. The onset is usually in early childhood with lesions involving primarily the hands and feet, forearms, legs, face, and scalp. Less often, the trunk and buttocks are affected, while the

Fig. 8.18. Elastosis perforans serpiginosa. Annular arcuate grouping of keratotic papules. (Courtesy of Dr. I. Zeligman)

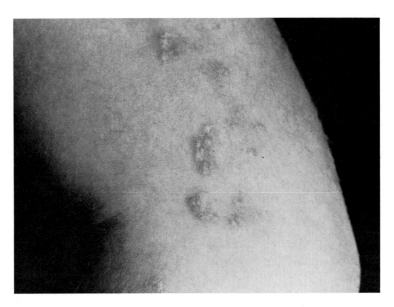

palms and soles are characteristically spared [5]. The initial lesion is a pinhead-sized, skin-colored papule that increases in size to about 4–6 mm, developing a central umbilication [1]. This central depression is filled with an adherent keratinous plug, the removal of which causes bleeding [4]. The maximum size is reached in about a month, after which the lesions regress spontaneously in 6–8 weeks [1, 4]. Slight atrophy and mild pigmentary changes may remain at the sites of the healed lesions [4, 5]. New lesions appear as older lesions involute [5]. The eruption is asymptomatic, but is accentuated by trauma [1–5] and atmospheric cold [5].

Pathology and Pathophysiology. The initial characteristic change is the appearance of a hematoxylinophilic mass of connective tissue in the upper dermis [1]. In the well-developed lesion, there is a cup-shaped depression in the epidermis filled with parakeratotic keratin, necrobiotic connective tissue, degenerating inflammatory cells, and some normal collagen bundles. These constituents of the plug eventually extrude through the disrupted epidermis [1]. This is the hallmark of the disease [5]. The process is provoked by superficial trauma to the skin, suggesting that the primary defect is in the pars papillaris of the dermis [5]. The collagen there undergoes necrobiotic changes that start the cycle whereby the altered connective tissue is eliminated via the epidermis [6].

Inheritance. Probably autosomal recessive [5].

Treatment. Avoidance of trauma is the mainstay of treatment.

References

1. Mehregan, A.H., Schwartz, O.D., Livingood, C.S.: Reactive perforating collagenosis. Arch. Derm. *96*, 277–282 (1967)
2. Mehregan, A.H.: Transepithelial elimination. Curr. Probl. Derm. *3*, 124 (1970)
3. Weiner, A.L.: Reactive perforating collagenosis. Arch. Derm. *102*, 540–544 (1970)
4. Nair, B.K.H., Sarojini, P.A., Basheer, A.M., Nair, C.H.K.: Reactive perforating collagenosis. Brit. J. Derm. *91*, 399–403 (1974)
5. Kanan, M.W.: Familial reactive perforating collagenosis and intolerance to cold. Brit. J. Derm. *91*, 405–414 (1974)
6. Malak, J.A., Kurban, A.K.: "Catharsis": an excretory function of the epidermis. Brit. J. Derm. *84*, 516–522 (1971)

Mucopolysaccharidoses

In 1917 Hunter [1] reported two brothers with physical and radiologic findings typical of the X-linked mucopolysaccharidosis (MPS) now called MPS II or the *Hunter syndrome*. In 1919 Hurler [2] described patients who probably suffered from the autosomal recessive form now referred to as MPS I or the *Hurler syndrome*. Since then, several syndromes with similar features have been published under the descriptive, but unnecessarily cruel, term "gargoylism" [3, 4]. In 1952 the Hurler syndrome was classified as a mucopolysaccharidosis after dermatan sulfate was isolated from the liver of two patients [5]. By 1966 six distinct mucopolysaccharidoses had been differentiated by combined clinical, genetic, and biochemical studies [6]. More have since been added to the list and, based on recent developments and studies, the mucopolysaccharidoses were reclassified in 1972 [7].

In 1970 the term *genetic mucolipidoses* was coined to designate disorders resembling mucopolysaccharidoses and sphingolipidoses [8]. Both the mucopolysaccharidoses and the mucolipidoses are *mucopolysaccharide storage diseases*. However, a *mucopolysaccharidosis* is deficient in a single enzyme, whereas in a *mucolipidosis* multiple lysosomal hydrolases are deficient in some cells and are elevated in body fluids [9–12].

Table 8.1 summarizes the new classification of the mucopolysaccharide storage diseases and their genetic and enzymatic defects. However, further discussion will concentrate only on the mucopolysaccharidoses.

Clinical Presentation. As the prototype mucopolysaccharidosis, MPS I H, or the Hurler syndrome, presents the following clinical features: lumbar gibbus, stiff joints, broad hands, deformity of the chest, dwarfism, clouding of the cornea, coarse facies, hepatosplenomegaly, mental retardation, and deafness (Figs. 8.19–8.22). The disease becomes clinically evident in infancy and is progressive. The usual causes of death are respiratory infection and cardiac failure.

A high concentration of mucopolysaccharides is found in the urine, along with metachromatic granules in the circulating lymphocytes or bone marrow cells. The excessive urinary mucopolysaccharides are dermatan sulfate and heparan sulfate.

Simple tests for excessive acid mucopolysaccharides in the urine have been devised. One of these uses the turbidity produced with acidified bovine serum albumin [15], while another uses a filter paper with metachromasia produced by toluidine blue [16].

The Skin in Mucopolysaccharidoses

MPS I H (Hurler syndrome). The skin is coarse, leathery, thick, inelastic, and hard (Fig. 8.23). Generalized hirsutism is usually present [17] (Figs. 8.19–8.22).

MPS I S (Scheie syndrome). There is excessive body hair along with the "carpal tunnel" syndrome bilaterally. The skin over the fingers appears taut and firmly bound to the underlying structures. A few, solitary spider telangiectases are found over the face, neck, chest, forearms, and hands.

MPS II (Hunter syndrome). The skin presents with grooving and either ridged or nodular thickening, especially over the upper arms and thorax, symmetrically distributed in an area of 6 by 10 cm from the angle of the scapula to the axillary line (Fig. 8.24). Hypertrichosis is usually striking [18, 19].

MPS III (Sanfilippo syndrome). Mild hypertrichosis.

MPS IV (Morquio syndrome). The skin is loose, thickened, tough, and inelastic, particularly over the limbs. Telangiectasia is found, especially on the face and extremities [20].

MPS VI (Maroteaux-Lamy syndrome). In two affected sisters the subcutaneous tissues of the volar surface of the second to fourth fingers were thickened [21].

Pathology and Pathophysiology. In 1964 the ultrastructure of hepatic cells in Hurler disease was described [22] and the mucopolysaccharidoses were classified as "lysosomal diseases" the following year [23, 24].

In vitro studies of fibroblasts have shown deficiencies in corrective factors in several of these disorders [25–27]. Subsequently, specific enzymatic deficiencies were discovered in most of them [28–36] (see Table 8.1). In the Hurler, Hunter, Sanfilippo A, and Maroteaux-Lamy syndromes, intrauterine diagnosis is possible [9, 37].

In the Hurler and Scheie diseases light microscopy of the skin reveals the diffusely vacuolated cytoplasm of basal and spinous cells. In some, a large perinuclear vacuole is present, displacing the nucleus, which assumes a crescent shape. Similar changes are present in the eccrine sweat duct and gland. The large, vacuolated, mononuclear cells just beneath the basement membrane contain large numbers of metachromatic granules in the vacuoles. Vacuolated cells, containing intensely metachromatic granules, are present throughout the dermis in perivascular and periappendageal locations. The hair follicles show some vacuolization in the outer root sheath cells [17].

Electron microscopic examination of the skin of patients with Hurler syndrome reveals that many prickle cells contain a single, very large vacuole indenting the nucleus. Dermal fibroblasts and macrophages contain large numbers of cytoplasmic vacuoles that are limited by a single membrane. It seems likely that these vacuoles contain secretory products, mainly acid mucopolysaccharides [38]. Similar changes have also been described in Hunter syndrome [39].

Inheritance. See Table 8.1.

Treatment. Clinical and chemical improvement with plasma infusions has been noted [40]. Therapy by enzyme replacement is promising.

Table 8.1. Mucopolysaccharide storage diseases[a]

Designation	Clinical presentation	Inheritance	Deficient enzyme
MPS I H Hurler syndrome	Early clouding of cornea, coarse features, mental retardation, death before age of 10 years	Autosomal recessive	α-L-Iduronidase
MPS I S Scheie syndrome	Stiff joints, cloudy cornea, aortic regurgitation, normal intelligence, normal lifespan	Autosomal recessive	α-L-Iduronidase
MPS I H/S Hurler-Scheie compound	Phenotype intermediate between Hurler and Scheie	Genetic compound of MPS I H and I S genes	α-L-Iduronidase
MPS II A Hunter syndrome, severe form	No clouding of cornea, milder course than in MPS I H, death before age of 15 years	X-linked recessive (the gene lyonizes) [13]	Iduronate sulfatase
MPS II B Hunter syndrome, mild form	Survival until age of 30–50 years, fair intelligence	X-linked recessive (allelic to MPS II A)	Iduronate sulfatase
MPS III A Sanfilippo syndrome A	Mild somatic and severe central nervous system signs	Autosomal recessive	Heparan N-sulfatase
MPS III B Sanfilippo syndrome B		Autosomal recessive	N-Acetyl-α-D-glucosaminidase
MPS IV A Morquio syndrome	Severe bone changes of distinctive type, cloudy cornea, aortic regurgitation	Autosomal recessive	Hexosamine 6-sulfatase
MPS IV B Morquio-like syndrome	Severe bone changes of distinctive type, cloudy cornea, aortic regurgitation	Autosomal recessive [14]	β-Galactosidase
MPS V	Vacant (formerly Scheie syndrome)		
MPS VI A Maroteaux-Lamy syndrome, classic form	Severe osseous and corneal changes, normal intellect	Autosomal recessive	Arylsulfatase B
MPS VI B Maroteaux-Lamy syndrome, mild form		Autosomal recessive (allelic to MPS VI A)	Arylsulfatase B
MPS VII β-Glucuronidase deficiency	Hepatosplenomegaly, dysostosis multiplex, white cell inclusions, mental retardation	Autosomal recessive	β-Glucuronidase
ML II Mucolipidosis II (I-cell disease)	Dysostosis multiplex with early onset (resembling MPS I H, but more severe), gingival hyperplasia; no mucopolysaccchariduria	Autosomal recessive	Multiple lysosomal hydrolases deficient in some cells, elevated in body fluids
ML III Mucolipidosis III (pseudo-Hurler polydystrophy)	Stiff joints, cloudy cornea, short stature, aortic valve disease; no mucopolysacchariduria	Autosomal recessive (? allelic with ML II)	Same as ML II
Multiple sulfatidosis (Austin variant of metachromatic leuko-dystrophy (MLD))	Progressive neurologic deterioration, hepatosplenomegaly, white blood cell inclusions; mucopolysacchariduria present	Autosomal recessive	Multiple sulfatases

[a] From McKusick et al. [9], with permission.

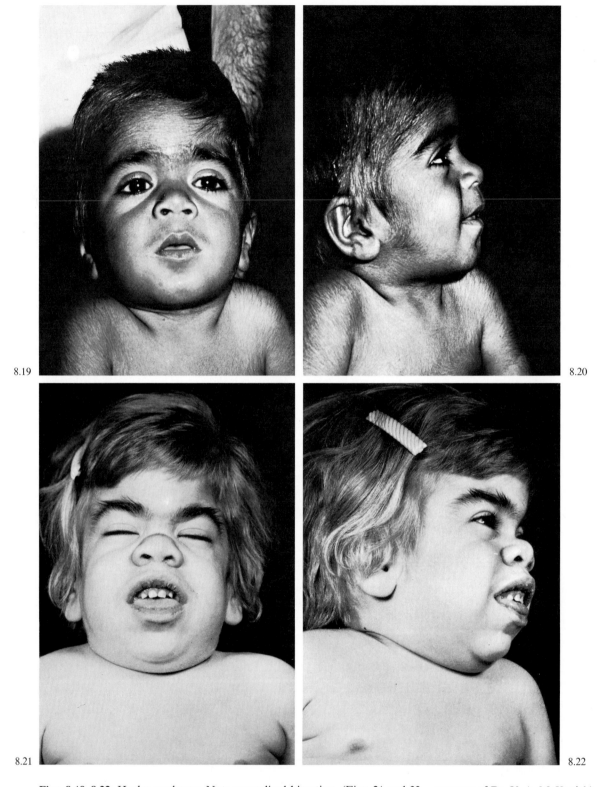

Figs. 8.19–8.22. Hurler syndrome. Note generalized hirsutism. (Figs. 21 and 22 – courtesy of Dr. V. A. McKusick)

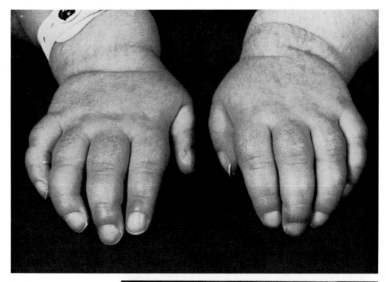

8.23

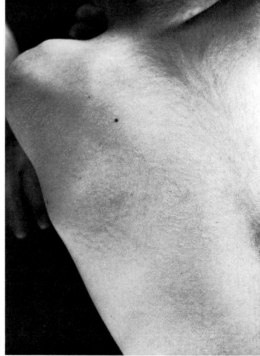

8.24

Fig. 8.23. Hurler syndrome. (Note leathery, thick skin of the hands with hirsutism)

Fig. 8.24. Hunter syndrome. Note mildly nodular thickening over the left scapular area

References

1. Hunter, C.: A rare disease in two brothers. Proc. roy. Soc. Med. *10*, 104–116 (1917)
2. Hurler, G.: Über einen Typ multipler Abartungen, vorwiegend am Skeletsystem. Z. Kinderheilk. *24*, 220–234 (1919)
3. Cockayne, E.A.: Gargoylism (chondro-osteodystrophy, hepatosplenomegaly, deafness) in two brothers. Proc. roy. Soc. Med. *30*, 104–107 (1936)
4. Ellis, R.W.B., Sheldon, W., Capon, N.B.: Gargoylism (chondro-osteo-dystrophy, corneal opacities, hepatosplenomegaly and mental deficiency). Quart. J. Med. *5*, 119–139 (1936)
5. Brante, G.: Gargoylism: a mucopolysaccharidosis? Scand. J. clin. lab. Invest. *4*, 43–46 (1952)
6. McKusick, V.A.: Heritable disorders of connective tissue, 3rd ed., pp. 325–399. Saint Louis: Mosby, C.V. Co. 1966
7. McKusick, V.A.: Heritable disorders of connective tissue, 4th ed., pp. 521–686. Saint Louis: Mosby, C.V. Co. 1972
8. Spranger, J.W., Wiedemann, H.R.: The genetic mucolipidoses. Diagnosis and differential diagnosis. Humangenetik *9*, 113–139 (1970)
9. McKusick, V.A., Neufeld, E.F., Kelly, T.E.: The mucopolysaccharide storage diseases. In: The metabolic basis of inherited disease. Stanbury, J.B., Wyngaarden, J.B., Fredrickson, D.S. (eds.), 4th ed., pp. 1282–1307. New York: McGraw-Hill Book Co. 1978
10. Glaser, J.H., McAlister, W.E., Sly, W.S.: Genetic heterogeneity in multiple lysosomal hydrolase deficiency. J. Pediat. *85*, 192–198 (1974)
11. Leroy, J.G., Ho, M.W., MacBrinn, M.X., Zielke, K., Jacob, J., O'Brien, J.S.: I-cell disease; biochemical studies. Pediat. Res. *6*, 752–757 (1972)

12. Liebaers, I., Neufeld, E.F.: Iduronate sulfatase activity in serum, lymphocytes, and fibroplasts – simplified diagnosis of the Hunter syndrome. Pediat. Res. 10, 733–736 (1976)

13. Danes, B.S., Bearn, A.G.: Hurler's syndrome: a genetic study of clones in cell culture with particular reference to the Lyon hypothesis. J. exp. Med. 126, 509–522 (1967)

14. Arbisser, A.I., Donelly, K.A., Scott, C.I., Jr., DiFerrante, N., Singh, J., Stevenson, R.E., Aylesworth, A.S., Howell, R.R.: Morquio-like syndrome with beta-galactose deficiency and normal hexosamine sulfatase activity: mucopolysaccharidosis IVB. Amer. J. med. Genet. 1, 195–205 (1977)

15. Dorfman, A., Ott, M.L.: A turbidimetric method for the assay of hyaluronidase. J. biol. Chem. 172, 367–375 (1948)

16. Berry, H.K., Spinanger, J.: A paper spot test useful in study of Hurler's syndrome. J. lab. clin. Med. 55, 136–138 (1960)

17. Hambrick, G.W., Jr., Scheie, H.G.: Studies of the skin in Hurler's syndrome. Mucopolysaccharidosis. Arch. Derm. 85, 455–470 (1962)

18. Cole, H.N., Jr., Irving, R.C., Lund, H.Z., Mercer, R.D., Schneider, R.W.: Gargoylism with cutaneous manifestations. Arch. Derm. Syph. 66, 371–383 (1952)

19. Andersson, B., Tandberg, O.: Lipochondrodystrophy (gargoylism, Hurler's syndrome) with specific cutaneous deposits. Acta paediat. 41, 162–167 (1952)

20. Greaves, M.W., Inman, P.M.: Cutaneous changes in the Morquio syndrome. Brit. J. Derm. 81, 29–36 (1969)

21. Spranger, J.W., Koch, F., McKusick, V.A., Natzschka, J., Wiedemann, H.-R., Zellweger, H.: Mucopolysaccharidosis VI (Maroteaux-Lamy's disease). Helv. paediat. Acta 25, 337–362 (1970)

22. Van Hoof, F., Hers, H.G.: L'ultrastructure des cellules hépatiques dans la maladie de Hurler (gargoylisme). C.R. Acad. Sci. [D] (Paris) 259, 1281–1283 (1964)

23. Hers, H.G.: Inborn lysosomal diseases. Gastroenterology 48, 625–633 (1965)

24. Van Hoof, F., Hers, H.G.: The abnormalities of lysosomal enzymes in mucopolysaccharidoses. Europ. J. Biochem. 7, 34–44 (1968)

25. Fratantoni, J.C., Hall, C.W., Neufeld, E.F.: Hurler and Hunter syndromes: mutual correction of the defect in cultured fibroblasts. Science 162, 570–572 (1968)

26. Barton, R.W., Neufeld, E.F.: A distinct biochemical deficit in the Maroteaux-Lamy syndrome (mucopolysaccharidosis VI). J. Pediat. 80, 114–116 (1972)

27. Cantz, M., Chrambach, A., Bach, G., Neufeld, E.F.: The Hunter corrective factor. Purification and preliminary characterization. J. biol. Chem. 247, 5456–5462 (1972)

28. Bach, G., Friedman, R., Weissmann, B., Neufeld, E.F.: The defect in the Hurler and Scheie syndromes: deficiency of α-L-iduronidase. Proc. nat. Acad. Sci. (Wash.) 69, 2048–2051 (1972)

29. Matalon, R., Dorfman, A.: Hurler's syndrome, an α-L-iduronidase deficiency. Biochem. biophys. Res. Commun. 47, 959–964 (1972)

30. Bach, G., Eisenberg, F., Jr., Cantz, M., Neufeld, E.F.: The defect in the Hunter syndrome: deficiency of sulfoiduronate sulfatase. Proc. nat. Acad. Sci. (Wash.) 70, 2134–2138 (1973)

31. Sjoberg, I., Fransson, L.A., Matalon, R., Dorfman, A.: Hunter's syndrome: a deficiency of L-idurono-sulfate sulfatase. Biochem. biophys. Res. Commun. 54, 1125–1132 (1973)

32. Kresse, H.: Mucopolysaccharidosis III A (Sanfilippo disease): deficiency of heparin sulfamidase in skin fibroblasts and leucocytes. Biochem. biophys. Res. Commun. 54, 1111–1118 (1973)

33. Matalon, R., Dorfman, A.: Sanfilippo A syndrome. Sulfamidase deficiency in cultured skin fibroblasts and liver. J. clin. Invest. 54, 907–912 (1974)

34. O'Brien, J.S.: Sanfilippo syndrome: profound deficiency of alpha-acetylglucosaminidase activity in organs and skin fibroblasts from type-B patients. Proc. nat. Acad. Sci. (Wash.) 69, 1720–1722 (1972)

35. Von Figura, K., Kresse, H.: The Sanfilippo B corrective factor: an N-acetyl-alpha-D-glucosaminidase. Biochem. biophys. Res. Commun. 48, 262–269 (1972)

36. Fluharty, A.L., Stevens, R.L., Sanders, D.L., Kihara, H.: Arylsulfatase B deficiency in Maroteaux-Lamy syndrome cultured fibroblasts. Biochem. biophys. Res. Commun. 59, 455–461 (1974)

37. Fratantoni, J.C., Neufeld, E.F., Uhlendorf, B.W., Jacobson, C.B.: Intrauterine diagnosis of the Hurler and Hunter syndrome. New Engl. J. Med. 280, 686–688 (1969)

38. DeCloux, R.J., Friederici, H.H.R.: Ultrastructural studies of the skin in Hurler's syndrome. Arch. Path. 88, 350–358 (1969)

39. Spicer, S.S., Garvin, A.J., Wohltmann, H.J., Simson, J.A.V.: Ultrastructure of skin in patients with mucopolysaccharidoses. Lab. Invest. 31, 488–502 (1974)

40. DiFerrante, N., Nichols, B.L., Donnelly, P.V., Neri, G., Hrgovcic, R., Berglund, R.K.: Induced degradation of glycosaminoglycans in Hurler's and Hunter's syndromes by plasma infusion. Proc. nat. Acad. Sci. (Wash.) 68, 303–307 (1971)

Heredity and Autoimmune Diseases

A number of observations have drawn attention to the relationship among individual connective tissue disorders and their common genetic background. These observations include: (a) overlapping of the signs and symptoms of the individual connective tissue diseases with each other and with agammaglobulinemia, Sjögren syndrome, thyroiditis, and others [1]; (b) familial occurrence of several of these diseases, especially systemic lupus erythematosus (SLE) (Figs. 8.25–8.27) [2] and rheumatoid arthritis [3]; (c) occurrence of connective tissue disorders in relatives of probands, often differing from that of the proband [1]; and (d) the presence of a large number of autoantibodies in patients with these disorders and in their families. These observations have led to the postulate that certain connective tissue disorders (lupus erythematosus, scleroderma, dermatomyositis, rheumatoid arthritis, polyarteritis nodosa) share a basic genetic diathesis which involves immunologic mechanisms. The exact nature of these mechanisms remains unclear. In SLE, using mathematical analyses of age and sex distribution, it has been suggested that probably three dominant X-linked alleles and autosomal factors at one or more loci are operative [4], and that SLE is a separate entity and has a genetic basis different from discoid lupus erythematosus [5].

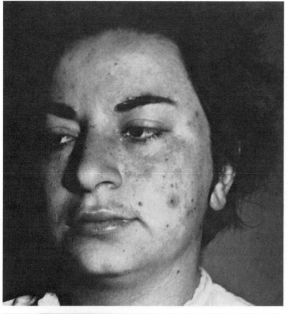

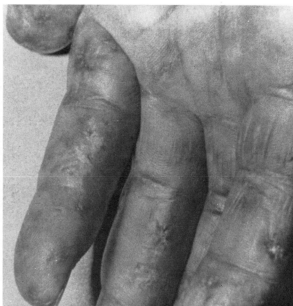

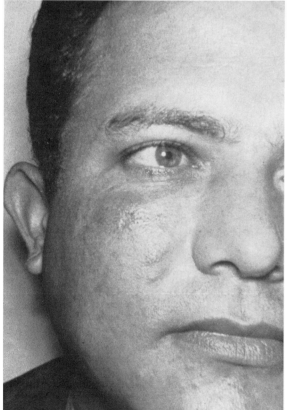

8.25

8.26

8.27

Figs. 8.25–8.27. Systemic lupus erythematosus

Fig. 8.25. Maculopapular erythematous eruptions on the face

Fig. 8.26. Characteristic infiltrative lesions on the palm. (Courtesy of Dr. I. Zeligman)

Fig. 8.27. Erythematous infiltrated plaque over the right cheek. (Courtesy of Dr. I. Zeligman)

References

1. Ziff, M.: Genetics, hypersensitivity and the connective tissue diseases. Amer. J. Med. *30*, 1–7 (1961)
2. Leonhardt, T.: Familial hypergammaglobulinaemia and systemic lupus erythematosus. Lancet *1957 II*, 1200–1203
3. Stecher, R.M., Hersh, A.H., Solomon, W.M., Wolpaw, R.: The genetics of rheumatoid arthritis: analysis of 224 families. Amer. J. hum. Genet. *5*, 118–138 (1953)
4. Burch, P.R.J., Rowell, N.R.: Systemic lupus erythematosus. Etiological aspects. Amer. J. Med. *38*, 793–801 (1965)
5. Beck, J.S., Rowell, N.R.: Discoid lupus erythematosus. A study of the clinical features and biochemical and serological abnormalities in 120 patients with observations on the relationship of this disease to systemic lupus erythematosus. Quart. J. Med. *35*, 119–136 (1966)

Chapter 9   Disorders of Hair

Contents

These disorders include either (a) coarser, longer, or more profuse growth of hair (hypertrichosis and hirsutism) [1] or (b) lacking or sparse growth of hair (alopecia) [2, 3].

Hereditary Hirsutism

Normal Subjects

Generalized: Racial and Familial Hirsutism

There are evident differences in hairiness among various races: Caucasians are much more hirsute than Orientals, Eskimos, American Indians, or Negroes [1]. Similarly, there may be marked intraracial differences. Thus, dark-haired, darkly pigmented Caucasians of either sex tend to be more hirsute than light-haired ones [1]. Hairiness of the beard, moustache area, sternal area, abdomen, arms, and legs seems to have a familial tendency in either sex (Fig. 9.1). Occasionally, even though the hair pattern is normal, the hairs are coarser and larger than normal. Facial hypertrichosis in women may have an autosomal dominant pattern of inheritance.

Localized Hypertrichosis

Midphalangeal Hair

Hypertrichosis of the middle phalanges of the fourth, third, fifth, and second fingers (in the order of frequency of the affection [1]) is not rare. Inheritance is autosomal dominant.

Hypertrichosis of Pinna
[Hairy Ears (Hypertrichosis Pinnae Auris)]

This trait consists of long hairs growing from the helix of the pinna (Fig. 9.2). Although Y-linked inheritance was suggested in 1964, there has been continuing controversy [4, 5]. More recently it was suggested that this trait is inherited as an autosomal dominant with a strong male influence [6].

Hypertrichosis Cubiti (Hairy Elbows Syndrome)

This type of inherited hypertrichosis has been reported in two of five siblings [7]. The condition is apparent at birth with hairiness of the elbows increasing until the age of five before starting to regress. The mode of inheritance is probably dominant, although inbreeding makes recessive inheritance a possible explanation for the findings [8].

Congenital Anomalies

Hypertrichosis Lanuginosa

This is an extremely rare condition in which the fetal pelage is not replaced by vellus and terminal hair but persists and is constantly renewed. Several varieties exist, of which the "dog-face" and "monkey-face" forms are better defined. In both forms, the increased hairiness is present at birth. In the former, the hair gradually lengthens and covers all of the body surface except the palms and soles [9], dorsal terminal phalanges, labia minora, prepuce, and glans penis. Dental abnormalities, especially anodontia, gingival fibromatosis, and deformities of the external ear may be associated findings. In the "monkey-face" form, hair terminals appear pigmented. Death may occur in early life. Both forms are inherited as autosomal dominant.

Cornelia de Lange Syndrome
(Brachmann–de Lange Syndrome)

In 1933 Cornelia de Lange [10] described two infants with brachycephaly, thick eyebrows, long eyelashes, micromelia, and syndactylism of the feet. More than 250 patients have been reported to date [11–13].

Clinical Presentation. The following are the most important features of this syndrome: short stature (usually below the third percentile); microcephaly with mental retardation; generalized hirsutism, which is more accentuated on the face; synophrys; hypertelorism; long and curly eyelashes; narrow palpebral fissures; strabismus; small nose with anteverted nostrils; longer than average philtrum; and small chin with the corners of the mouth curved downward [11, 14] (Figs. 9.3 and 9.4). The voice is growling and low-pitched. The ears are usually low-set.

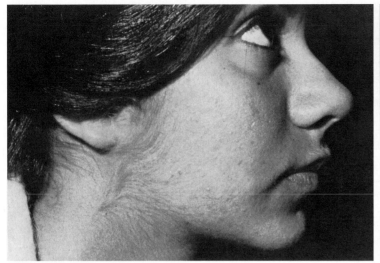

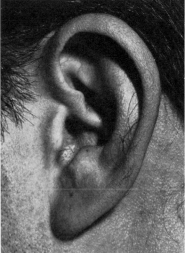

Fig. 9.1. Familial hirsutism

Fig. 9.2. Hypertrichosis of pinna

Most of these patients have a low birth weight for their gestational age. About 20% of the patients have limb malformations which may consist of shortened arms, small hands and feet, tapering digits, clinodactyly, phocomelia, or oligodactyly [11].

The most important dermatologic finding is the hirsutism, which is usually marked on the forehead, nape of the neck, upper lip, forearms, back, and sacral area. The hair is coarse and dry [11, 15]. Vascular lability and cutis marmorata may be present [16]. The marmoration is generalized except for the palms and soles. The branching pattern is pink-red with normal-colored skin between the arborizations [15]. The dermal ridges of the hypothenar areas of the palms and soles are hypoplastic and simian creases are commonly present.

Occasional anomalies include myopia, optic atrophy, cleft palate, congenital heart defects [17], and defects of the gastrointestinal tract (hiatus hernia, duplication of the gut, malrotation of the colon, pyloric stenosis). There may be hypoplasia of the external genitalia (in both sexes) and undescended testes. However, usually normal secondary sex characteristics develop in both sexes and menstruation in females is normal [18].

Episodes of aspiration in infancy and recurrent infections are the major causes of death. These patients rarely attain adulthood.

Pathology and Pathophysiology. There is a striking delay in maturation of most organ systems [19]. The severe mental retardation is due to a small brain and abnormalities of cerebral convolutions and demyelinization. Most patients have normal chromosomal karyotypes [18]. However, in certain reports [19], anomalies have been detected in a high percentage of cases where the chromosomes were studied. The chromosomal anomalies do not reveal any consistency that could be significant in elucidating the pathophysiology of the condition.

The main histopathologic features of the skin involve the small blood vessels of the subpapillary layer. The endothelial lining is prominent and the vessels are surrounded by a zone of edema [15].

Inheritance. Much controversy still exists over the mode of inheritance of this syndrome. In 1963 an autosomal dominant pattern of inheritance was suggested [20]. In 1967 a familial occurrence and parental consanguinity were noted, thus favoring the autosomal recessive mode [21]. In a more recent report [22], 54 families were studied and the recurrence rate among siblings was estimated to be between 2.2 and 5.1%. Based on this, the possibility of a polygenic inheritance was favored. Finally, in 1971, in the light of additional data, the autosomal recessive mode of inheritance was considered to be the more probable [12].

Treatment. There is no definitive treatment.

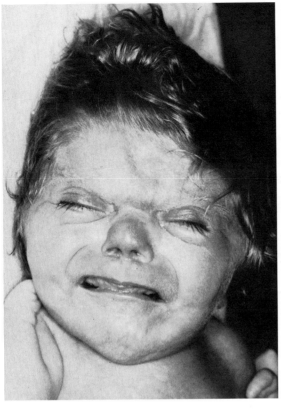

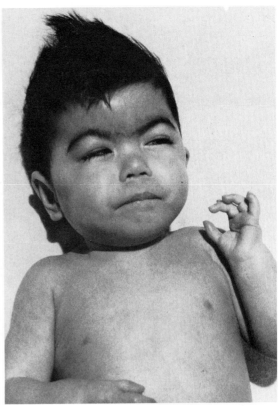

9.3

9.4

Fig. 9.3. Cornelia de Lange syndrome. Note hirsutism of the forehead and abnormality of the right upper limb. (From Pashayan, H., et al.: Birth defects original article series. Vol. XI, No. 5, pp. 147–156. National Foundation-March of Dimes 1975)

Fig. 9.4. Cornelia de Lange syndrome. Note the synophrys and the narrow palpebral fissures. (Courtesy of Dr. F.C. Fraser)

Hereditary Alopecias

Abnormalities of Hair Follicles

Aplasia

Universal: Congenital Universal Alopecia (Hypotrichosis, "Hairlessness")

Clinical Presentation. The scalp hair may be normal at birth but it may be lost within a few months or the scalp may be hairless from the onset [23]. Axillary and pubic hair, eyebrows, and eyelashes are scanty. Teeth, nails, and general health are normal (Fig. 9.5).

In two sibs, hypotrichosis was associated with syndactyly (and partial ectrodactyly in one) and retinitis pigmentosa [24].

Pathology and Pathophysiology. The main feature is absence of hair follicles.

Inheritance. Autosomal recessive.

Treatment. There is no treatment.

Alopecia-Epilepsy-Oligophrenia Syndrome of Moynahan (Familial Congenital Alopecia, Epilepsy, Mental Retardation, and Abnormal EEG)

One family has been reported with this syndrome. At birth there is hairlessness; later scant, downy hair of the scalp and eyelashes appears. Mental retardation, grand mal seizures, and abnormal EEG (gross generalized abnormality of an unusual kind) are other features of the syndrome. Histologically, the scalp shows small scanty hair follicles, some with a rim of keratin but no hair [25]. Inheritance is probably autosomal recessive.

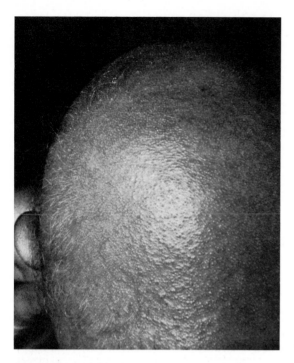

Fig. 9.5. Congenital alopecia and keratosis pilaris

Hypoplasia

Hereditary Hypotrichosis (Marie Unna Type)

Clinical Presentation. Affected individuals are born with little or no eyebrows, eyelashes, or body hair. The scalp hair grows more profuse in early childhood and becomes coarse and twisted. This is followed by alopecia at puberty especially over the vertex [26]. Milia may be present. A hereditary hypotrichosis limited to the skull has been described in a large kindred in Spain. Retardation of hair growth appears at 5–12 years and is complete by 20–25 years. The inheritance is autosomal dominant [27].

Pathology and Pathophysiology. The abnormal hairs are flat, ribbonlike, and twisted. Electron microscopy reveals intracellular fractures of cuticular and medullary cells, increased interfibrillar matrix, and fractures of cortical cell fibrils [28].

Inheritance. Autosomal dominant.

Treatment. There is no treatment.

Hypotrichosis with Light-Colored Hair and Facial Milia

A pedigree with this syndrome has recently been described [29]. Affected individuals have milia and sparseness and hypopigmentation of hairs. The milia are confined to the face. With increasing age the abnormalities are less severe. Hairs have normal mechanical properties, X-ray diffraction patterns, and electrophoretic patterns for the matrix and filament proteins [29]. Inheritance is autosomal dominant.

Various Syndromes in Which Hypotrichosis Is Less Constant or Less Well-Defined

Autosomal Recessive Conditions

Cartilage-Hair Hypoplasia (Metaphyseal Chondrodysplasia, McKusick Type). In 1964 McKusick [30] discovered this syndrome for the first time in an inbred Amish population. However, it has more recently been identified in other groups as well.

Clinical Presentation. The characteristic features of the disease are small stature and abnormalities of the skeleton, hair, and immune system.

The dwarfism is of the short-limbed variety and superficially resembles classic achondroplasia. Adult heights vary from 105–145 cm (Figs. 9.6 and 9.7). However, the head is normal in size without bulging of the forehead or exaggerated nasal saddling. Loose-jointedness in the hands and feet is striking. Bending of the ribs at the costochondral junction and symmetrical depression resembling Harrison's grooves occur in several patients and marked sternal deformity is present in some. Additional skeletal anomalies include mild bowing of the legs; short tibia in relation to fibula; short hands, fingernails, and toenails; decreased height of vertebrae; incomplete extension of the elbow; lumbar lordosis; and small pelvic inlet. The condition is already evident at birth because of the reduced crown-to-heel measurement and abnormally high upper segment-lower segment ratio [31].

The hair is fine, sparse, and silky on the scalp as well as the eyebrows and eyelashes. In some patients the hair is lighter in color and has an abnormally small caliber [31] (Figs. 9.8–9.10).

In the adult the radiologic features are not diagnostic. However, classic achondroplasia can be excluded because the skull is normal and the lumbar spine does not show caudad tapering of the interpeduncular distances typical of achondroplasia [31]. Changes are of the type which radiologists call metaphyseal dysostosis. The nature of the skeletal disorder is demonstrated by radiologic studies performed before closure of the epiphyses. The ossification centers of the epiphyses have a normal appearance. The metaphyseal ends of most tubular

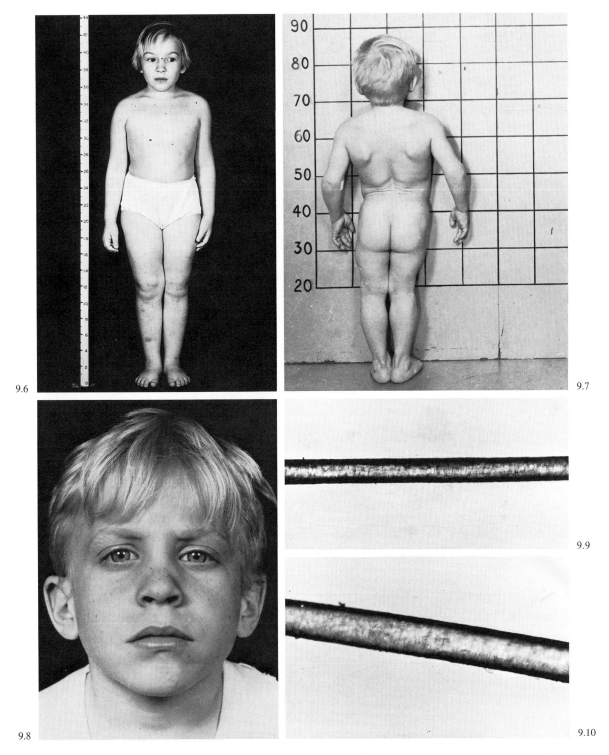

9.6

9.7

9.9

9.8

9.10

Figs. 9.6–9.10. Cartilage-hair hypoplasia

Figs. 9.6 and 9.7. General view of the body. (Fig. 6 – from Lowry, R.B., et al.: Clin. Pediat. *9*, 44–46, 1970. Fig. 7 – courtesy of Dr. V.A. McKusick)

Fig. 9.8. Note fine hair of light color. (Courtesy of Dr. V.A. McKusick)

Figs. 9.9 and 9.10. Light microscopy of the hair. Fig. 9 – patient's hair. Fig. 10 – control of the same age and sex. Note the small caliber of patient's hair. (Courtesy of Dr. R.B. Lowry)

bones are scalloped and irregularly sclerotic, often with cystic areas which appear to represent poorly ossified cartilage or cartilaginous inclusions. All of the tubular bones of the extremities including those of the hands participate in the process, as do the ribs, which at the costochondral junction show flaring, cupping, and cystic changes. "Bone age" is irregular [31].

There is a severe or fatal response to smallpox vaccination, varicella, and recurrent respiratory tract infections [32].

Pathology and Pathophysiology. Children with cartilage-hair hypoplasia (CHH) have chronic, non-cyclic neutropenia and lymphopenia, diminished delayed skin hypersensitivity, diminished responsiveness of lymphocytes in vitro to phytohemagglutinin (PHA), and delayed rejection of the skin allografts. Immunoglobulin levels in serum and saliva are normal or elevated. The findings suggest that patients with CHH have a functional defect of the small lymphocytes that mediate cellular immunity. Such dysfunction may be the result of an abnormality of the thymus or of the lymphocytes themselves. Some patients with CHH appear to have a decline in cellular immune function with age [32].

The hair shafts are only half as thick as the normal. They are weaker than normal hair. There may be decreased reactivity of some disulfide bonds in the hair leading to its abnormal biophysical and biochemical characteristics [33].

Inheritance. Autosomal recessive with reduced penetrance when dwarfism is taken as the phenotype for ascertainment.

Treatment. Thymus transplants have been attempted as treatment for CHH [34].

Trichorhinophalangeal Syndrome. Giedion, in 1966, described this entity which involves abnormalities of the hair, nose, and phalanges [35]. The scalp and body hair is sparse and slow-growing. There is sparsity of the lateral eyebrows and baldness is early. The nose is pear-shaped with a long philtrum. The phalanges of the fingers and toes may be crooked and shortened and may show cone-shaped epiphyses. There may also be hypoplasia of the midface. Inheritance is autosomal dominant [36], although a recessive form may also exist [37].

Dysplasia

Generalized Alopecia Due to Hamartomas of Hair Follicles

A female patient with progressive generalized alopecia was found, on investigation, to have occult hair follicle hamartomas [38]. A familial incidence was suspected (Fig. 9.11).

Universal Atrichia with Papular Lesions

Widespread papular lesions were associated with generalized alopecia in four females who had no other ectodermal defects [39,40]. Histologically, the papules were malformed follicles with follicular cysts and other malformations of the pilosebaceous apparatus. In one case the condition affected two siblings. Inheritance is autosomal recessive.

Abnormalities of Hair Shaft

Pili Torti

Clinical Presentation. The hair may appear normal at birth, but by the second or third year the abnormality becomes clinically evident. Occasionally, there may be alopecia at birth [2]. The affected hairs are brittle and break off 4–5 cm from the scalp to give a stubblelike appearance. Friction, as from a pillow, may contribute to the alopecia (Fig. 9.12). There may be improvement with puberty or the condition may persist into adulthood [3]. Axillary and pubic hairs, the eyebrows, and eyelashes may also be involved.

Pili torti may be associated with other hair defects: trichorrhexis nodosa, trichorrhexis invaginata, and monilethrix [3]. The condition may also be associated with keratosis pilaris, seborrhea, ichthyosis, and ectodermal dysplasia [3]. Mental retardation and cerebral degeneration have been reported in association with pili torti [3], as well as sensorineural hearing loss (Björnstad syndrome) [41].

Pathology and Pathophysiology. The hair shafts are twisted 180°. The cuticle appears normal with scanning electron microscopy [42] (Fig. 9.13).

Inheritance. Probably autosomal recessive.

Treatment. The mainstay of treatment is avoidance of trauma.

Fig. 9.11. General-
ized alopecia due
to hair follicle ha-
martoma

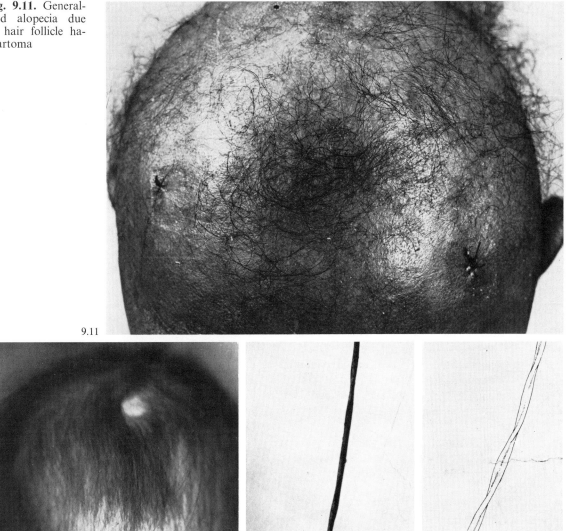

9.11

9.12

9.13a
9.13b

Fig. 9.12. Pili torti. Sparse hair with stubblelike appearance at areas of friction. (From Nichamin, S.J.: Amer. J. Dis. Child. *95*, 612–615, 1958)

Fig. 9.13a and b. Pili torti. Microscopy of hair with diagrammatic illustration. (From Nichamin, S.J.: Amer. J. Dis. Child. *95*, 612–615, 1958)

Monilethrix

Clinical Presentation. At birth the hair usually appears normal but within a few months it is lost. There may be some regrowth of hair at puberty or the alopecia may persist. Erythematous, follicular, papular, and pustular lesions appear on the forehead, face, scalp, and nape of the neck. Through these emerge the brittle, beaded hairs which break 1 cm above the skin surface (Figs. 9.14–9.17). The body hair may also be affected. The severity of the affection varies widely within the same pedigree. Other hair shaft defects, nail and teeth abnormalities, physical retardation, syndactyly, and juvenile cataracts may be associated with monilethrix [3]. It may also be associated with mental retardation, epilepsy, schizophrenia, and neurodegenerative disease [43]. Keratosis pilaris and argininosuccinicaciduria with an elevated plasma glutamic acid have also been noted [3].

Pathology and Pathophysiology. The hair shaft shows elliptical nodes, 0.7–1 mm apart, separated by constricted internodes, and an absent medulla through which the hair fractures [3]. Longitudinal ridging of the internodes can be demonstrated with the scanning electron microscope [42].

Inheritance. Autosomal dominant. Some reports claim that a recessive mode of inheritance is present in one out of five families with monilethrix [44].

Treatment. There is no definitive treatment. Griseofulvin may be helpful.

Pseudomonilethrix

In members of five families a new hair shaft defect has been described [45, 46].
The age of onset is in childhood with progressive thinning of scalp hair. The skin is normal, but formes frustes of pili torti and trichorrhexis nodosa are noted. The affected hairs show irregular spacing with the nodes thicker than in the normal shaft, while the internodes remain the same. No abnormalities are noted with the scanning electron microscope. The disease is inherited as autosomal dominant.

Trichorrhexis Nodosa

Most often this is an acquired abnormality of the shaft due to physical or chemical trauma. Occasionally, the condition may be inherited.
The defect is in the form of a nodelike swelling with segmental longitudinal splitting of the fiber through which the hair fractures. This defect is found in sex-linked neurodegenerative diseases and sibs with mental and physical retardation [3, 47]. The hair has a low sulfur content with a defective cuticle (Pollitt syndrome) [3, 47] (Figs. 9.18 and 9.19). Inheritance is probably autosomal recessive.

Trichorrhexis Invaginata (Bamboo Hair)

There is intussusception of the hair shaft within the follicle, and as the hair grows the defect appears as bamboolike nodes. This abnormality is most frequently associated with Netherton syndrome (see p. 40).

Pili Annulati (Ringed Hair)

Clinical Presentation. The abnormality is present at birth or appears during the second year. Affected hairs, which may be few or include the entire scalp, are characterized by light and dark bands on the shafts in reflected light [3]. There may be no increased fragility or the hairs may break off at a length of 15–20 cm.

Pathology and Pathophysiology. The light bands, which are about 1 mm wide, are due to air spaces in the cortex [3]. Scanning electron microscopy shows surface irregularity of the abnormal bands [42]. In one patient, a decrease in the sulfur content of the affected hair was found [3].

Inheritance. Autosomal dominant. Many sporadic cases exist.

Treatment. If the condition is associated with hair fragility, avoidance of trauma is stressed.

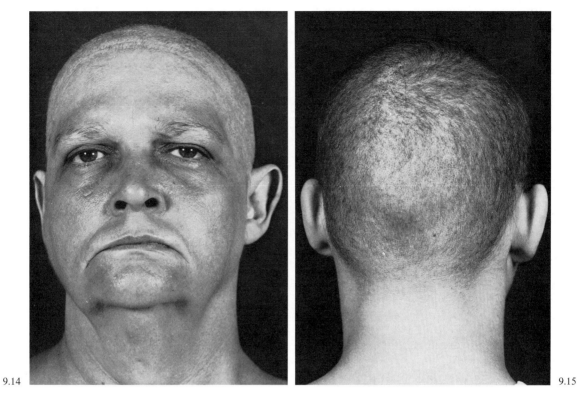

9.14   9.15

Figs. 9.14 and 9.15. Monilethrix. Varying degrees of alopecia. (Courtesy of Dr. V.A. McKusick. Fig. 15 – from Penchaszadeh, V.B.: In: The clinical delineation of birth defects. Bergsma, D. (ed.), Vol. VII, No. 8, pt. XII, pp. 262–264. Baltimore: Williams & Wilkins Co. 1971)

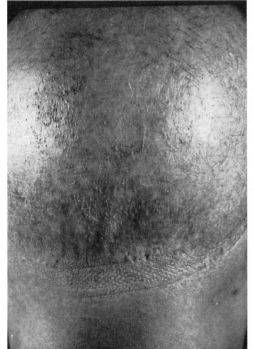

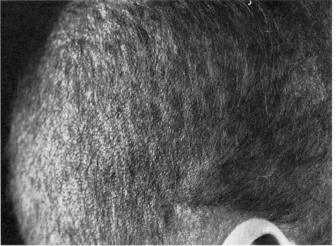

9.17

16

Figs. 9.16 and 9.17. Monilethrix. Note short hair and follicular eruption. (Courtesy of Dr. V. A. McKusick. Fig. 17 – from Penchaszadeh, V.B.: In: The clinical delineation of birth defects. Bergsma, D. (ed.), Vol. VII, No. 8, pt. XII, pp. 262–264. Baltimore: Williams & Wilkins Co. 1971)

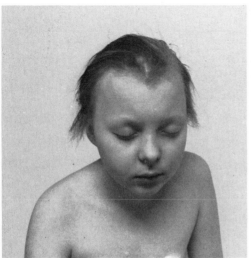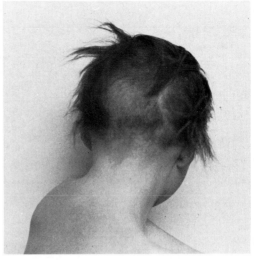

9.18

9.19

Figs. 9.18 and 9.19. Alopecia due to low sulfur content of hair. (Courtesy of Dr. A.C.Brown)

Kinky Hair Disease (Menkes Syndrome)

In 1962 Menkes et al. [48] described this disease characterized by stubby hair, neurologic deterioration in infancy, and growth retardation.

Clinical Presentation. The infant is normal during the first 2 or 3 months of life. Later, severe psychomotor retardation is evident and seizures are noted. Other important features of the disease are abnormal hair, micrognathia, high-arched palate, an equinovarus deformity, short stature, spasticity [49, 50], and a horizontal nystagmus with slight pallor of the optic discs [51] (Figs. 9.20 and 9.21). There may also be temperature instability, scorbutic bone changes, excessive wormian bone formation, low or absent plasma copper and ceruloplasmin, and increased susceptibility to infection.

The hair is sparse, coarse, stubby, light brown in color, and displays an abnormal autofluorescence. A wiry texture is noted at birth or during the first 3 months of life (Fig. 9.22).

Death occurs between the first and fourth years.

Pathology and Pathophysiology. Microscopic examination of the hair displays varying shaft diameters (monilethrix), twisting of the shafts (pili torti), and fractures (trichorrhexis nodosa).

The brain is severely atrophied. Patchy abnormality of systemic arteries with stenosis or obliteration is observed. There is evidence of a defect in the intestinal absorption of copper [52]. The defect probably lies in transport within the intestinal cells or across the membrane on the serosal surface of the cells [53]. The hair changes are probably the result of defective formation of disulfide bonds in keratin, since this process is copper-dependent. Cultured skin fibroblasts from patients with Menkes disease consistently exhibit elevated copper concentrations when compared to control fibroblast cultures. Menkes cells can be differentiated from cultured fibroblasts of controls, of presumed heterozygotes, and of Wilson disease patients by copper concentration. This finding provides a genetic marker, a defect in metal metabolism demonstrated in human fibroblasts, that should prove valuable in the diagnosis of Menkes disease and in the study of its fundamental defect and its prenatal detection [54].

Inheritance. X-linked recessive.

Treatment. There is no effective treatment. Intravenous copper therapy permits normal ceruloplasmin synthesis and catabolism but no clinical improvement results.

Woolly Hair

Woolly hair, a distinctive Negroid racial characteristic, has occurred in Caucasoids in whom the possibility of mixed blood was remote. Affected individuals have tight curls in childhood and very wavy hair as adults [55] (Fig. 9.23). There are no associated abnormalities. Microscopically, there is torsion of the hair around the long axis, an ovoid cross section, and decrease in the hair diameter. Hair density, growth rate, and anagen-telogen ratio are normal [55]. A large proportion of dysplastic

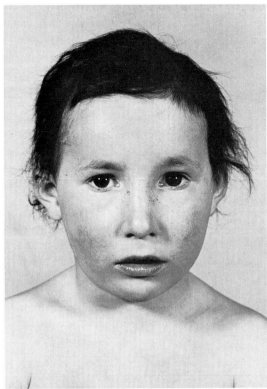 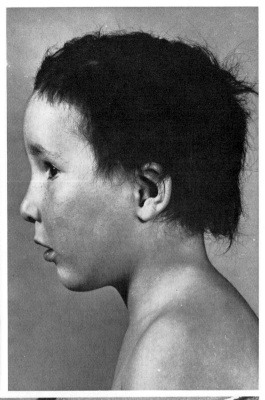

9.20   9.21

Figs. 9.20 and 9.21. Kinky hair disease. Note coarse, stubby hair and micrognathia. (From Robinson, G.C., Johnston, M.M.: J. Pediat. *70*, 621–623, 1967)

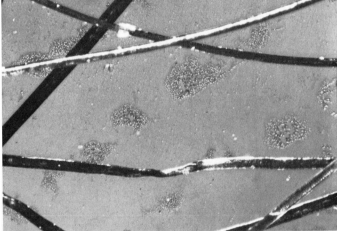

Fig. 9.22. Kinky hair disease. Microscopy of hair showing varied diameters and twisting of the shafts. (From Robinson, G.C., Johnston, M.M.: J. Pediat. *70*, 621–623, 1967)

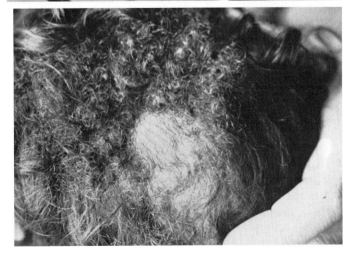

Fig. 9.23. Woolly hair

hair is found [55]. The inheritance is autosomal dominant [55]. In an affected family with very fair color, there was an autosomal recessive inheritance [55].

Brittle Hair (Hair-Brain Syndrome, Amish Brittle Hair Syndrome)

In this syndrome, which is found among the Amish, there is brittle hair, mild impairment of growth and intellect, and decreased fertility. The hairs have an irregular grooved surface with absence of scales and marked decrease in sulfur content [56]. Inheritance is autosomal recessive.

Miscellaneous Alopecias

Baldness (Male-Pattern Alopecia, Patterned Baldness)

Clinical Presentation. The completely hairy scalp with no frontoparietal recession of the hairline is characteristic of most affected children until puberty when hair is lost in both sexes [1]. With advancing age, baldness occurs with increasing frequency in males, with a peak in the seventh decade; in females the incidence does not increase beyond the fifth decade [57]. Advanced stages of baldness are not found in women [57]. The mildest form of baldness is a symmetric triangular recession in the frontoparietal regions. Sparseness of hair on the crown and loss of hair as a broad band along the anterior border of the hairline occur with increased frontoparietal recession. With advancing age, men tend to acquire extensive frontoparietal and frontal recessions as well as loss of hair on the crown, until these areas coalesce to form an area of alopecia which has the outline of a horseshoe when viewed from above. The bald scalp appears thin and smooth. Tiny vellus hairs are seen.

Pathology and Pathophysiology. With aging, the scalp undergoes thinning of the epidermis and disappearance of the capillary loops supplying the epidermis [58]. The normal grouping of hair follicles is lost, and there is progressive transformation of growing hair follicles into lanugo types [58]. The sebaceous glands become multilobular and the eccrine glands become larger.
The pathogenesis of baldness is dependent on genetic predisposition, androgenic stimulation, and aging. Males castrated before puberty do not develop baldness; if eunuchs are given testosterone, baldness appears only in those whose relatives tend to be bald [59]. The influence of aging is shown by the progressive extension of the bald area with increasing age; testosterone-treated eunuchs develop baldness commensurate with the extent of baldness of males of a similar age [59]. Baldness affects only hair follicles of the scalp and not those of the beard, axillae, or pubic area. Racial variation is important: baldness is most frequent in Caucasoids, rare in Mongoloids.

Inheritance. Autosomal dominant, sex-influenced.

Treatment. There is no effective treatment for baldness or its prevention. Artificial hairpieces may be used. Major plastic surgical procedures and implantation of nylon filaments have not been very successful [60]. The Orentreich technique of multiple punch scalp autografts could be very rewarding [60].

Alopecia Areata

Clinical Presentation. The characteristic manifestation is the appearance of asymptomatic, single or multiple, circular or oval areas of hair loss without scarring (Figs. 9.24–9.27). The scalp is most commonly affected but other hairy areas may also be involved. Usually there is regrowth of hair within a few months but other alopecia areas may develop with progression to universal alopecia. Periods of regrowth and recurrence of alopecia are common. Initial attempts produce fine nonpigmented hair. The disease may appear at any age but usually affects both sexes in the third and fourth decades. The severer forms tend to affect younger individuals [2]. The skin in areas of alopecia appears normal although at times it may be faintly erythematous. At the margins of the bald areas, distinctive, short, pigmented, tapering-down hairs (exclamation point hairs) are seen [2].
Pitting and brittleness of the nails, mainly fingernails, and occasionally shedding of the nails may be seen [61]. Other associated disorders include posterior subcapsular cataracts, neuropsychiatric problems (17–22%), thyroid abnormalities (8%), diabetes mellitus (2%), vitiligo (4%), and atopic manifestations.

Pathology and Pathophysiology. There is an increase in the percentage of telogen hairs at the margins of the areas of alopecia [62]. The shedding of these hairs is followed by the appearance of early anagen

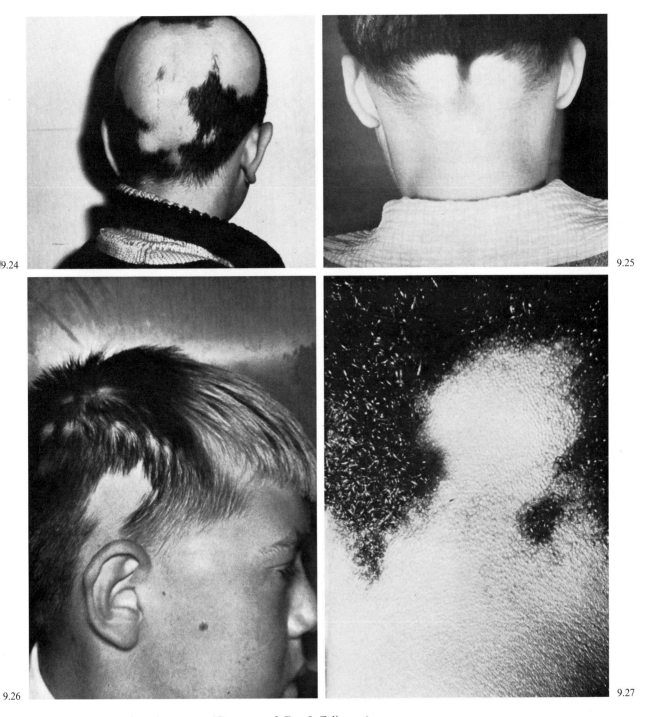

9.24

9.25

9.26

9.27

Figs. 9.24–9.27. Alopecia areata. (Courtesy of Dr. I. Zeligman)

hairs that seem to be restrained from further maturation [62]. The hair bulbs are superficially located in the dermis and are enveloped by a connective tissue sheath infiltrated with lymphocytes.

Recent evidence suggests an autoimmune mechanism in this disorder. The incidence of thyroid disease in patients with alopecia areata and of diabetes mellitus in relatives of patients with alopecia areata is greater than in control groups [63]. In patients with alopecia there is a significant correlation with circulating antibodies against thyroglobulin and parietal, adrenal, and thyroid cells [64].

Inheritance. Familial incidence occurs in 10% of cases [61]. Inheritance may be autosomal dominant.

Other Conditions

Abnormalities of Pattern

Catatrichy (Forelock)

In this abnormality, a forelock made up of hair finer and more wavy than the rest of the head is present [65]. It is probably inherited as autosomal dominant.

Hair Whorl ("Crown")

The whorl of the occipital scalp hair shows a clockwise or counterclockwise rotation. It is probable that the former is the dominant characteristic. Double whorls may also be familial.

Widow's Peak

In this anomaly there is a downward projection of the anterior scalp hair in a V-shaped manner. When severe, this abnormality may be associated with ocular hypertelorism [66]. Widow's peak is inherited as probable autosomal dominant.

Abnormalities of Color

Red Hair

The pigment that is responsible for the red color in human hair is trichosiderin, which consists of protein, iron, and a chromophore group and differs in all major respects from the black melanins [67]. The mode of inheritance of red hair is not settled as some favor an autosomal recessive mode [68] and others suggest that the presence of red pigment in the hair is dominant to its absence and hypostatic to brown or black [69].

Similarly, strikingly blond hair may be recessive.

Abnormalities of Structure

Some of these abnormalities have been discussed under the particular hair shaft defect. In one instance, however, a structural abnormality detected by electrophoresis has been characterized in hairs that show no abnormality of thickness, texture, or color.

The abnormality is a variant polypeptide of the α-fibrous proteins of human hair [70]. This abnormality is inherited as autosomal codominant.

References

1. Muller, S.A.: Hirsutism: a review of the genetic and experimental aspects. J. invest. Derm. *60*, 457–474 (1973)
2. Muller, S.A.: Alopecia: syndromes of genetic significance. J. invest. Derm. *60*, 475–492 (1973)
3. Brown, A.C.: Congenital hair defects. In: The clinical delineation of birth defects. Bergsma, D. (ed.), Vol. VII, No. 8, pt, XII, pp. 52–68. Baltimore: Williams & Wilkins Co. 1971
4. Dronamraju, K.R.: Y-linkage in man. Nature (Lond.) *201*, 424–425 (1964)
5. Stern, C., Centerwall, W.R., Sarkr, S.S.: New data on the problem of Y-linkage of hairy pinnae. Amer. J. hum. Genet. *16*, 455–471 (1964)
6. McKusick, V.A.: Mendelian inheritance in man, 4th ed., p. xvi. Baltimore: Johns Hopkins University Press 1975
7. Beighton, P.: Familial hypertrichosis cubiti: hairy elbows syndrome. J. med. Genet. 7, 158–160 (1970)
8. McKusick, V.A.: Mendelian inheritance in man, 5th ed., p. 139. Baltimore: Johns Hopkins University Press 1978
9. Beighton, P.: Congenital hypertrichosis lanuginosa. Arch. Derm. *101*, 669–672 (1970)
10. de Lange, C.: Sur un type nouveau de dégénération (typus amstelodamensis). Arch. Méd. Enf. *36*, 713–719 (1933)
11. Berg, J.M., McCreary, B.D., Ridler, M.A.C., Smith, G.F.: The de Lange syndrome, p. 127. Oxford: Pergamon Press 1970
12. Motl, M.L., Opitz, J.M.: Studies of malformation syndromes XXVA. Phenotypic and genetic studies of the Brachmann-de Lange syndrome. Hum. Heredity *21*, 1–16 (1971)
13. Beratis, N.G., Hsu, L.Y., Hirschhorn, K.: Familial de Lange syndrome. Report of three cases in a sibship. Clin. Genet. *2*, 170–176 (1971)

14. Nicholson, D.H., Goldberg, M.F.: Ocular abnormalities in the de Lange syndrome. Arch. Ophthal. 76, 214–220 (1966)

15. Salazar, F.N.: Dermatological manifestations of the Cornelia de Lange syndrome. Arch. Derm. 94, 38–43 (1966)

16. Abraham, J.M., Russell, A.: de Lange syndrome. A study of nine examples. Acta paediat. scand. 57, 339–353 (1968)

17. Syamasundar Rao, P., Sissman, N.J.: Congenital heart disease in the de Lange syndrome. J. Pediat. 79, 674–677 (1971)

18. McArthur, R.G., Edwards, J.H.: de Lange syndrome: report of 20 cases. Canad. med. Ass. J. 96, 1185–1198 (1967)

19. Craig, A.P., Luzzatti, L.: Translocation in de Lange's syndrome? Lancet 1965II, 445–446

20. Ptacek, L.J., Opitz, J.M., Smith, D.W., Gerritsen, T., Waisman, H.A.: The Cornelia de Lange syndrome. J. Pediat 63, 1000–1020 (1963)

21. Pearce, P.M., Pitt, D.B., Roboz, P.: Six cases of de Lange's syndrome; parental consaguinity in two. Med. J. Aust. 1, 502–506 (1967)

22. Pashayan, H., Whelan, D., Guttman, S., Fraser, F.C.: Variability of the de Lange syndrome: report of 3 cases and genetic analysis of 54 families. J. Pediat. 75, 853–858 (1969)

23. Tillman, W.G.: Alopecia congenita: report of two families. Br. med. J. 1952II, 428

24. Albrectsen, B., Svendsen, I.B.: Hypotrichosis, syndactyly, and retinal degeneration in two siblings. Acta derm.-venereol. (Stockh.) 36, 96–101 (1956)

25. Moynahan, E.J.: Familial congenital alopecia, epilepsy, mental retardation with unusual electroencephalograms. Proc. roy. Soc. Med. 55, 411–412 (1962)

26. Peachey, R.D.G., Wells, R.S.: Hereditary hypotrichosis (Marie Unna type). Trans. St. Johns Hosp. derm. Soc. 57, 157–166 (1971)

27. Toribio, J., Quiñones, P.A.: Hereditary hypotrichosis simplex of scalp: evidence for autosomal dominant inheritance. Brit. J. Derm. 91, 687–696 (1974)

28. Solomon, L.M., Esterly, N.B., Medenica, M.: Hereditary trichodysplasia: Marie Unna's hypotrichosis. J. invest. Derm. 57, 389–400 (1971)

29. Parrish, J.A., Baden, H.P., Goldsmith, L.A., Matz, M.H.: Studies of the density and the properties of the hair in a new inherited syndrome of hypotrichosis. Ann. hum. Genet. 35, 349–356 (1972)

30. McKusick, V.A.: Metaphyseal dysostosis and thin hair: a "new" recessively inherited syndrome? Lancet 1964I, 832–833

31. McKusick, V.A., Eldridge, R., Hostetler, J.A., Ruangwit, U., Egeland, J.A.: Dwarfism in the Amish. II. Cartilage-hair hypoplasia. Bull. Johns Hopk. Hosp. 116, 285–326 (1965)

32. Lux, S.E., Johnston, R.B., Jr., August, C.S., Say, B., Penchaszadeh, V.B., Rosen, F.S., McKusick, V.A.: Chronic neutropenia and abnormal cellular immunity in cartilage-hair hypoplasia. New Engl. J. Med. 282, 231–236 (1970)

33. Kelling, C., Goldsmith, L.A., Baden, H.P.: Biophysical and biochemical studies of the hair in cartilage-hair hypoplasia. Clin. Genet. 4, 500–506 (1974)

34. Hong, R., Ammann, J., Haung, S.W., Levy, R.L., Davenport, G., Bach, M.L., Bach, F.H., Bortin, M.M., Kay, H.E.M.: Cartilage-hair hypoplasia: effect of thymus transplants. Clin. Immunol. Immunopathol. 1, 15–25 (1972)

35. Giedion, A.: Das tricho-rhino-phalangeale syndrom. Helv. pediat. Acta 21, 475–482 (1966)

36. McKusick, V.A.: Heritable disorders of connective tissue, 4th ed., p. 807. Saint Louis: Mosby, C.V. Co. 1972

37. Giedion, A., Burdea, M., Fruchter, Z., Meloni, T., Trosc, V.: Autosomal-dominant transmission of the tricho-rhino-phalangeal syndrome. Report of 4 unrelated families, review of 60 cases. Helv. paediat. Acta 28, 249–259 (1973)

38. Brown, A.C., Crounse, R.G., Winkelmann, R.K.: Generalized hair-follicle hamartoma. Associated with alopecia, aminoacidura (sic), and myasthenia gravis. Arch. Derm. 99, 478–493 (1969)

39. Damsté, T.J., Prakken, J.R.: Atrichia with papular lesions; a variant of congenital ectodermal dysplasia. Dermatologica (Basel) 108, 114–121 (1954)

40. Loewenthal, L.J.A., Prakken, J.R.: Atrichia with papular lesions. Dermatologica (Basel) 122, 85–89 (1961)

41. Reed, W.B., Stone, V.M., Boder, E., Ziprkowski, L.: Hereditary syndromes with auditory and dermatological manifestations. Arch. Derm. 95, 456–461 (1967)

42. Dawber, R., Comaish, S.: Scanning electron microscopy of normal and abnormal hair shafts. Arch. Derm. 101, 316–322 (1970)

43. Bray, P.F.: Sex-linked neurodegenerative disease associated with monilethrix. Pediatrics 36, 417–420 (1965)

44. Salamon, T., Schnyder, U.W.: Über die Monilethrix. Arch. klin. exp. Derm. 215, 105–136 (1962)

45. Bentley-Phillips, B., Bayles, M.A.H.: A previously undescribed hereditary hair anomaly (pseudo-monilethrix). Brit. J. Derm. 89, 159–167 (1973)

46. Bentley-Phillips, B., Bayles, M.A.H.: Pseudo-monilethrix. Brit. J. Derm. 92, 113–115 (1975)

47. Pollitt, R.J., Jenner, F.A., Davies, M.: Sibs with mental and physical retardation and trichorrhexis nodosa with abnormal amino acid composition of the hair. Arch. Dis. Child. 43, 211–216 (1968)

48. Menkes, J.H., Alter, M., Steigleder, G.K., Weakley, D.R., Sung, J.H.: A sex-linked recessive disorder with retardation of growth, peculiar hair, and focal cerebral and cerebellar degeneration. Pediatrics 29, 764–779 (1962)

49. Aguilar, M.J., Chadwick, D.L., Okuyama, K., Kamoshita, S.: Kinky hair disease. I. Clinical and pathological features. J. Neuropathol. exp. Neurol. 25, 507–522 (1966)

50. Billings, D.M., Degman, M.: Kinky hair syndrome. A new case and a new review. Amer. J. Dis. Child. 121, 447–449 (1971)

51. Seelenfreund, M.H., Gartner, S., Vinger, P.F.: The ocular pathology of Menkes' disease (kinky hair disease). Arch. Ophthal. 80, 718–720 (1968)

52. Danks, D.M., Campbell, P.E., Stevens, B.J., Mayne, V., Cartwright, E.: Menkes' kinky hair syndrome. An inherited defect in copper absorption with widespread effects. Pediatrics 50, 188–201 (1972)

53. Danks, D.M., Cartwright, E., Stevens, B.J., Townley, R.R.W.: Menkes' kinky hair disease: further definition of the defect in copper transport. Science 179, 1140–1142 (1973)

54. Horn, N.: Copper incorporation studies on cultured cells for prenatal diagnosis of Menkes' disease. Lancet 1976I, 1156–1158

55. Hutchinson, P.E., Cairns, R.J., Wells, R.S.: Woolly hair: clinical and general aspects. Trans. St. John's Hosp. derm. Soc. 60, 160–177 (1974)

56. Jackson, C.E., Weiss, L., Watson, J.H.L.: "Brittle" hair with short stature, intellectual impairment, and decreased fertility: an autosomal recessive syndrome in an Amish kindred. Pediatrics 54, 201–207 (1974)

57. Hamilton, J.B.: Patterned loss of hair in man: types and incidence. Ann. N.Y. Acad. Sci. 53, 708–728 (1950–1951)

58. Ellis, R.A.: Ageing of the human male scalp. In: The biology of hair growth. Montagna, W., Ellis, R.A. (eds.), pp. 469–485: New York: Academic Press 1958

59. Hamilton, J.B.: Male hormone stimulation is prerequisite and an incitant in common baldness. Amer. J. Anat. 71, 451–480 (1942)

60. Ayres, S., III: Conservative surgical management of male pattern baldness. An evaluation of current techniques. Arch. Derm. *90*, 492–499 (1964)

61. Muller, S.A., Winkelmann, R.K.: Alopecia areata. An evaluation of 736 patients. Arch. Derm. *88*, 290–297 (1963)

62. Van Scott, E.J.: Morphologic changes in pilosebaceous units and anagen hairs in alopecia areata. J. invest. Derm. *31*, 35–43 (1958)

63. Cunliffe, W.J., Hall, R., Stevenson, C.J., Weightman, D.: Alopecia areata, thyroid disease and autoimmunity. Brit. J. Derm. *81*, 877–881 (1969)

64. Kern, F., Hoffman, W.H., Hambrick, G.W., Jr., Blizzard, R.M.: Alopecia areata. Immunologic studies and treatment with prednisone. Arch. Derm. *107*, 407–412 (1973)

65. Stoddard, S.E.: Inheritance of "natural bangs": catatrichy, new character dependent upon dominant autosomal gene. J. Heredity *30*, 543–545 (1939)

66. Smith, D.W., Coben, M.M.: Widow's peak scalp-hair anomaly and its relation to ocular hypertelorism. Lancet *1973 II*, 1127–1128

67. Flesch, P.: The epidermal iron pigments of red species. J. invest. Derm. *51*, 337–343 (1968)

68. Neel, J.V.: Concerning inheritance of red hair. J. Heredity. *34*, 93–96 (1943)

69. Rife, D.C.: The inheritance of red hair. Acta Genet. med. (Roma) *16*, 342–349 (1967)

70. Baden, H.P., Lee, L.D.: Polymorphism in hair α-proteins. Clin. Res. *22* (Abstr.), 325 (1974)

Table 9.1 Disorders of eyelashes and eyebrows

Name	Inheritance	Clinical presentation	Ref.
Absent eyebrows and eyelashes with mental retardation	Autosomal recessive (suspected)	Absence of eyebrows and eyelashes associated with mental retardation, progressive spastic quadriplegia, microcephaly, glaucoma, and small, beaked nose	[1]
Alacrimia congenita	Autosomal recessive (suspected)	Distichiasis with ptosis, conjunctivitis, keratitis, and alacrimia congenita	[2]
Distichiasis	Autosomal dominant	"Distichiasis" and "districhiasis" are used interchangeably to mean 2 rows of eyelashes, although the terms "districhiasis" and "tristrichiasis" refer to 2 and 3 hairs per follicle, respectively (Figs. 9.28 and 9.29)	[3]
Distichiasis with lymphedema	Autosomal dominant	This gene mutation is most probably at a different locus from that of distichiasis alone. Irritation from eyelashes may result in corneal ulceration (Fig. 9.30) The lymphedema is always of late onset (Fig. 9.31).	[3]
Hyperlysinemia (persistent)	Autosomal recessive	Lax ligaments and synophrys Severe mental retardation; petit mal convulsions in many cases	[4]
Trichomegaly	Autosomal dominant (probable)	Unusually long eyelashes May be associated with cataracts and hereditary spherocytosis	[5]
Trichomegaly with mental retardation, dwarfism, and pigmentary degeneration	Autosomal recessive (probable)	Unusually long eyelashes May be associated with mental retardation, dwarfism, and pigmentary degeneration of the retina	[6]
Tristichiasis	Autosomal dominant (probable)	Three rows of eyelashes	[7]
Whorl in eyebrow	Autosomal dominant (probable)	Whorl in the hair of left eyebrow near nose	[8]

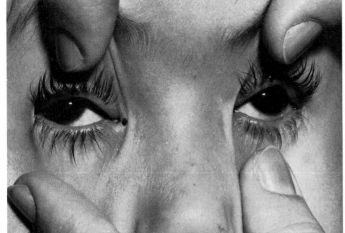

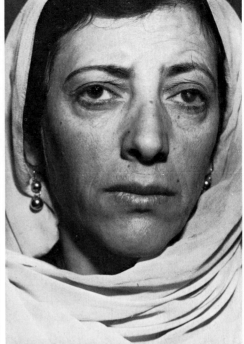

9.28

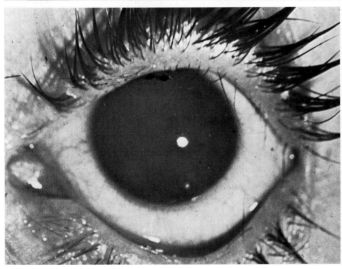

9.29

9.30

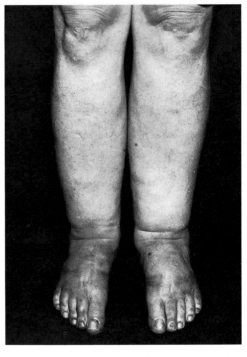

Figs. 9.28 and 9.29. Distichiasis. Note two rows of eyelashes on the upper lid

Fig. 9.30. Distichiasis. Note scarring of the cornea of the left eye

Fig. 9.31. Distichiasis with lymphedema

9.31

References

1. Hall, B.D., Berg, B.O., Rudolph, R.S., Epstein, C.J.: Pseudo-progeria-Hallermann-Streiff (PHS) syndrome. In: The clinical delineation of birth defects. Bergsma, D. (ed.), Vol. X, No. 7, pp. 137–146 (1974)
2. Krüger, K.E.: Angeborenes Fehlen der Tränensekretion in einer Familie. Klin. Mbl. Augenheilk. *124*, 711–713 (1954)
3. Robinow, M., Johnson, G.F., Verhagen, A.D.: Distichiasis-lymphedema. A hereditary syndrome of multiple congenital defects. Amer. J. Dis. Child. *119*, 343–347 (1970)
4. Ghadimi, H.: The hyperlysinemias. In: The metabolic basis of inherited disease. Stanbury, J.B., Wyngaarden, J.B., Fredrickson, D.S. (eds.), 4th ed., pp. 387–396. New York: McGraw-Hill Book Co. 1978
5. Goldstein, J.H., Hutt, A.E.: Trichomegaly, cataract, and hereditary spherocytosis in two siblings. Amer. J. Ophthal. *73*, 333–335 (1972)
6. Corby, D.G., Lowe, R.S., Jr., Haskins, R.C., Hebertson, L.M.: Trichomegaly, pigmentary degeneration of the retina and growth retardation. A new syndrome originating in utero. Amer. J. Dis. Child. *121*, 344–345 (1971)
7. Danforth, C.H.: Studies on hair. With special reference to hypertrichosis. Arch. Derm. Syph. *11*, 494–508 (1925)
8. Virchow, H.: Stellung der Haare im Brauenkopf. Z. Ethnol. *44*, 402–403 (1912)

Chapter 10   Disorders of Nails

Contents

The nails are involved in a number of heritable disorders affecting the skin in general, particularly when the process of keratinization is affected. Such nail abnormalities that are part of well-established entities are discussed under those entities. In this chapter, abnormalities that affect predominantly the nails will be discussed.

Anonychia and Onychoatrophy

Anonychia or absence of nails from birth is a very rare disorder. Frequently anonychia is not complete and there may be rudimentary fragile nails on some of the fingers or toes. Such a condition may be referred to as onychoatrophy [1] (Figs. 10.1 and 10.2). The disorder is apparent at birth with absence of all or most of the nails of the fingers and toes. The nail beds are present. The symptoms are mainly cosmetic, but at times there is discomfort in handling small things and a tendency of the nail rudiments to stick to woven clothing [1]. The inheritance is autosomal recessive [2].

Reports of anonychia with other abnormalities are recorded. Anonychia with ectrodactyly is inherited as autosomal dominant [3]; rudimentary nails associated with congential deafness are probably recessively inherited [4]; anonychia with bizarre pigmentation of axillae and groin and other skin and hair abnormalities is dominantly inherited [5]; and anonychia with onychodystrophy is probably dominantly inherited [6].

Koilonychia (Spoon Nails)

This common nail deformity is due to loss of the normal contour. The nail becomes flat or concave (Fig. 10.3). The majority of cases are either idiopathic or associated with a variety of systemic disorders, the most frequent of which is hypochromic anemia [7]. The affected nails are thin and concave with everted edges. The concavity is most obvious when viewed laterally. The thumbnails are predominantly involved, but the index and middle fingers and some toes may be affected as well. Inheritance is autosomal dominant.

Leukonychia

Leukonychia, or white nails, may be congenital or acquired; if congenital, it may be total, partial, or striate. The texture of the affected nails is normal [8]. The condition is present at birth. There are many postulates to explain the pathogenesis of this condition, the most probable being a defect in keratinization with retention of nuclei and nuclear material [8]. There are no definite associated abnormalities other than epidermal cysts. The disorder is inherited as autosomal dominant.

The association of leukonychia, knuckle pads, and deafness comprises a distinct syndrome. The hear-

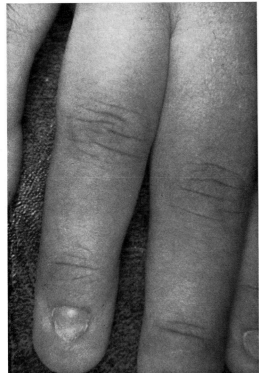

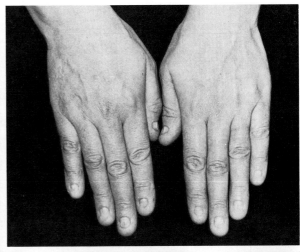

10.2

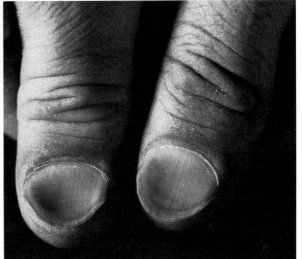

10.1

10.3

Figs. 10.1 and 10.2. Onychoatrophy and anonychia congenita. (Fig. 1 – courtesy of Dr. I. Zeligman. Fig. 2 – from Hopsu-Havu, V.K., Jansén, C.T.: Arch. Derm. *107*, 752–753, 1973)

Fig. 10.3. Koilonychia. (Courtesy of Dr. I. Zeligman)

ing loss is due to a lesion in the cochlea, sometimes with a superimposed conductive loss. Palmoplantar keratodermia may also be a feature of this syndrome [9]. Inheritance is autosomal dominant [9].

Nail-Patella Syndrome (Hereditary Osteo-Onychodysplasia)

The syndrome involves ectodermal and mesodermal abnormalities and is manifested by absence or hypoplasia of the nails and patella, iliac horns, abnormalities of the elbows, and, frequently, kidney changes. The nails are grossly defective, usually greatly reduced in size and never reaching the fingertips. The thumbnails are most frequently affected and these may be completely absent or, in mild cases, the ulnar half of the nail is missing. The

changes in the other nails diminish progressively from the index to the little finger. A V-shaped half-moon is a characteristic abnormality in some nails. Fingernails are involved more frequently than toenails.

The patella may be absent or reduced in size. Dislocation of the patella is common. The elbow joints may show limited supination and incomplete extension. Iliac horns (bony spines) are present in the pelvis. Other abnormalities are thickened scapulae, absent skin creases on distal fingers, webbing of the elbows, heterochromia of the iris with cloverleaf deformity, and cataracts [10]. Renal abnormalities are fairly common. By electron microscopy, the affected kidneys show thickening of the glomerular basement membrane due to the presence of the fibrillar collagen [11].

The disease is inherited as autosomal dominant with linkage between the locus controlling this gene and that of the AB0 blood group [12]. The grade of severity shows a much higher correlation between affected sibs than between offspring and affected parent. This is due to the wild-type isoalleles (see p. 7).

Pachyonychia Congenita

In 1906 Jadassohn and Lewandowsky [13] first described this rare disorder characterized by hypertrophy of the nail bed, palmoplantar hyperkeratosis, follicular keratosis, and oral leukokeratosis.

Clinical Presentation. The fingernails and the toenails are usually affected at birth or shortly thereafter [14, 15]. Marked thickening and discoloration of the nails, which appear lusterless and folded longitudinally, have been noted. Subungual keratosis is marked resulting in raised nail edges. The nail abnormalities may be the only manifestations of the syndrome in some families (Figs. 10.4 and 10.5).

Palmoplantar keratodermia may appear and is most marked at sites of pressure. This hyperkeratosis may be quite painful. Often there is hyperhidrosis of the palms and soles. Occasionally, bullae may appear over the toes, ankles, and sides of the feet. Keratosis pilaris is frequently seen especially on the knees, elbows, buttocks, and occasionally the face [16] (Figs. 10.6 and 10.7).

The leukokeratoses are frequently present at birth. The oral lesions are commonly seen as whitish plaques on the tongue [17]. Occasionally there is involvement of the buccal mucosa, larynx, nose, cornea, and anus. In some cases the teeth may be abnormal. The hair is usually normal, but may be unusually profuse or scanty.

Pathology and Pathophysiology. The affected nails exhibit hyperkeratosis with dyskeratosis of the nail matrix [15]. The skin lesions show hyperkeratosis with focal parakeratosis, acanthosis, hypergranulosis, and occasional dyskeratosis. The mucosal lesions are characterized by a uniform intracellular vacuolization, the absence of intercellular bridges in the prickle cell layer, and the absence of Schiff-positive material in the epithelium [17].

The complications arising from the various lesions are a decrease in manual dexterity, repeated infections around the nails with shedding of the nails, corneal opacities, and partial blindness. The mucosal lesions are not premalignant.

Inheritance. Autosomal dominant.

Treatment. Surgical ablation of the nails and special shoes to diminish plantar keratodermia have been suggested [18].

Other Nail Disorders

Periodic Shedding of Nails

This is a rare disorder in which one or more nails are shed periodically. There is replacement of the shed nails but the new nails are frequently imperfect. It is inherited as autosomal dominant.

Racket Nail (Pouce en Raquette, Brachydactyly Type D, Stub Thumb)

This is not an uncommon abnormality of the thumbs. The distal phalanx is shorter and wider than normal. The nail conforms to the altered shape of the thumb and is short and wide with loss of the lateral curvature. One or both thumbs may be affected. This condition may be distinguished from two others: one in which all the fingernails are racket-shaped and the other in which the thumbnails are short without corresponding shortening of the distal phalanx [19]. The disease is inherited as autosomal dominant.

Brachydactyly Type A5 with Nail Dysplasia

In one kindred, absence of the middle phalanges of the fingers and duplication of the terminal phalanx of the thumb are associated with nail dysplasia [20]. An autosomal dominant mode of inheritance is recorded.

CHANDS (Curly Hair-Ankyloblepharon-Nail Dysplasia Syndrome)

In another kindred, curly hair, ankyloblepharon, and nail dysplasia (hypoplasia) seem to form an autosomal recessive syndrome [21, 22] (Fig. 10.8).

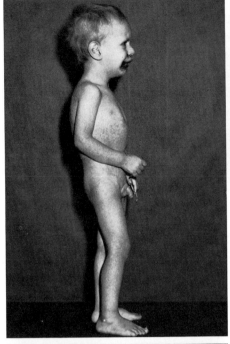

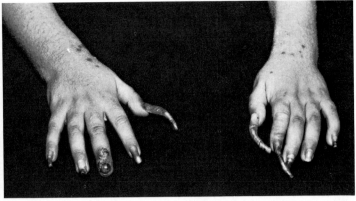

10.4

10.5

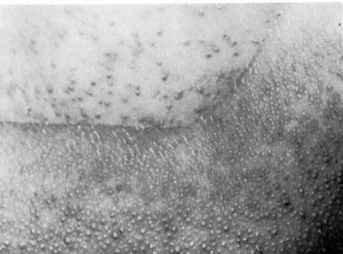

10.7

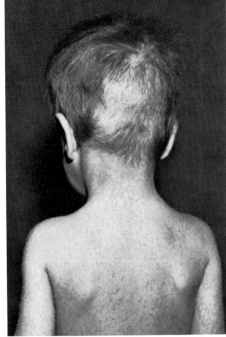

10.6

Figs. 10.4–10.7. Pachyonychia congenita

Fig. 10.4. General appearance

Fig. 10.5. Involvement of the nails

Fig. 10.6. Keratosis pilaris and scanty hair

Fig. 10.7. Close view of keratosis pilaris lesions

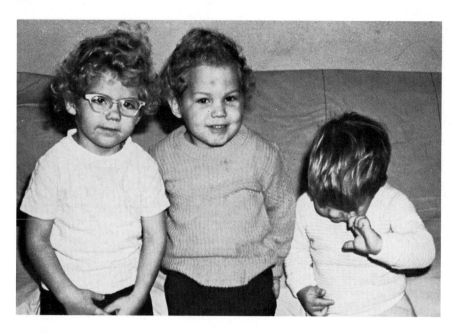

Fig. 10.8. CHANDS (*C*urly *H*air, *A*nkyloblepharon, *N*ail *D*ysplasia *S*yndrome). Note the curly hair of the affected siblings. (From Baughman, F.A., Jr.: In: The clinical delineation of birth defects. Bergsma, D. (ed.), Vol. VII, No. 8, pt. XII, pp. 100–102. Baltimore: Williams & Wilkins Co. 1971)

Onycholysis and Scleronychia

The association in a kindred of partial onycholysis (distal fingernails) with thickened, hardened nails has been described and is probably dominantly inherited [23].

Nail Dysplasia with Hypodontia (Tooth-and-Nail Syndrome)

In this syndrome the main features are hypodontia and dysplastic nails, especially those of the toes. Sweating is normal. Scalp hair may be fine, but eyebrows and eyelashes are normal [24]. Inheritance is probably autosomal dominant.

Onychodystrophy and Deaf-Mutism

The association of onychodystrophy with hereditary sensorineural deafness has been described in several families [25, 26]. Other features that may be present are bi- or triphalangic thumbs. Inheritance is autosomal recessive.

References

1. Hopsu-Havu, V.K., Jansén, C.T.: Anonychia congenita. Arch. Derm. *107*, 752–753 (1973)
2. Mahloudji, M., Amidi, M.: Simple anonychia. Further evidence for autosomal recessive inheritance. J. med. Genet. *8*, 478–480 (1971)
3. Lees, D.H., Lawler, S.D., Renwick, J.H., Thoday, J.M.: Anonychia with ectrodactyly: clinical and linkage data. Ann. hum. Genet. *22*, 69–79 (1957)
4. Feinmesser, M., Zelig, S.: Congenital deafness associated with onychodystrophy. Arch. Otolaryng. *74*, 507–508 (1961)
5. Verbov, J.: Anonychia with bizarre flexural pigmentation – an autosomal dominant dermatosis. Brit. J. Derm. *92*, 469–474 (1975)
6. Timerman, I., Museteanu, C., Simionescu, N.N.: Dominant anonychia and onychodystrophy. J. med. Genet. *6*, 105–106 (1969)
7. Bergeron, J.R., Stone, O.J.: Koilonychia. A report of familial spoon nails. Arch. Derm. *95*, 351–353 (1967)
8. Albright, S.D., Wheeler, C.E., Jr.: Leukonychia. Total and partial leukonychia in a single family with a review of the literature. Arch. Derm. *90*, 392–399 (1964)
9. Bart, R.S., Pumphrey, R.E.: Knuckle pads, leukonychia and deafness. A dominantly inherited syndrome. New Engl. J. Med. *276*, 202–207 (1967)
10. Silverman, M.E., Goodman, R.M., Cuppage, F.E.: The nail-patella syndrome. Clinical findings and ultrastructural observations in the kidney. Arch. intern. Med. *120*, 68–74 (1967)
11. Bennett, W.M., Musgrave, J.E., Campbell, R.A., Elliot, D., Cox, R., Brooks, R.E., Lovrien, E.W., Beals, R.K., Porter, G.A.: The nephropathy of the nail-patella syndrome. Clinicopathologic analysis of 11 kindreds. Amer. J. Med. *54*, 304–319 (1973)
12. Jameson, R.D., Lawler, S.D., Renwick, J.H.: Nail-patella syndrome: clinical and linkage data on family. Ann. hum. Genet. *20*, 348–353 (1956)

13. Jadassohn, J., Lewandowsky, F.: Pachyonychia congenita. Ikonograph. Dermatologica (Basel) *1*, 29–31 (1906)
14. Buckley, W.R., Cassuto, J.: Pachyonychia congenita. Arch. Derm. *85*, 397–402 (1962)
15. Joseph, H.L.: Pachyonychia congenita. Arch. Derm. *90*, 594–603 (1964)
16. Soderquist, N.A., Reed, W.B.: Pachyonychia congenita with epidermal cysts and other congenital dyskeratoses. Arch. Derm. *97*, 31–33 (1968)
17. Gorlin, R.J., Chaudhry, A.P.: Oral lesions accompanying pachyonychia congenita. Oral Surg. *11*, 541–544 (1958)
18. Garb, J.: Pachyonychia congenita. Regression of plantar lesions on patients wearing specially made rubber base foot molds and shoes. Arch. Derm. Syph. *62*, 117–124 (1950)
19. Basset, M.R.H.: Trois formes génotypiques d'ongles courts: le pouce en raquette, les ongles courts simples. Bull. Soc. franç. Derm. Syph. *69*, 15–20 (1962)
20. Bass, H.N.: Familial absence of middle phalanges with nail dysplasia: a new syndrome. Pediatrics *42*, 318–323 (1968)
21. Baughman, F.A., Jr.: CHANDS: the curly hair-ankyloblepharon-nail dysplasia syndrome. In: The clinical delineation of birth defects. Bergsma, D. (ed.), Vol. VII, No. 8, pt. XII, pp. 100–102. Baltimore: Williams & Wilkins Co. 1971
22. Baughman, F.A., Jr.: Personal communication (1977)
23. Schulze, H.D.: Hereditäre Onycholysis partialis mit Skleronychie. Derm. Wschr. *152*, 766–775 (1966)
24. Giansanti, J.S., Long, S.M., Rankin, J.L.: The "tooth and nail" type of autosomal dominant ectodermal dysplasia. Oral Surg. *37*, 576–582 (1974)
25. Goodman, R.M., Lockareff, S., Gwinup, G.: Hereditary congenital deafness with onychodystrophy. Arch. Otolaryng. *90*, 474–477 (1969)
26. Moghadam, H., Statten, P.: Hereditary sensorineural hearing loss associated with onychodystrophy and digital malformations. Canad. med. Ass. J. *107*, 310–312 (1972)

Chapter 11 Oral Mucosal Lesions

Contents

Table 11.1. Syndromes with cleft lip[a]

Name	Genetics	Clinical presentation	Ref.
Cleft lip and/or palate with mucous cysts of lower lip	Autosomal dominant	Malformations of the lower lip with symmetric lumps The syndrome may be expressed only by pits Cleft lip and/or palate may be present	[3]
Cleft lip-palate with split hand and foot	Autosomal dominant (irregular)	Split hand and/or foot and cleft lip-palate Atresia of the lacrimal puncta	[4]
Waardenburg syndrome (see also p. 64)	Autosomal dominant	Deafness, white forelock, dystopia canthorum Cleft lip and palate	
Cleft lip-palate, mucous cysts of the lower lip, popliteal pterygium, digital and genital anomalies	Autosomal dominant	Cleft lip and palate Webbing from ischeal tuberosities to heels Bifid scrotum and cryptorchidism in males, hypoplasia of labia majora in females	[5]
EEC syndrome (see also p. 110)	Autosomal dominant	Ectrodactyly of both hands and one foot Ectodermal dysplasia with severe keratitis Cleft lip-palate	[6, 7]
Nevoid basal cell carcinoma syndrome (see also p. 213)	Autosomal dominant	Basal cell nevus, palmar pits, jaw cysts, kyphoscoliosis, fused ribs, characteristic lamellar calcification of the falx cerebri Lip and/or palatal clefts occur with increased frequency	
Postaxial polydactyly with median cleft of upper lip	Autosomal dominant (suspected)	Unilateral or double harelip Polydactyly	[8, 9]
Rapp-Hodgkin ectodermal dysplasia syndrome (see also p. 110)	Autosomal dominant (X-linked dominant not excluded)	Thin skin with hypohidrosis and sparse fine hair; small, narrow, dysplastic nails Hypodontia with reduced, conical teeth Small mouth, variable cleft of lip, palate, uvula	
Oculodentodigital syndrome	Autosomal dominant with variable expressivity Many are new mutations	Hair is fine, dry, sparse, slow growing Syndactyly of fourth and fifth fingers, third and fourth toes Eyes have microcornea and porous iris Teeth have enamel hypoplasia	
Opitz syndrome	? Autosomal dominant with sex limitation	Ocular hypertelorism, widow's peak, hypospadias, cryptorchidism, hernias, mental deficiency, cardiac anomaly Cleft lip with or without cleft palate	

[a] After McKusick [1] and Gorlin et al. [2].

Table 11.1 (continued)

Name	Genetics	Clinical presentation	Ref.
Cleft lip with or without cleft palate	Multifactorial	As isolated malformation, cleft lip with or without cleft palate behaves as a distinct entity with complex genetics	[10]
Cleft lip-palate with abnormal thumbs and microcephaly	Autosomal recessive (probable)	Cleft lip and palate Microcephaly Hypoplasia and distal displacement of the thumbs Elbow deformities limiting extension	[11]
Ectodermal dysplasia, cleft lip and palate, hand and foot deformity, and mental retardation (see also p. 110)	Autosomal recessive (probable)	Anhidrosis, hypotrichosis, microdontia, dysplasia of nails Cleft lip and palate Deformities of fingers and toes Malformation in the genitourinary system	[12]
Roberts syndrome (see also p. 105)	Autosomal recessive	Severe absence deformities of long bones Oxycephalic skull with prominent eyes Cleft lip-palate Syndactyly	[13]
Cryptophthalmia (see also p. 97)	Autosomal recessive	Both eyes covered with skin, total or partial soft tissue syndactyly of fingers or toes, coloboma of alae nasi, abnormal hairline, 10% have cleft lip and palate	
Meckel syndrome	Autosomal recessive	Polycystic kidneys, exencephalocele, polydactyly, microcephaly, microphthalmia, and cleft lip and/or palate	
Orofaciodigital II (OFD II) syndrome-Mohr (see also p. 105)	Autosomal recessive	Lobed tongue, polydactyly of hands, polysyndactyly of the halluces Midline partial cleft of lip	
Orofaciodigital I (OFD I) syndrome (see also p. 105)	Autosomal or X-linked dominant (lethal in hemizygous male)	Clefts of jaw, lip, and tongue in area of lateral incisors and canines Other malformations of face and skull Malformations of hands, especially syndactyly Mental retardation and familial trembling Hypertrophied frenuli	[14]
Aase syndrome	Unknown, X-linked recessive suggested	Triphalangeal thumbs, mild radial hypoplasia, narrow shoulders, cardiac defects One patient had cleft lip and palate	
4p$^-$ syndrome	Chromosomal	Ocular hypertelorism with broad or beaked nose Microcephaly and/or cranial asymmetry Low-set simple ear with preauricular dimple Cleft lip and/or palate with "fishlike" mouth Deletion of the short arm of chromosome no. 4	
5p$^-$ (Cri du Chat) syndrome	Chromosomal	Catlike cry in infancy, microcephaly Cleft lip and palate occasionally Deletion of the short arm of chromosome no. 5	
Trisomy 13 syndrome (see also p. 293)	Chromosomal	Microphthalmia, coloboma of iris Defects of nose and forebrain of holoprosencephaly type Cleft lip (60–80%), cleft palate, or both	
Trisomy 18 syndrome (see also p. 293)	Chromosomal	Mental deficiency, hypertonicity Tendency for index finger to overlap third Cleft lip, cleft palate, or both occur in 10–50% of cases	
Triploidy syndrome	Chromosomal	Usually aborted or born prematurely with a large placenta Cleft lip occurs in less than 50% of cases Low-set, malformed ears Syndactyly of third and fourth fingers Microphthalmia, coloboma of iris	

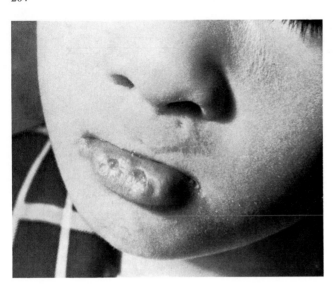

Fig. 11.1. Lip pits. Note paired depressions of lower lip. (From Nora, J.J., Fraser, F.C.: Medical genetics, p. 113. Philadelphia: Lea & Febinger 1974)

References to Table 11.1

1. McKusick, V.A.: Mendelian inheritance in man, 5th ed. Baltimore: Johns Hopkins University Press 1978
2. Gorlin, R.J., Červenka, J., Pruzansky, S.: Facial clefting and its syndromes. In: The clinical delineation of birth defects. Bergsma, D. (ed.), Vol. VII, No. 7, pt. XI, pp. 3–49. Baltimore: Williams & Wilkins Co. 1971
3. Červenka, J., Gorlin, R.J., Anderson, V.E.: The syndrome of pits of the lower lip and cleft lip and/or palate. Genetic considerations. Amer. J. hum. Genet. *19*, 416–432 (1967)
4. Walker, J.C., Clodius, L.: The syndromes of cleft lip, cleft palate, and lobster-claw deformities of hands and feet. Plast. reconstr. Surg. *32*, 627–636 (1963)
5. Gorlin, R.J., Sedano, H.O., Červenka, J.: Popliteal pterygium syndrome. A syndrome comprising cleft lip-palate, popliteal and intercrural pterygia, digital and genital anomalies. Pediatrics *41*, 503–509 (1968)
6. Rüdiger, R.A., Haase, W., Passarge, E.: Association of ectrodactyly, ectodermal dysplasia, and cleft lip-palate. The EEC syndrome. Amer. J. Dis. Child. *120*, 160–163 (1970)
7. Pashayan, H.M., Pruzansky, S., Solomon, L.: The EEC syndrome. Report of six patients. In: The clinical delineation of birth defects. Bergsma, D. (ed.), Vol. X, No. 7, pp. 105–120. Baltimore: Williams & Wilkins Co. 1974
8. Thurston, E.O.: A case of median hare-lip associated with other malformations. Lancet *1909 II*, 996–997
9. Rischbieth, H.: Hare-lip and cleft palate. In: Treasury of human inheritance, Vol. I, pt. IV, Plate J. London: Cambridge University Press 1918
10. Curtis, E.J., Fraser, F.C., Warburton, D.: Congenital cleft lip and palate. Risk figures for counseling. Amer. J. Dis. Child. *102*, 853–857 (1961)
11. Juberg, R.C., Hayward, J.R.: A new familial syndrome of oral, cranial, and digital anomalies. J. Pediat. *74*, 755–762 (1969)
12. Rosselli, D., Gulienetti, R.: Ectodermal dysplasia. Brit. J. plast. Surg. *14*, 190–204 (1961)
13. Roberts, J.B.: A child with double cleft of lip and palate, protrusion of the intermaxillary portion of the upper jaw and imperfect development of the bones of the four extremities. Ann. Surg. *70*, 252 (1919)
14. Gorlin, R.J., Anderson, V.E., Scott, C.R.: Hypertrophied frenuli, oligophrenia, familial trembling and anomalies of the hand. Report of four cases in one family and a *forme fruste* in another. New Engl. J. Med. *264*, 486–489 (1961)

Lip Pits or Fistulas

Commissural pits or angular fistulas occur at the angles of the mouth. Most often these are asymptomatic, but occasionally may present as angular cheilitis. The lesions are 1–4 mm deep [1]. Sometimes preauricular pits are associated findings. Commissural lip pits are inherited probably as autosomal dominant.

Congenital fistulas of the lower lip appear as paired or slightly slitlike depressions on either side of the center of the lower lip [2] (Fig. 11.1). The pits are on the vermilion border and the depressions are surrounded by a slightly elevated wall, 2–4 mm high. The fistulous tracts may extend 5–25 mm and end blindly in the orbicularis oris muscle [2]. Mucus may be forced through the orifices. The tract is lined by stratified squamous epithelium. There is a high incidence of lower lip fistulas associated with cleft lip or palate. Inheritance of the lower lip fistulas is probably autosomal dominant [2].

References

1. Everett, F.G., Weskott, W.B.: Commissural lip pits. Oral Surg. *14*, 202–209 (1961)
2. Taylor, W.B., Lane, D.K.: Congenital fistulas of the lower lip. Associations with cleft lip-palate and anomalies of the extremities. Arch. Derm. *94*, 421–424 (1966)

Gingival Fibromatosis

Benign Intraepithelial Dyskeratosis

This rare disorder usually appears with the eruption of permanent dentition and occasionally with the eruption of deciduous dentition. It is rarely present at birth [1]. There is firm, painless, mild to severe hypertrophy of the gums, especially evident in the anterior maxillary region. The teeth may be partially buried by the hypertrophied gums which may be smooth or stippled.

The gingival abnormality may be an isolated finding [2] or it may be associated with other defects, the commonest of which is hypertrichosis. Gingival fibromatosis with hypertrichosis is a separate entity. The hypertrichosis may be present at birth or appears at puberty [1]. The age of onset of hypertrichosis is unrelated to that of the gingival fibromatosis [1]. The eyebrows are bushy and coarse and terminal hairs appear on the cheeks, chin, forehead, arms, legs, and back. Mental retardation is the second most frequent association [1]. Other less commonly encountered associations are epilepsy [3], doughy hyperelastic skin [1], and cherubism [3]. The association of gingival fibromatosis with hepatosplenomegaly, enlargement of the soft tissues of the ears and nose, hypermobility of joints, shortening of terminal phalanges, and reduction of nail size has been described in several kindreds [4] and is considered a separate genetic disease.

Pathology and Pathophysiology. There is proliferation of connective tissue with thick collagen fibers. Varying degrees of edema and inflammation are present. The overlying epithelium may be hyperplastic.

Inheritance. Autosomal dominant for all three types.

Treatment. Oral hygiene is important. Recurrences are frequent after surgical excision.

This recently described syndrome exhibits white plaques of the oral mucosa and hyperemic conjunctiva [1, 2].

Clinical Presentation. Oral lesions usually appear in early infancy and increase in severity with age until adolescence. They consist of asymptomatic soft white plaques involving the commissures of the mouth, buccal and labial mucosae, vermilion border of the lips, floor of the mouth, and the ventral and lateral surfaces of the tongue (Fig. 11.2). The dorsum of the tongue and the pharynx are usually uninvolved. When severe, the lesions appear folded but lack induration.

The ocular lesions appear in early infancy as foamy gelatinous plaques overlying a hyperemic bulbar conjunctiva (Fig. 11.3). They range from small pingueculae to large plaques. Photophobia is common, especially in summer. All the lesions are benign, but permanent blindness may result after vascularization of the cornea.

Pathology and Pathophysiology. The oral and ocular lesions are similar histologically. There is acanthosis with large vacuolated prickle cells and benign dyskeratotic cells. The latter are characterized by waxy eosinophilic cells and a "cell-within-cell" pattern. These diagnostic features are demonstrable by biopsy and exfoliative cytology [2, 3].

Inheritance. Autosomal dominant [2].

Treatment. No treatment is indicated.

References

1. Anderson, J., Cunliffe, W.J., Roberts, D.F., Close, H.: Hereditary gingival fibromatosis. Brit. med. J. *1969 III*, 218–219
2. Witkop, C.J., Jr.: Heterogeneity in gingival fibromatosis. In: The clinical delineation of birth defects. Bergsma, D. (ed.), Vol. VII, No. 7, pt. XI, pp. 210–221. Baltimore: Williams & Wilkins Co. 1971
3. Ramon, Y., Berman, W., Bubis, J.J.: Gingival fibromatosis combined with cherubism. Oral Surg. *24*, 435–448 (1967)
4. Laband, P.F., Habib, G., Humphreys, G.S.: Hereditary gingival fibromatosis. Report of an affected family with associated splenomegaly and skeletal and soft-tissue abnormalities. Oral Surg. *17*, 339–351 (1964)

References

1. Von Sallmann, L., Paton, D.: Hereditary benign intraepithelial dyskeratosis. I. Ocular manifestations. Arch. Ophthal. *63*, 421–429 (1960)
2. Witkop, C.J., Jr., Shankle, C.H., Graham, J.B., Murray, M.R., Rucknagel, D.L., Byerly, B.H.: Hereditary benign intraepithelial dyskeratosis. II. Oral manifestations and hereditary transmission. Arch. Path. *70*, 696–711 (1960)
3. Witkop, C.J., Jr., Gorlin, R.J.: Four hereditary mucosal syndromes. Comparative histology and exfoliative cytology of Darier-White's disease, hereditary benign intraepithelial dyskeratosis, white sponge nevus, and pachyonychia congenita. Arch. Derm. *84*, 762–771 (1961)

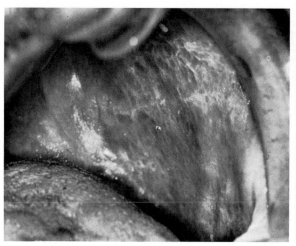

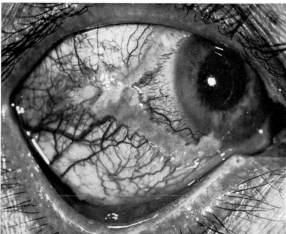

Fig. 11.2. Benign intraepithelial dyskeratosis. Soft, white plaques on the buccal mucosa. (From Witkop, C.J., Jr., et al.: Arch. Path. *70*, 696–711, 1960)

Fig. 11.3. Benign intraepithelial dyskeratosis. Gelatinous plaques overlying the hyperemic conjunctiva. (From Witkop, C.J., Jr., et al.: Arch. Path. *70*, 696–711, 1960)

Melkersson-Rosenthal Syndrome

Melkersson, in 1928, described the association of recurrent facial palsy and labial edema [1]. Rosenthal, in 1931, added scrotal tongue to the syndrome and emphasized its hereditary nature [2].

Clinical Presentation. The main features are chronic swelling of the face, peripheral facial palsy, and in some cases lingua plicata. The disease may start in childhood [3].

The earliest skin manifestation is repeated swelling of the face simulating angioneurotic edema. This swelling involves the upper lip, lower lip, cheeks, or other parts of the face [4]. The edema subsides initially but with repeated attacks it persists, giving the affected parts a firm, rubbery feel (Fig. 11.4).

Facial paralysis may precede the swelling or may develop later (Fig. 11.5). Characteristically, the paralysis is recurrent, partial or complete, and occasionally is accompanied by sensory defects in taste [4]. Scrotal tongue (lingua plicata), if present, usually precedes the facial swelling and/or paralysis (Fig. 11.6).

Frequently formes frustes occur, with combinations of any two of the three findings [4].

Pathology and Pathophysiology. The histologic findings in the skin are nonspecific and consist of edema and lymphocytic infiltration.

Inheritance. Autosomal dominant.

Treatment. There is no effective treatment.

References

1. Melkersson, E.: Ett fall av recidiverande facialispares i samband med angioneurotiskt ödem. Hygiea *90*, 737–741 (1928)
2. Rosenthal, C.: Klinisch-erbbiologischer Beitrag zur Konstitutionspathologie: Gemeinsames Auftreten von (rezidivierender familiärer) Facilislähmung, Angioneuroticischen Gesichtsödem und Lingua plicata in Arthritismus-Familien. Z. Neurol. Psychol. *131*, 475–501 (1931)
3. Kunstadter, R.H.: Melkersson's syndrome. A case report of multiple recurrence of Bell's palsy and episodic facial edema. Amer. J. Dis. Child. *110*, 559–561 (1965)
4. Klaus, S.N., Brunsting, L.A.: Melkersson's syndrome (persistent swelling of the face, recurrent facial paralysis, and lingua plicata): report of a case. Proc. Staff Mayo Clin. *34*, 365–370 (1959)

Mucosal Neuromas with Endocrine Tumors

Clinical Presentation. Mucosal neuromas appear early in life and involve mainly the lips and tongue but may also affect the buccal, gingival, nasal, and conjunctival mucosae and other sites [1]. The involvement of the lips causes diffuse hypertrophy with a "negroid" appearance. Usually the anterior two-thirds of the tongue is involved and the neuromas here appear pinkish and pedunculated [1] or as firm, sessile nodules [2, 3]. Pedunculated nodules on the eyelids are common [1] and involvement of the cornea, traversed by medullated nerve fibers, has been reported [1]. Occasionally, cutaneous neuromas are present [4]. Other findings are pigmentation of the hands, feet, and circumoral area,

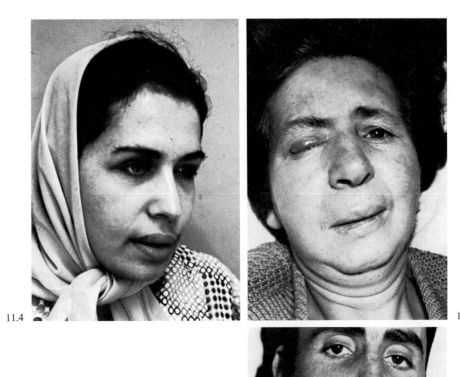

Figs. 11.4–11.6. Melkersson-Rosenthal syndrome

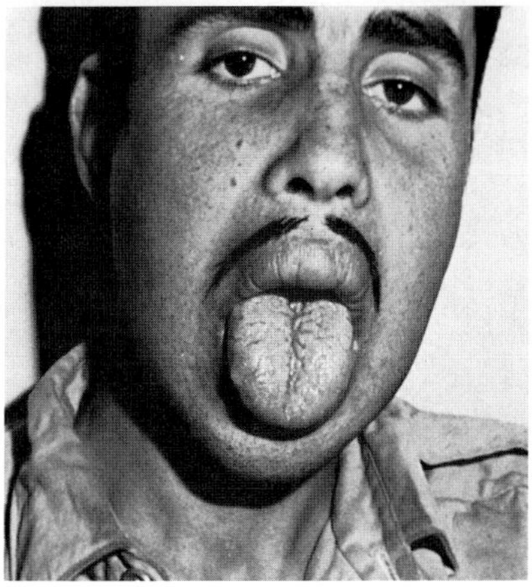

Fig. 11.4. Swelling of the lips

Fig. 11.5. Right facial paralysis. (Courtesy of Dr. W. Frain-Bell)

Fig. 11.6. Edema of the lip and scrotal tongue

11.4

11.5

11.6

proximal myopathy, and production of thyrocalcitonin [5]. The multiple mucosal neuromas are associated relatively frequently with pheochromocytomas, usually bilateral, and medullary thyroid carcinomas known to elaborate amyloid. Marfanoid features and diverticulosis may also be associated findings [1].

Pathology and Pathophysiology. The mucosal lesions are plexiform neuromas – unencapsulated masses of convoluted nerves [1]. Of the several postulates that have been advanced to explain the association of mucosal neuromas and endocrine tumors, one emphasizes the neural crest origin of the components of the syndrome [2].

Inheritance. Autosomal dominant.

Treatment. The presence of the characteristic mucosal neuromas should alert the physician to the possibility of endocrine tumors. Prophylactic thyroidectomies have been advocated.

References

1. Gorlin, R.J., Sedano, H.O., Vickers, R.A., Červenka, J.: Multiple mucosal neuromas, pheochromocytoma and medullary carcinoma of the thyroid – a syndrome. Cancer *22*, 293–299 (1968)
2. Schimke, R.N., Hartmann, W.H., Prout, T.E., Rimoin, D.L.: Syndrome of bilateral pheochromocytoma, medullary thyroid carcinoma and multiple neuromas. A possible regulatory defect in the differentiation of chromaffin tissue. New Engl. J. Med. *279*, 1–7 (1968)
3. Walker, D.M.: Oral mucosal neuroma – medullary thyroid carcinoma syndrome. Brit. J. Derm. *88*, 599–603 (1973)
4. Ljungberg, O., Cederquist, E., von Studnitz, W.: Medullary thyroid carcinoma and phaeochromocytoma: a familial chromaffinomatosis. Brit. med. J. *1967 I*, 279–281
5. Cunliffe, W.J., Black, M.M., Hall, R., Johnston, I.D.A., Hudgson, P., Shuster, S., Gudmundsson, T.V., Joplin, G.F., Williams, E.D., Woodhouse, N.J.Y., Galante, L., MacIntyre, I.: A calcitonin-secreting thyroid carcinoma. Lancet *1968 II*, 63–66

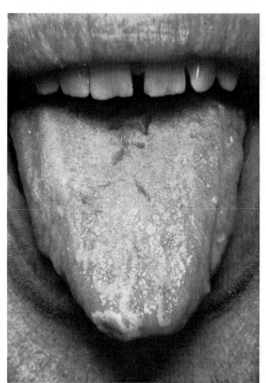

Fig. 11.7. Geographic tongue. (Courtesy of Dr. I. Zeligman)

Fig. 11.8. Scrotal tongue. (Courtesy of Dr. I. Zeligman)

11.7

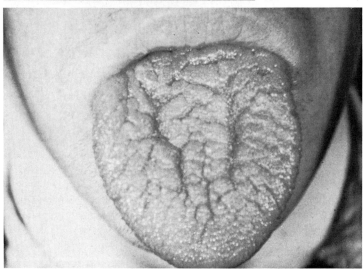

11.8

Tongue Abnormalities

Geographic Tongue
(Benign Migratory Glossitis)

This disorder is seen mainly in children. It is characterized by the appearance of multiple red patches, with slightly elevated borders, on the dorsum of the tongue. Characteristically, there is continuous migration of the patches with changing configuration (Fig. 11.7). Occasionally, the lips and palate are similarly affected. A burning sensation may be present, but otherwise the condition is asymptomatic. Geographic and scrotal tongue may coexist in the same individuals. Inheritance is probably autosomal dominant [1]. No treatment is needed or effective.

Reference

1. Dawson, T.A.J., Pielou, W.D.: Geographical tongue in three generations. Brit. J. Derm. *79*, 678–681 (1967)

Scrotal Tongue
(Lingua Plicata, Fissured Tongue)

This is a rather common disorder which increases in incidence with age, reaching over 14% in the seventh decade [1]. There is usually a deep, longitudinal groove with radiating grooves imparting a cerebriform or scrotal appearance to the surface of the tongue [2]. The ordinary markings of the tongue surface are exaggerated and the fungiform papillae are prominent [2] (Fig. 11.8). Usually the condition is asymptomatic. It may be associated with geographic tongue. The condition occurs with a high incidence in Down syndrome (see p. 290) and is also frequently present in Melkersson-Rosenthal syndrome (see p. 206). Inheritance is autosomal dominant. There is no effective treatment.

References

1. Halperin, V., Kolas, S., Jefferis, K., Huddleston, S., Robinson, H.B.G.: The occurrence of Fordyce spots, benign migratory glossitis, median rhomboid glossitis, and fissured tongue in 2,478 dental patients. Oral. Surg. 6, 1072–1077 (1953)
2. Tobias, N.: Scrotal tongue and its inheritance. Arch. Derm. Syph. *52*, 266 (1945)

Pigmented Tongue

This peculiar form of tongue pigmentation, seen particularly in Negroes, is spotty and occurs mainly on the tip and lateral edges of the tongue [1]. The pigmentation is in the distribution of the fungiform papillae of the tongue. These are red in color, smooth-surfaced, and cone-shaped [2]. In this condition, the fungiform papillae are enlarged and the melanin pigmentation is at their tips [2]. The condition is asymptomatic. In one family, pigmentation of the fungiform papillae of the tongue was associated with pigmentation of the nail beds [3]. The trait for pigmentation is recessive (while the normal allele is dominant over the "pigmented" allele) [4, 5].

References

1. Kaplan, B.J.: The clinical tongue. Lancet *1961I*, 1094–1097
2. Koplon, B.S., Hurley, H.J.: Prominent pigmented papillae of the tongue. Arch. Derm. *95*, 394–396 (1967)
3. Norum, R.A.: Association of pigmented nails, pigmented fungiform papillae of tongue, and apocrine chromidrosis. In: The clinical delineation of birth defects. Bergsma, D. (ed.), Vol. X, No. 4, pt. XVI, pp. 351–352. Baltimore: Williams & Wilkins Co. 1974
4. Rao, D.C.: Tongue pigmentation in man. Hum. Heredity *20*, 8–12 (1970)
5. Rao, D.C.: Formal segregation analysis for tongue pigmentation in man. Hum. Heredity *23*, 308–312 (1973)

White Sponge Nevus
(Familial White Folded Dysplasia
of the Mucous Membrane,
White Folded Gingivostomatitis)

Cannon first described this syndrome in 1935 [1].

Clinical Presentation. The lesions may appear at birth, in early infancy, or during adolescence. The oral mucosa appears white, deeply folded or corrugated, soft, and spongy. The buccal and labial mucosae are usually involved; occasionally, the greater part or all of the oral mucosa may be involved. The labia, vagina, anus, and rectum may be similarly affected. The lesions are asymptomatic and benign [1–3].

Pathology and Pathophysiology. There is marked acanthosis, with vacuolation of the granular and prickle cells. Parakeratosis is frequent. There are dyskeratotic cells with a rigid-appearing eosinophilic cytoplasm. These cells are also demonstrable by exfoliative cytology [3].

Inheritance. Autosomal dominant [3].

Treatment. No treatment is indicated.

References

1. Cannon, A.B.: White sponge nevus of the mucosa (naevus spongiosus albus mucosae). Arch. Derm. Syph. *31*, 365–370 (1935)
2. Zegarelli, E.V., Everett, F.G., Kutscher, A.H., Gorman, J., Kupferberg, N.: Familial white folded dysplasia of the mucous membranes. Arch. Derm. *80*, 59–65 (1959)
3. Witkop, C.J., Jr., Gorlin, R.J.: Four hereditary mucosal syndromes. Comparative histology and exfoliative cytology of Darier-White's disease, hereditary benign intraepithelial dyskeratosis, white sponge nevus, and pachyonychia congenita. Arch. Derm. *84*, 762–771 (1961)

Chapter 12 Proliferative Disorders

Contents

Collagenoma and Connective Tissue Nevus

Familial Cutaneous Collagenoma

One report describes three brothers with this condition [1].

Clinical Presentation. At about the age of 15 years,
cutaneous nodules appear over the back, especially
the upper two-thirds, and less frequently over the
shoulders and abdomen. The nodules are discrete,
0.5–4.5 cm, slightly elevated, and movable (Figs.
12.1 and 12.2). The overlying skin surface has a *peau
d'orange* effect [1, 2] or is normal [2]. Associated
findings in the reported cases are idiopathic
myocardiopathy, atrophy of the left iris, profound
high-frequency sensorineural hearing loss, and recurrent vasculitis [1].

Pathology and Pathophysiology. There is a marked
increase in collagen in the dermis [1, 2]. The elastic
fibers are essentially normal [1] or decreased [2].

Inheritance. Probably autosomal recessive [2].

Treatment. No treatment is needed.

References

1. Henderson, R.R., Wheeler, C.E., Jr., Abele, D.C.: Familial
   cutaneous collagenoma. Report of cases. Arch. Derm. *98*,
   23–27 (1968)
2. Hegedus, S.I., Schorr, W.F.: Familial cutaneous collagenoma.
   Cutis *10*, 283–288 (1972)

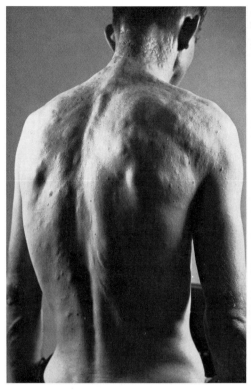

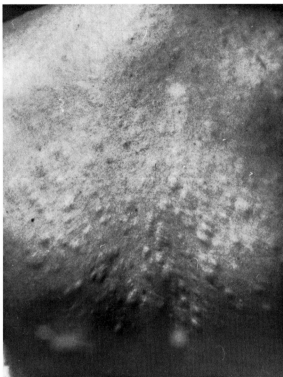

Fig. 12.1. Familial cutaneous collagenoma. Note the distribution over the back and the shoulders. (From Henderson, R.R., et al.: Arch. Derm. *98*, 23–27, 1968)

Fig. 12.2. Familial cutaneous collagenoma. Closer view of the lesions. (From Hegedus, S.I., Schorr, W.F.: Cutis *10*, 283–288, 1972)

Osteopoikilosis (Dermatofibrosis Lenticularis Disseminata, Connective Tissue Nevus-Osteopoikilosis Syndrome)

Osteopoikilosis refers to circumscribed sclerotic areas found incidentally on radiologic examination as densities in the epiphyses or metaphyses of the long bones, pelvis, and bones of the hands and feet [1]. The term "dermatofibrosis lenticularis disseminata" refers to a type of connective tissue nevus associated with osteopoikilosis [1]. Either the skin or the bone lesions may be absent in individual members of families that have both [2, 3].

Clinical Presentation. Osteopoikilosis is a harmless malformation. The skin lesions usually appear in childhood and are symmetric or asymmetric in distribution, firm, slightly raised, skin-colored or yellowish papules [1]. The papules are usually set close together to give a cobblestone pattern or a linear configuration [1]. Orange-red plaques with pseudopodlike extensions may appear [3, 4]. The sites usually involved are the upper back, arms, forearms, lumbar region, buttocks, and thighs.

Occasionally, the flexural folds are also involved [5] (Figs. 12.3 and 12.4).

Other associated findings are small stature, supernumerary ribs, supernumerary vertebrae, mental deficiency, neuropathy, and infantilism [1].

Pathology and Pathophysiology. The cutaneous lesions show an increase in collagen fibers that appear normal [1, 4] or frayed and twisted with irregular cross-striations [4]. The elastic fibers may be absent [1] or coarse, irregular [3], smudgy, or thickened [4, 5], especially deep in the dermis [1]. Within the same family affected individuals may show a considerable spectrum of changes in collagen and elastic fibers [4].

Inheritance. Autosomal dominant [2].

Treatment. No treatment is required, except excision of individual lesions for cosmetic purposes.

References

1. Raque, C.J., Wood, M.G.: Connective-tissue nevus. Dermatofibrosis lenticularis disseminata with osteopoikilosis. Arch. Derm. *102*, 390–396 (1970)
2. Berlin, R., Hedensiö, B., Lilja, B., Linder, L.: Osteopoikilosis – a clinical and genetic study. Acta med. scand. *181*, 305–314 (1967)

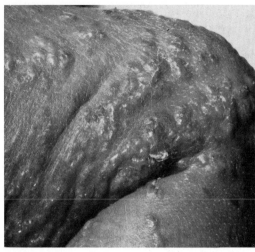
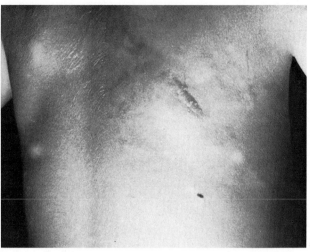

12.3

12.4

Figs. 12.3 and 12.4. Osteopoikilosis. Aggregated, skin-colored papules. (Fig. 3 – courtesy of Dr. W. F. Frain-Bell.

Fig. 4 – from Schorr, W.F., et al.: Arch. Derm. *106*, 208–214, 1972)

3. Smith, A.D., Waisman, M.: Connective tissue nevi. Familial occurrence and association with osteopoikilosis. Arch. Derm. *81*, 249–252 (1960)
4. Schorr, W.F., Opitz, J.M., Reyes, C.N.: The connective tissue nevus-osteopoikilosis syndrome. Arch. Derm. *106*, 208–214 (1972)
5. Danielsen, L., Midtgaard, K., Christensen, H.E.: Osteopoikilosis associated with dermatofibrosis lenticularis disseminata. Arch. Derm. *100*, 465–470 (1969)

Epidermal Proliferative Disorders

Self-Healing Squamous Epithelioma (Ferguson Smith Type)

J. Ferguson Smith first described this tumor in 1934 [1]. The condition is considered to be the generalized or multiple form of keratoacanthoma [2].

Clinical Presentation. The mean age of onset of the tumors is 25.5 years [3]. No tumor has been observed to develop before puberty. The sites of predilection are the exposed areas [2, 3], especially the nose, ears, and circumoral region. The number of tumors varies from 1–90 [3]. The lesions start as macules or papules, enlarge gradually, and form central keratinous plugs (Figs. 12.5–12.7). There is spontaneous involution leaving a pitted or smooth scar [2]. Deep infiltration is more frequent than in solitary keratoacanthoma and thus scarring is more evident. As lesions involute, new lesions appear. Recurrence after excision or destruction is uncom-

mon and no case of metastasis has been reported [2]. Pruritus may be a prominent feature [4].

Pathology and Pathophysiology. Characteristically, there is a keratin-filled central crater, overhung by epidermis. The epidermis is hyperplastic with nests of epithelial cells invading the dermis or showing dyskeratosis and keratin pearl formation. A heavy inflammatory infiltrate surrounds the tumor. The basal cell layer is often intact [2, 4]. It is assumed that the tumors arise within a pilosebaceous follicle [3]. No viral particles have been detected in this tumor [3].

Inheritance. Autosomal dominant.

Treatment. Once the diagnosis is established, the majority of lesions may be safely observed without treatment, as there is spontaneous involution. The lesions that continue to enlarge or become cosmetically unacceptable are best excised [2].

References

1. Ferguson Smith, J.: A case of multiple primary squamous-celled carcinomata of the skin in a young man with spontaneous healing. Brit. J. Derm. *46*, 267–272 (1934)
2. Epstein, N.N., Biskind, G.R., Pollack, R.S.: Multiple primary self-healing squamous-cell "epitheliomas" of the skin. Generalized keratoacanthoma. Arch. Derm. *75*, 210–223 (1957)
3. Ferguson-Smith, M.A., Wallace, D.C., James, Z.H., Renwick, J.H.: Multiple self-healing squamous epithelioma. In: The clinical delineation of birth defects. Bergsma, D. (ed.), Vol. VII, No. 8, pt. XII, pp. 157–163. Baltimore: Williams & Wilkins Co. 1971
4. Ereaux, L.P., Schopflocher, P.: Familial primary self-healing squamous epithelioma of skin. Ferguson-Smith type. Arch. Derm. *91*, 589–594 (1965)

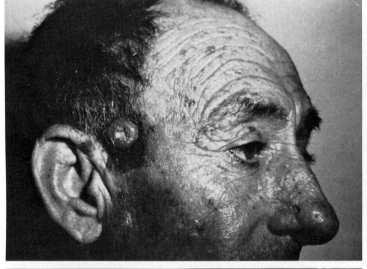

12.5

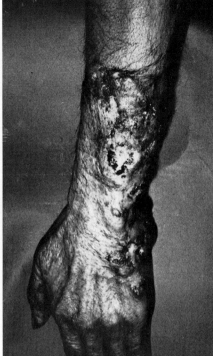

12.7

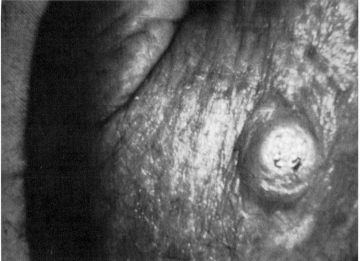

12.6

Figs. 12.5 and 12.6. Self-healing squamous epithelioma. Individual nodules with the characteristic central keratinous plugs

Fig. 12.7. Self-healing squamous epithelioma. Coalesced multiple lesions over the forearm

Basal Cell Nevus Syndrome (Gorlin Syndrome, Nevoid Basal Cell Carcinoma)

Jarisch is credited with the first case report in 1894 [1]; Nomland distinguished the nevoid character of the tumors in 1932 [2]. Binkley and Johnson pointed out the multiple defects in this syndrome [3].

Clinical Presentation. The syndrome affects not only the skin but also the skeletal, central nervous, and endocrine systems, as well as the eyes. The main cutaneous lesions are multiple basal cell epitheliomas (Figs. 12.8 and 12.9). These are usually numerous and appear between puberty and the mid-thirties [4, 5]. The early lesions appear as flesh-colored or brownish dome-shaped papules on the face, neck, upper trunk, and upper limbs [5]. The older lesions frequently ulcerate. Other skin findings are milia, comedones, epithelial and sebaceous cysts, lipomas, and palmoplantar pits. The pits are usually shallow holes (1–3 mm), discrete or confluent, with red bases [6].

The main osseous abnormalities are multiple mandibular cysts and mild mandibular prognathism [5]. These usually contribute to the characteristic facies with frontal and temporoparietal bossing, sunken eyes, and broad nasal root [5]. Other skeletal abnormalities are rib anomalies (bifurcation, splaying synostosis, partial agenesis, or cervical rudimentary); scoliosis; cervical or upper thoracic vertebral fusion; bridging of the sella; spina bifida occulta; syndactyly or oligodactyly or both; a short fourth metacarpal; Sprengel deformity of the scapula; medial hooking of the scapula; defective medial clavicle; pectus excavatum or cari-

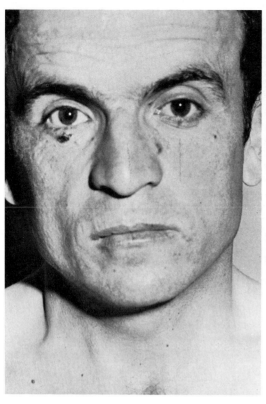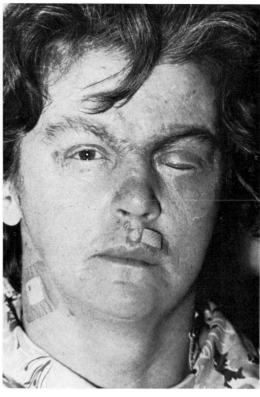

12.8   12.9

Figs. 12.8 and 12.9. Basal cell nevus syndrome. Multiple basal cell tumors

natum; pes planus; and hallux valgus [5]. Calcification of the dura, choroid, and petroclinoid
ligaments is frequent. Mental retardation, schizophrenia, congenital hydrocephalus, nerve deafness,
and agenesis of corpus callosum have been
reported.

The eye findings include dystopia canthorum, hypertelorism, congenital blindness (due to corneal
opacity, cataract, glaucoma, or colobomas of the
choroid and optic nerve), and chalazion. Ovarian
fibroma or cyst (or both), hypogonadism, and pelvic
calcification may also occur. Other findings are
lymphomesenteric cysts, kidney malformations, and
inguinal hernia. Fibrosarcoma of the jaw, amelob-
lastoma, and medulloblastoma have been reported
in a few patients.

Pathology and Pathophysiology. The basal cell epitheliomas in this condition are histologically indistinguishable from the various morphologic types
of nonhereditary tumors [4]. Probably, the nevoid
tumors are more often associated with an inflammatory infiltrate [5]. The pits result from absence
of dense palmar or plantar keratin [6]. At the base
of the pit are loose keratin flakes and small parakeratotic areas with attenuation of the granular cell
layer. The rete ridges are irregular and are popu-

lated by small basaloid cells with varying degrees of
vacuolization [6]. Electron microscopy reveals
poor development of the tonofibrils, small keratohyalin granules, and incomplete discharge of ce-
mentsomes [7].

The mandibular cysts are lined by simple epithelium [4].

Some patients are thought to have hyporesponsive-
ness to parathyroid hormone [4]. Recent evidence,
however, has refuted this [8].

Inheritance. Autosomal dominant.

Treatment. The epitheliomas should be treated by
curettage or surgery.

References

1. Jarish, A.: Zur Lehre von den Hautgeschwülsten. Arch.
   Derm. Syph. (Berl.) *28*, 163–222 (1894)
2. Nomland, R.: Multiple basal cell epitheliomas originating
   from congenital pigmented basal cell nevi. Arch. Derm. Syph.
   25, 1002–1008 (1932)
3. Binkley, G.W., Johnson, H.H., Jr.: Epithelioma adenoides
   cysticum: basal cell nevi, agenesis of the corpus callosum, and
   dental cysts. Arch. Derm. Syph. *63*, 73–84 (1951)
4. Clendenning, W.E., Block, J.B., Radde, I.C.: Basal cell nevus
   syndrome. Arch. Derm. *90*, 38–53 (1964)

5. Gorlin, R.J., Sedano, H.O.: The multiple nevoid basal cell carcinoma syndrome revisited. In: The clinical delineation of birth defects. Bergsma, D. (ed.), Vol. VII, No. 8, pt. XII, pp. 140–148. Baltimore: Williams & Wilkins Co. 1971
6. Howell, J.B., Mehregan, A.H.: Pursuit of the pits in the nevoid basal cell carcinoma syndrome. Arch. Derm. *102*, 586–597 (1970)
7. Hashimoto, K., Howell, J.B., Yamanishi, Y., Holubar, K., Bernhard, R., Jr.: Electron microscopic studies of palmar and plantar pits of nevoid basal cell epithelioma. J. invest. Derm. *59*, 380–393 (1972)
8. Kaufman, R.L., Chase, L.R.: Basal cell nevus syndrome: normal responsiveness to parathyroid hormone. In: The clinical delineation of birth defects. Bergsma, D. (ed.), Vol. VII, No. 8, pt. XII, pp. 149–155. Baltimore: Williams & Wilkins Co. 1971

Cylindromatosis (Turban Tumors, Spiegler-Brooke Tumors)

Cylindromas may be solitary (nonhereditary) or multiple (hereditary).

Clinical Presentation. The lesions usually appear in early adulthood and gradually increase in number and size. They are predominantly on the scalp, rarely on the face, trunk, or extremities. The tumors are smooth, dome-shaped, firm, pink to red nodules. They may be numerous and occasionally pedunculated (Figs. 12.10–12.13). Malignant degeneration in these tumors is rare.

The frequent association of multiple lesions of cylindroma with multiple lesions of trichoepithelioma suggests that these tumors may represent a single entity [1].

Pathology and Pathophysiology. The tumors are dermal and are made up of masses and columns of cells surrounded by a hyaline sheath and a narrow band of stroma. The cells are of two types: those with small, darkly staining nuclei at the periphery and those with larger, central nuclei. Lumenlike structures are present, and these may contain hyaline material.

The hyaline sheath is PAS-positive, distase-resistant, and does not stain with Alcian blue, making it a neutral mucopolysaccharide [2]. The material in the lumina contains acid as well as neutral mucopolysaccharides. There is controversy as to the origin of these tumors and the direction of differentiation (apocrine [3] or eccrine [4]).

Inheritance. Probably autosomal dominant with stronger expression in the female [5]. The possibility of X-linkage with dominance in a small proportion of families is not completely excluded [5].

Treatment. Surgical excision is the treatment of choice.

References

1. Welch, J.P., Wells, R.S., Kerr, C.B.: Ancell-Spiegler cylindromas (turban tumors) and Brooke-Fordyce trichoepitheliomas: evidence for a single genetic entity. J. med. Genet. *5*, 29–35 (1968)
2. Fusaro, R.M., Goltz, R.W.: Histochemically demonstrable carbohydrates of appendageal tumors of the skin. II. Benign apocrine gland tumors. J. invest. Derm. *38*, 137–142 (1962)
3. Hashimoto, K., Lever, W.F.: Histogenesis of skin appendage tumors. Arch. Derm. *100*, 356–369 (1969)
4. Crain, R.C., Helwig, E.B.: Dermal cylindroma (dermal eccrine cylindroma). Amer. J. clin. Path. *35*, 504–515 (1969)
5. McKusick, V.A.: Mendelian inheritance in man, 5th ed., pp. 114 and 799. Baltimore: Johns Hopkins University Press 1978

Trichoepithelioma (Multiple Benign Cystic Epithelioma, Epithelioma Adenoides Cysticum of Brooke)

Brooke [1] and Fordyce [2] independently described this tumor in 1892. The term trichoepithelioma is preferred because it indicates the differentiation of the tumor cells toward hair structures. Trichoepithelioma may be solitary (nonhereditary) or multiple (hereditary).

Clinical Presentation. Multiple trichoepithelioma is characterized by multiple lesions which usually appear before puberty and rarely after the third decade, grow in size for a while, and then remain stationary [3]. They are predominantly on the face, especially the nasolabial folds and upper lip, but the back and scalp [3], neck, trunk, and extremities [4] may also be affected. The lesions on the face usually measure 0.2–0.5 cm in diameter, whereas those on the back are larger [3]. The tumors are flesh-colored, firm, and translucent with, occasionally, surface telangiectasia [3] (Figs. 12.14–12.17). The lesions often coalesce. Ulceration is rare [5]. The lesions are usually asymptomatic. One affected individual developed a basosquamous carcinoma [4]. Lesions of trichoepithelioma and cylindroma may coexist. Some believe that these two tumors represent a single entity [6]. No other associated findings have been recorded [4, 5].

Pathology and Pathophysiology. The tumors are usually well-circumscribed and occupy the upper and middermis. There are lobules and a lacelike network of tracts of basaloid cells. Keratinous cysts

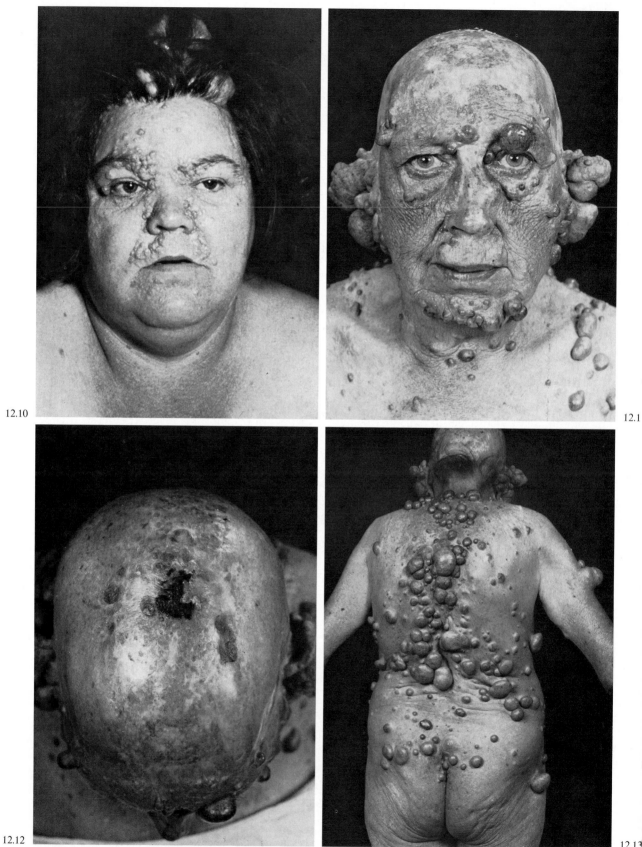

12.10

12.1

12.12

12.13

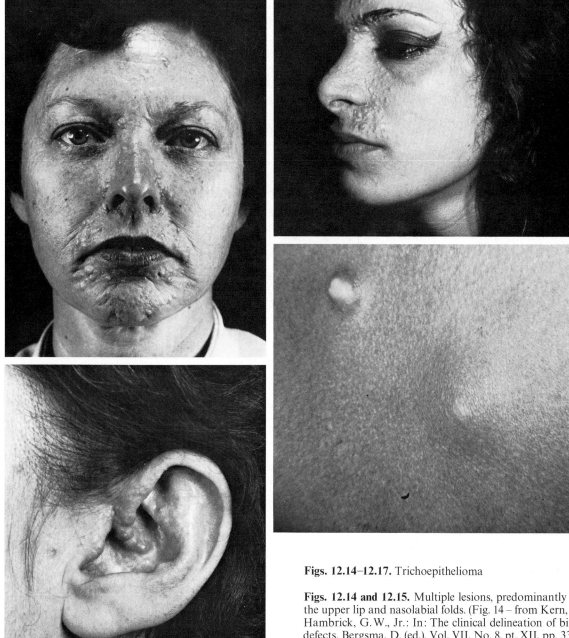

12.14

12.15

12.17

12.16

Figs. 12.14–12.17. Trichoepithelioma

Figs. 12.14 and 12.15. Multiple lesions, predominantly on the upper lip and nasolabial folds. (Fig. 14 – from Kern, F., Hambrick, G.W., Jr.: In: The clinical delineation of birth defects. Bergsma, D. (ed.), Vol. VII, No. 8, pt. XII, pp. 332–333. Baltimore: Williams & Wilkins Co. 1971)

Fig. 12.16. Involvement of the pinna. (From Kern, F., Hambrick, G.W., Jr.: In: The clinical delineation of birth defects. Bergsma, D. (ed.), Vol. VII, No. 8, pt. XII, pp. 332–333. Baltimore: Williams & Wilkins Co. 1971)

Fig. 12.17. Close-up view

◄ **Figs. 12.10–12.13.** Cylindromatosis. Smooth, dome-shaped nodules over the face, scalp, and trunk. (Courtesy of Dr. V. A. McKusick, from Harper, P.S.: In: The clinical delineation of birth defects. Bergsma, D. (ed.), Vol. VII, No. 8, pt. XII, pp. 338–341. Baltimore: Williams & Wilkins Co. 1971)

are prominent and, characteristically, keratinization is abrupt. The stroma of the tumor is sharply demarcated from the surrounding dermis [3]. Foreign body reactions of epithelioid and giant cells are common, with occasional calcium deposits [3]. The origin of these tumors is believed to be from a pluripotential cell with differentiation directed toward hair structures [3].

Inheritance. Autosomal dominant.

Treatment. There is no satisfactory mode of treatment. Surgical excision, electrodesiccation, curettage, and X-ray irradiation have been unrewarding.

References

1. Brooke, H.G.: Epithelioma adenoides cysticum. Brit. J. Derm. *4*, 269–286 (1892)
2. Fordyce, J.A.: Multiple benign cystic epithelioma of the skin. J. cutaneous genito-urin. Dis. *10*, 459–473 (1892)
3. Gray, H.R., Helwig, E.B.: Epithelioma adenoides cysticum and solitary trichoepithelioma. Arch. Derm. *87*, 102–114 (1963)
4. Ziprkowski, K., Schewach-Millet, M.: Multiple trichoepithelioma in a mother and two children. Dermatologica (Basel) *132*, 248–256 (1966)
5. Gaul, L.E.: Heredity of multiple benign cystic epithelioma. "The Indiana family". Arch. Derm. *68*, 517–524 (1953)
6. Welch, J.P., Wells, R.S., Kerr, C.B.: Ancell-Spiegler cylindromas (turban tumors) and Brooke-Fordyce trichoepitheliomas: evidence for a single genetic entity. J. med. Genet. *5*, 29–35 (1968)

Pilomatrixoma (Benign Calcifying Epithelioma of Malherbe)

Clinical Presentation. Pilomatrixomas are single tumors that often occur in young people, the median age being 23 years [1]. Both sexes are affected. The arms, face, and neck are the sites most frequently involved, but other areas like thighs, scalp, shoulders, and trunk may be affected [1]. The tumors appear as asymptomatic nodules, reddish or bluish in color, firm to stony-hard, and lobular (Fig. 12.18). Pain on pressure may be a presenting symptom. Occasionally these tumors may be inflamed. Familial occurrence of this tumor is rare; isolated reports have appeared: five affected persons in two generations of a family [2], an affected father and daughter [3], and two affected sisters [4]. Association with myotonia atrophica [4, 5] may indicate more than a coincidental finding.

Pathology and Pathophysiology. The lesions are round or oval, well-circumscribed dermal masses. These masses are composed of sheets and bands of small basophilic epithelial cells with scanty cytoplasm and indistinct cell margins, separated by connective tissue [1]. Centrally, the cells have more abundant eosinophilic cytoplasm with visible cell margins. Pyknosis then develops and shadow cells with translucent glassy cytoplasm and well-defined cell borders are formed [1]. Small masses of keratin are seen and calcification is frequent. Occasionally ossification is noted. Foreign body reactions are usual. Ultrastructural [6] and histochemical [1, 6] studies show that this is an appendageal tumor of the hair and its follicle, composed mainly of hair cortex cells with differentiation toward mature hair structures, hence the term "pilomatrixoma." The course is benign.

Inheritance. Probably autosomal dominant.

Treatment. If the tumors are painful or subject to periodic inflammation, surgical excision is indicated.

References

1. Forbis, R., Jr., Helwig, E.B.: Pilomatrixoma (calcifying epithelioma). Arch. Derm. *83*, 606–618 (1961)
2. Duperrat, B., Albert, N.I.: Forme familiale de l'épithélioma de Malherbe. Bull. Soc. franç. Derm. Syph. *55*, 196–197 (1948)
3. Geiser, J.D.: Forme familiale d'épithélioma (calcifié) de Malherbe. Dermatologica (Basel) *120*, 361–365 (1960)
4. Harper, P.S.: Calcifying epithelioma of Malherbe and myotonic dystrophy in sisters. In: The clinical delineation of birth defects. Bergsma, D. (ed.), Vol. VII, No. 8, pt. XII, pp. 343–345. Baltimore: Williams & Wilkins Co. 1971
5. Cantwell, A.R.,Jr., Reed, W.B.: Myotonia atrophica and multiple calcifying epithelioma of Malherbe. Acta derm.-venereol. (Stockh.) *45*, 387–390 (1965)
6. Hashimoto, K., Nelson, R.G., Lever, W.F.: Calcifying epithelioma of Malherbe. Histochemical and electron microscopic studies. J. invest. Derm. *46*, 391–408 (1966)

Seborrheic Keratoses (Seborrheic Warts)

This common epidermal tumor usually appears after the fourth or fifth decade in both sexes. Some reports have stressed its familial occurrence [1].

Clinical Presentation. The commonest sites of involvement are the trunk, face, and scalp; rarely are other areas involved. The lesions are multiple and start as well-defined, yellowish plaques. These gradually darken in color and assume a stuck-on appearance. The surface is verrucous and greasy and the color varies from tan to brown or black (Figs. 12.19 and 12.20). Usually they are asymptomatic, but occasionally they may be pruritic.

Fig. 12.18. Pilomatrixoma. Well-circumscribed, reddish blue, firm nodule

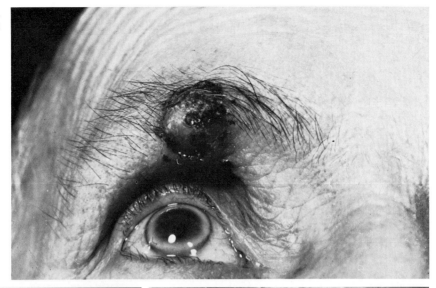

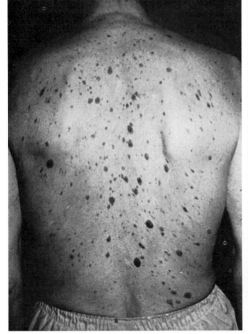

Fig. 12.19. Seborrheic keratoses. Usual distribution

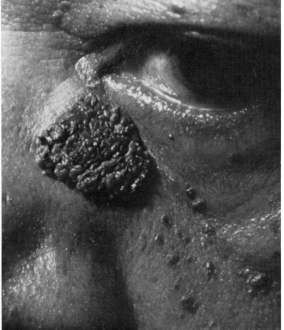

Fig. 12.20. Seborrheic keratoses. Close-up view, showing a greasy, verrucous surface

Pathology and Pathophysiology. There is hyperkeratosis, papillomatosis, and acanthosis. The latter is due to proliferation of basaloid cells, which is mainly upward. Horn cysts and pseudohorn cysts are common. The amount of melanin pigment is variable.

Inheritance. In the familial type, inheritance is probably autosomal dominant [1].

Treatment. No treatment is needed except for cosmetic purposes or if the lesions are irritated and inflamed. Treatment with curettage after freezing with fluoroethyl or light desiccation gives good results.

Reference

1. Reiches, A.J.: Seborrheic keratoses. Are they delayed hereditary nevi? Arch. Derm. Syph. *65*, 596–600 (1952)

Dermatosis Papulosa Nigra

This is a rather common disorder among American blacks, affecting 35% of the adult population [1].

Clinical Presentation. Starting around puberty and increasing with age, firm, pigmented, nontender, smooth papules appear on the face (Figs. 12.21 and 12.22). In many instances, the trunk may also be involved [1].

Pathology and Pathophysiology. The histologic picture is similar to that of seborrheic keratosis (see p. 219). There is hyperkeratosis, acanthosis, and horn cysts [1].

Inheritance. Although the predominant occurrence of this disorder in blacks is consistent with a genetic basis, its pattern of inheritance has not been clearly established.

Treatment. There is no need for treatment unless cosmetically indicated. Then, curettage after freezing with fluoroethyl or light desiccation gives good results.

Reference

1. Hairston, M.A., Jr., Reed, R.J., Derbes, V.J.: Dermatosis papulosa nigra. Arch. Derm. *89*, 655–658 (1964)

Familial Cutaneous Papillomatosis

A pedigree has been described with this condition [1]. The eruption starts in the late teens. The lesions slowly enlarge, darken, and then remain stationary. The affected sites are the back and arms, and less often the chest and knees. The lesions are 1–2 mm, brownish black hyperkeratotic papules, discrete, or arranged in a reticulate pattern or coalesced to form plaques [1]. Histologically, there is hyperkeratosis, acanthosis, papillomatosis, and increased pigment in the basal cell layer [1]. Inheritance is probably autosomal dominant.

Reference

1. Baden, H.P.: Familial cutaneous papillomatosis. Arch. Derm. *92*, 394–395 (1965)

Multiple Fibrofolliculomas

A condition with pilar hamartomas has been recently described in a kindred [1]. The skin tumors are small and dome-shaped and appear at around the age of 25 years. Associated skin findings were trichodiscomas and acrochordons. Histologically, the pilar hamartomas consist of a circumscribed proliferation of loose connective tissue surrounding an abnormal hair follicle. Epithelial strands from the hair follicle extend into this connective tissue zone. The inheritance is thought to be autosomal dominant [1].

Reference

1. Birt, A.R., Hogg, G.R., Dube, W.J.: Hereditary multiple fibrofolliculomas with trichodiscomas and acrochordons. Arch. Derm. *113*, 1674–1677 (1977)

Multiple Hamartoma Syndrome (Cowden Disease)

This syndrome was first described in 1963 by Lloyd and Dennis [1] and named Cowden disease from the surname of the probands.

Clinical Presentation. The organ system that most consistently manifests this syndrome is the skin. The cutaneous changes include dome-shaped, flesh-colored papules; flat-topped, lichenoid papules with a central keratotic plug; punctate keratodermia of the palms; and verrucous lesions strikingly similar to those of verruca vulgaris, verruca plana, and acrokeratotic lesions of keratosis follicularis (Darier disease). The verrucous lesions at the angles of the mouth and on the oral mucosa may mimic hypertrophic perleche, benign gingival hyperplasia, or ectopic or recurrent lymphoreticular tissue. These skin lesions behave as benign hamartomas [2].

The syndrome is important because of the associated abnormalities of the thyroid gland, breasts, gastrointestinal, nervous, and other organ systems. Thyroid tumors (goiter, adenoma, carcinoma) and acute thyroiditis may develop. Fibrocystic disease of the breast has been found in all the female patients, with a significant association of carcinoma of the breast. Gastrointestinal tract abnormalities include colonic polyps, diverticulae of the colon, and ganglioneuromas. Neuromas and ganglioneuromas are found incidentally in the middle and lower dermis in association with cutaneous lesions.

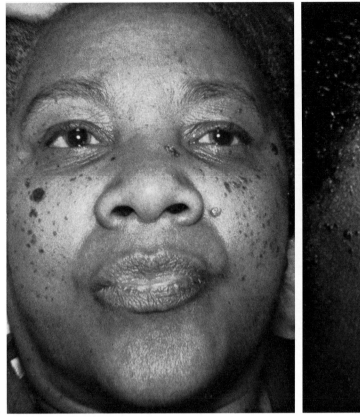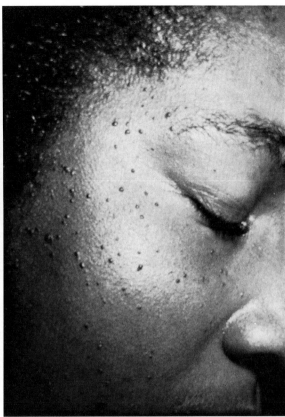

2.21   12.22

Figs. 12.21 and 12.22. Dermatosis papulosa nigra. Firm, pigmented papules

Central nervous system affection may be manifested by mental dullness or retardation, intention tremor, electroencephalographic changes, and meningioma formation. Female genital tract abnormalities may also occur [2].

Pathology and Pathophysiology. Light microscopic examination shows nonspecific changes such as hyperkeratosis acanthosis simulating pseudoepitheliomatous hyperplasia, and a mild perivascular infiltrate of lymphocytes, histiocytes, polymorphonuclear leukocytes, and rare plasma cells [2]. Electron microscopy reveals dense accumulations of collagen immediately beneath the basement membrane. Within the keratinocytes deep in the epidermis, there is clumping of tonofilaments. Vacuoles are seen in the keratinocyte cytoplasm. Keratinosomes appear to be reduced in number in the upper epidermis [2].

Inheritance. Autosomal dominant [2].

Treatment. The skin lesions are recalcitrant to the usual modalities employed in the treatment of common verrucae. Therapy should be directed mainly to the abnormalities of the thyroid, breasts, gastrointestinal, nervous, and other organ systems [2].

References

1. Lloyd, K.M., Dennis, M.: Cowden's disease. A possible new symptom complex with multiple system involvement. Ann. intern. Med. *58*, 136–142 (1963)
2. Gentry, W.C.,Jr., Eskritt, N.R., Gorlin, R.J.: Multiple hamartoma syndrome (Cowden disease). Arch. Derm. *109*, 521–525 (1974)

Steatocystoma Multiplex (Sebocystomatosis, Hereditary Epidermal Polycystic Disease)

Clinical Presentation. Onset is usually in adolescence, although lesions may appear at birth. The eruption consists of multiple cysts, a few millimeters to 2 cm in diameter, involving the face, scalp, trunk, and proximal extremities (Fig. 12.23). The anterior central chest is more often involved. The cysts have a rubbery feel and are usually elevated and movable.

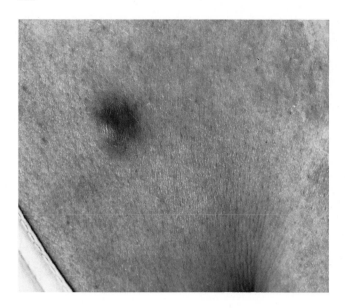

Fig. 12.23. Steatocystoma multiplex. Multiple small cysts. (Courtesy of Dr. V. A. McKusick)

No punctum is visible but, if punctured, an odorless oily fluid appears. A common complication is infection of the cysts with subsequent scarring.

Pathology and Pathophysiology. The cysts are lined by keratinizing epithelium in which lobules of sebaceous glands may be present. Lanugo hairs may be seen in the lumen. The cysts are connected to the overlying epidermis by a band of undifferentiated epithelial cells [1].

Inheritance. Autosomal dominant.

Treatment. Individual cysts may be incised, drained, and phenolized or excised.

Reference

1. Kligman, A.M., Kirschbaum, J.D.: Steatocystoma multiplex: a dermoid tumor. J. invest. Derm. *42*, 383–387 (1964)

Multiple Eruptive Milia

A father and son have been reported with this condition [1]. The lesions appear in childhood as multiple, nonpigmented, 1–3-mm papules over the face (especially the malar region), shoulders, upper trunk, and axillae. Many of the papules have a central folliclelike depression; some have a papillomatous extension [1] (Figs. 12.24 and 12.25). Histologically, there is evidence of nevoid disturbance within the epidermis and dermis as well as dilatation and keratin plugging of the follicular infundibulum [1]. Inheritance is autosomal dominant.

Reference

1. Heard, M.G., Horton, W.H., Hambrick, G.W., Jr.: The familial occurrence of multiple eruptive milia. In: The clinical delineation of birth defects. Bergsma, D. (ed.), Vol. VII, No. 8, pt. XII, pp. 333–337. Baltimore: Williams & Wilkins Co. 1971

Fibrous Proliferative Disorders

Congenital Generalized Fibromatosis

Stout, in 1954, described this entity among the various juvenile fibromatoses [1]. The disorder seems to be very rare [2]. It is characterized by the appearance, at birth, of multiple, rubbery to firm nodules, 0.5–2.5 cm in diameter. These are widely distributed on the skin, especially on the trunk, thighs, and shoulders [2]. The larger nodules may ulcerate. The tumors may involve the skin and subcutaneous tissue or there may also be visceral involvement (muscle, heart, lungs, gastrointestinal tract, liver, pancreas, thyroid, etc.) [3]. With involvement of the viscera, the outcome is fatal. Histologically, there is fibroblastic proliferation in the form of scattered fibrocellular islands composed of plump fibroblasts with reticulin, fibroglia, and collagen fibrils [2]. Inheritance is probably autosomal dominant.

References

1. Stout, A.P.: Juvenile fibromatoses. Cancer *7*, 953–978 (1954)
2. Shnitka, T.K., Asp, D.M., Horner, R.H.: Congenital generalized fibromatosis. Cancer *11*, 627–639 (1958)
3. Kauffman, S.L., Stout, A.P.: Congenital mesenchymal tumors. Cancer *18*, 460–476 (1965)

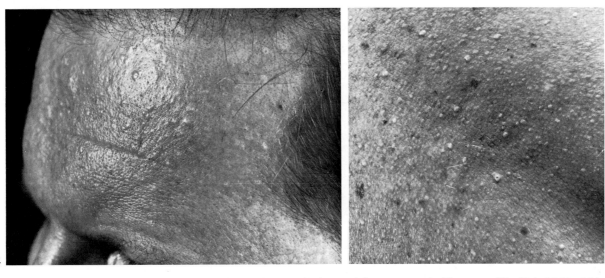

Figs. 12.24 and 12.25. Multiple eruptive milia. Lesions on the face and the upper trunk. (Courtesy of Dr. V. A. McKusick)

Juvenile Fibromatosis

Drescher et al. [1] were the first to describe this rare entity in 1967. At around 2 years of age nodules appear, predominantly on the head and less so on the shoulders, trunk, extremities, face, and hands [1]. The growths start as flat plaques which gradually reach the size of 5 cm or more. They are painless, elastic, and adherent to the overlying skin. Hypertrophy of gums and nail beds is present [1]. Contractures of the joints of the extremities and radiologic evidence of destruction of the proximal parts of the humeri and punched-out osteolytic lesions in the femur and tibia may be present [2]. General health is preserved. Histologically, there is an abundant, homogeneous, amorphous, acidophilic, and PAS-positive ground substance in which spindle cells are embedded and form minute streaks [1]. These cells have abundant frothy cytoplasm. Ultrastructurally, the tumor cells have fibril-filled balls around the Golgi apparatus and peculiar microfibrils in the stroma [3]. Inheritance is autosomal recessive. Treatment is by surgical excision. A few recur.

References

1. Drescher, E., Woyke, S., Markiewicz, C., Tegi, S.: Juvenile fibromatosis in siblings (fibromatosis hyalinica multiplex juvenilis). J. pediat. Surg. 2, 427–430 (1967)
2. Kitano, Y.: Juvenile hyalin fibromatosis. Arch. Derm. 112, 86–88 (1976)
3. Woyke, S., Domagala, W., Olszewski, W.: Ultrastructure of a fibromatosis hyalinica multiplex juvenilis. Cancer 26, 1157–1168 (1970)

Keloids

Clinical Presentation. Many kinds of trauma to the skin may result in an overgrowth of connective tissue which gives rise to hypertrophic scars and keloids. Such a scar hypertrophy may be apparent a few weeks after injury in the form of a raised, thickened, erythematous plaque. Keloids are characterized by being painful and irritative and by the progression of the scar tissue beyond the site of the original trauma. They tend to reach maturity in 6–18 months when the erythema fades [1]. They have a smooth surface and a firm consistency (Figs. 12.26 and 12.27). They seldom disappear spontaneously. Keloids are more frequent in dark-skinned races and involved sites are mainly the ears, face, and neck, less so the abdomen and scalp [2]. Keloids may be the site of development of malignancies. Familial occurrence has been reported [2, 3].

Keloids have also been found in a kindred associated with congenital torticollis, cryptorchidism, and renal dysplasia [4]. The mode of inheritance in this kindred is consistent with X-linked recessive.

Pathology and Pathophysiology. The distinguishing histologic features of keloids are thick, glassy, pale-staining collagen bundles [1, 2] with abundant mucinous ground substance [1].

Inheritance. Not clearly established. Probably autosomal dominant.

Treatment. Intralesional corticosteroids may be helpful in early keloids. In well-established cases, excision followed by radiotherapy gives the lowest recurrence rate.

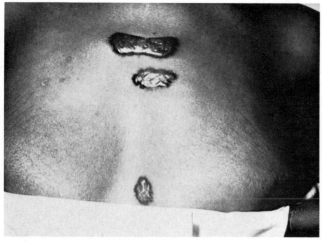
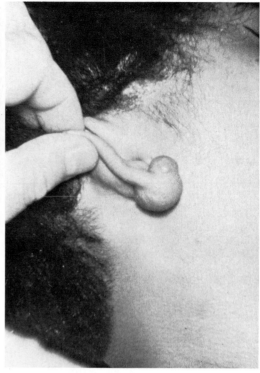

12.26

12.27

Figs. 12.26 and 12.27. Keloids

References

1. Mackenzie, D.H.: Keloids and hypertrophic scars. In: The differential diagnosis of fibroblastic disorders. pp. 32–38. Oxford: Blackwell Scientific Publications 1970
2. Cosman, B., Crikelair, G.F., Ju, D.M.C., Gaulin, J.C., Lattes, R.: The surgical treatment of keloids. Plast. reconstr. Surg. 27, 335–358 (1961)
3. Bloom, D.: Heredity of keloids: review of the literature and report of a family with multiple keloids in five generations. N.Y. State J. Med. 56, 511–519 (1956)
4. Goeminne, L.: A new probably X-linked inherited syndrome. Congenital muscular torticollis, multiple keloids, cryptorchidism and renal dysplasia. Acta Genet. med. (Roma) 17, 439–467 (1968)

Hemangiomas

Multiple Glomus Tumors

Glomus tumors are generally of two types, solitary and multiple. Only multiple glomus tumors are heritable [1, 2].

Clinical Presentation. Multiple glomus tumors usually appear before the age of 21 years; some have been noted at birth [1]. The number of tumors varies, usually being less than ten. The lesions can be grouped in one area, like the hand or foot [3], or they can be generalized [4]. The localized form has an earlier age of onset [3]. Lesions do not occur periungually. Usually they are asymptomatic, although occasionally there may be pain or tenderness [1]. The tumors are usually small, bluish nodules. Occasionally they may be large, soft, and compressible. When they are very numerous, thrombocytopenia may be a complication as in the case of cavernous hemangiomas [4].

Pathology and Pathophysiology. Multiple glomus tumors characteristically are nonencapsulated and are composed of large, wide, irregularly shaped blood-filled cavities [1]. Well-organized thrombi may be seen within these cavities, which are lined by a single layer of flat endothelial cells. Small glomus cells, one to three layers thick, are peripheral to the endothelial lining. Some channels may not show any glomus cells [3]. Ultrastructurally, the glomus cells are shown to be vascular smooth muscle cells [5]. Glomus tumors do not seem to show any abnormal blood flow patterns [5].

Inheritance. Autosomal dominant [1].

Treatment. If tender or painful or associated with thrombocytopenia, excision is recommended.

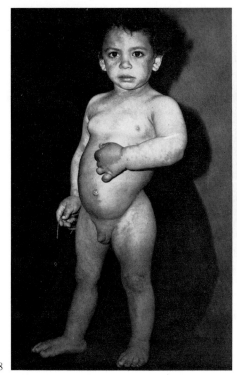

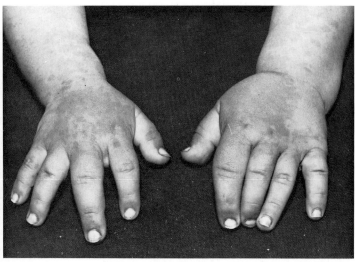

2.28

12.29

Figs. 12.28 and 12.29. Klippel-Trénaunay-Weber syndrome. Note the nevus flammeus and the underlying hypertrophy of the soft tissue

References

1. Gorlin, R.J., Fusaro, R.M., Benton, J.W.: Multiple glomus tumor of the pseudocavernous hemangioma type. Report of a case manifesting a dominant inheritance pattern. Arch. Derm. *82*, 776–778 (1960)
2. Schnyder, U.W.: Über Glomustumoren. Dermatologica (Basel) *131*, 83–88 (1965)
3. Laymon, C.W., Petersen, W.C., Jr.: Glomangioma (glomus tumor). A clinicopathologic study with special reference to multiple lesions appearing during pregnancy. Arch. Derm. *92*, 509–514 (1965)
4. McEvoy, B.F., Waldman, P.M., Tye, M.J.: Multiple hamarto-matous glomus tumors of the skin. Arch. Derm. *104*, 188–191 (1971)
5. Goodman, T.F., Abele, D.C.: Multiple glomus tumors. A clinical and electron microscopic study. Arch. Derm. *103*, 11–23 (1971)

Klippel-Trénaunay-Weber Syndrome (Osteohypertrophic Varicose Nevus)

Klippel and Trénaunay in 1900 [1] and Weber in 1907 [2] described this syndrome with vascular nevus and hypertrophic changes. A better designation would be hemangiectatic osteohypertrophy in view of the variability of the associated vascular component.

Clinical Presentation. At birth a nevus flammeus type of hemangioma may be present on the extremities, trunk, or head. With time, there may be a local overgrowth of soft tissue and hypertrophy of the whole or part of the bone in an extremity, associated with phlebectasias and arteriovenous aneurysms (Figs. 12.28 and 12.29).

Other developmental defects such as syndactyly or polydactyly may be associated with the syndrome. Venous abnormalities of an internal organ may be seen [3].

Pathology and Pathophysiology. The osteohypertrophy is assumed to be the result of venous hypertension caused by varicosities or an arteriovenous fistula.

The cutaneous lesions simulate Kaposi sarcoma and are referred to as pseudo-Kaposi sarcomas. There is proliferation of capillaries and fibroblasts, extravasation of red cells, and deposition of hemosiderin in the dermis [4].

Inheritance. Suggestions of a genetic etiology are meager [5].

Treatment. There is no drastic treatment. The nevi may be cosmetically camouflaged. In cases of gangrene or recurrent ulceration, amputation of the involved part may be necessary.

References

1. Klippel, M., Trénaunay, P.: Nevus variqueux ostéo-hypertro-phique. Arch. Gen. méd. *3*, 641–672 (1900)
2. Weber, F.P.: Angioma formation in connection with hyper-trophy of limbs and hemi-hypertrophy. Brit. J. Derm. *19*, 231–235 (1907)
3. Owens, D.W., Garcia, E., Pierce, R.R., Castrow, F.F.: Klippel-Trenaunay-Weber syndrome with pulmonary vein varicosity. Arch. Derm. *108*, 111–113 (1973)
4. Waterson, K.W., Jr., Shapiro, L., Dannenberg, M.: Develop-mental arteriovenous malformation with secondary angio-dermatitis. Report of a case. Arch. Derm. *100*, 297–302 (1969)
5. McKusick, V.A.: Mendelian inheritance in man, 5th ed., p. 233. Baltimore: Johns Hopkins University Press 1978

Maffucci Syndrome (Dyschondroplasia with Cavernous Angiomas)

In this rare syndrome there is an association be-tween dyschondroplasia (Ollier disease) and hemangiomas.

Clinical Presentation. The affected individual is normal at birth, but during early life one or more soft, bluish nodules appear, usually on a finger or toe [1]. Dilated venous satellites or phlebectasias frequently develop either connected to these nod-ules or elsewhere. Irregular bending and dwarfing of a limb may occur. As the bone extends in length, islands of nonossifying cartilage persist in the met-aphysis [1, 2]. The long bones of the arms, legs, hands, and feet are commonly involved. Grotesque deformities result from the multiple enchondromas. Pathologic fractures are common and healing is slow and incomplete (Figs. 12.30 and 12.31). Skewing and warping of the body result from unequal growth of the two sides. Cartilaginous tumors appear near the epiphyseal line.
Many patients succumb to a variety of neoplasms: chondrosarcoma, angiosarcoma, malignant lymph-angioma, glioma, and ovarian teratoma [1]. The association of the Maffucci syndrome with the blue rubber bleb nevus has been reported [3].

Pathology and Pathophysiology. The vascular le-sions are essentially cavernous hemangiomas, lined with a single layer of endothelial cells. In a few instances, there is endothelial cell proliferation. In one case, cutaneous lymphangiomas were as-sociated with dyschondroplasia [4]. The skeletal lesions show persistence of cartilage in the meta-physis and intermingled areas of distorted cartilage and bone without the normal orderly process of ossification [1, 2].

Inheritance. Not definite.

Treatment. There is no treatment except possible surgical intervention, with amputation of a severely deformed extremity [2].

References

1. Bean, W.B.: Vascular spiders and related lesions of the skin, pp. 166–176. Springfield: Charles C Thomas 1958
2. Carleton, A., Elkington, J.S.C., Greenfield, J.G., Robb-Smith, A.H.T.: Maffucci's syndrome (dyschondroplasia with haem-angeiomata). Quart. J. Med. *11*, 203–228 (1942)
3. Sakurane, H.F., Sugai, T., Saito, T.: The association of blue rubber bleb nevus and Maffucci's syndrome. Arch. Derm. *95*, 28–36 (1967)
4. Suringa, D.W.R., Ackerman, A.B.: Cutaneous lymph-angiomas with dyschondroplasia (Maffucci's syndrome). A unique variant of an unusual syndrome. Arch. Derm. *101*, 472–474 (1970)

Blue Rubber Bleb Nevus

Bean, in 1958, proposed the name of this syndrome [1].

Clinical Presentation. The syndrome is character-ized by the association of cutaneous hemangiomas with hemangiomas of the gastrointestinal tract. The cutaneous lesions appear at birth or in early infancy and increase in size and number. There may be large, disfiguring, cavernous angiomas, or a blood sac looking like a blue rubber nipple covered with thin white skin, or irregular blue marks sometimes with punctate blackish spots merging with the adjacent normal skin [1]. They may be few in number or numerous and occur predominantly on the limbs and trunk [2]. They vary in size from a few millimeters to several centimeters. Some lesions may be painful.
The gastrointestinal lesions are manifested by re-current bleeding and anemia. These lesions are usually multiple, submucosal, and involve the small intestine more often than the colon [2]. Pulmonary hypertension may be a feature of this syndrome [3].

Pathology and Pathophysiology. Essentially, the hemangiomas are of the cavernous type.

Inheritance. Although most cases are sporadic, autosomal dominant inheritance is well-established [2, 4] with perhaps increased penetrance in males [3].

Treatment. In cases of severe intestinal bleeding, resection of the heavily involved bowel may be necessary.

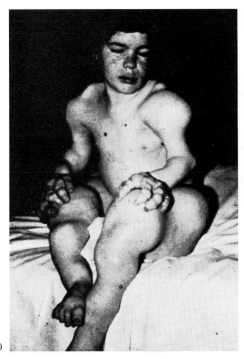

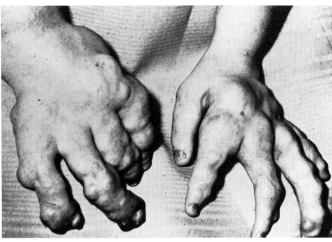

12.31

Figs. 12.30 and 12.31. Maffucci syndrome. Note the nodularities over the extremities and the resulting distortions

12.30

References

1. Bean, W.B.: Vascular spiders and related lesions of the skin, pp. 178–185. Springfield: Charles C Thomas 1958
2. Berlyne, G.M., Berlyne, N.: Anaemia due to "blue-rubber-bleb" naevus disease. Lancet *1960II*, 1275–1277
3. Talbot, S., Wyatt, E.H.: Blue rubber bleb naevi (report of a family in which only males were affected). Brit. J. Derm. *82*, 37–39 (1970)
4. Walshe, M.M., Evans, C.D., Warin, R.P.: Blue rubber bleb naevus. Brit. med. J. *1966II*, 931–932

Lipomatoses

Angiolipoma

Clinical Presentation. Usually shortly after puberty, painful subcutaneous nodules appear. These gradually increase in number. The overlying skin is normal and unattached to the nodules. The pain is inconstant, dull, and elicited by pressure or palpation. The trunk and extremities are the usual sites of involvement. The face, scalp, palms, and soles are not involved [1].

Pathology and Pathophysiology. The nodules are encapsulated, sometimes lobulated, 0.8–3.8 cm in diameter. Histologically, there is proliferation of adipose and vascular tissues. There is no tendency to recur, invade, or metastasize [1].

Inheritance. The majority of cases are not familial. In some reports an autosomal dominant inheritance is suspected [2].

Treatment. Surgical excision is advised when the nodules are painful, or for cosmetic purposes.

References

1. Howard, W.R., Helwig, E.B.: Angiolipoma. Arch. Derm. *82*, 924–931 (1960)
2. Klem, K.K.: Multiple lipoma-angiolipomas. Acta chir. scand. *97*, 527–532 (1949)

Familial Lipomatosis

There are two main types of familial lipomatosis: familial multiple lipomatosis and familial benign symmetric (cervical) lipomatosis.

Familial Multiple Lipomatosis

The lesions are usually apparent between puberty and the age of 30 years [1]. There are multiple, lobulated nodules, soft and rubbery, varying in size from 1–6 cm. The overlying skin is normal. The tumors are occasionally painful when they are developing but asymptomatic when fully grown [1]. The sites of involvement are usually the back and upper extremities and less so the chest and lower extremities.

Multiple lipomas may be a feature of Gardner syndrome (see p. 136) or they may be associated with neurofibromatosis (see p. 255) or visceral lipomas.

Histologically, the nodules are made up of normal fat cells with connective tissue septa and capsule. Inheritance is autosomal dominant. No treatment is necessary. If the lipomas are large or symptomatic, surgical excision is indicated.

Familial Benign Symmetric (Cervical) Lipomatosis

This form is characterized by the presence of large, coalescent, nontender lipomas, especially in the neck region and less so in other areas [2]. Histologically, they are indistinguishable from regular lipomas. Inheritance is probably autosomal dominant.

References

1. Kurzweg, F.T., Spencer, R.: Familial multiple lipomatosis. Amer. J. Surg. 82, 762–765 (1951)
2. Greene, M.L., Glueck, C.J., Fujimoto, W.Y., Seegmiller, J.E.: Benign symmetric lipomatosis (Launois-Bensaude adenolipomatosis) with gout and hyperlipoproteinemia. Amer. J. Med. 48, 239–246 (1970)

Adiposis Dolorosa (Dercum Disease)

This rare disorder was first described by Dercum in 1892 [1].

Clinical Presentation. The disease usually affects menopausal women between 35 and 50 years of age [2]. At the time of onset, the patients are obese, although weight loss and asthenia appear as the disease progresses [2]. There are noninflammatory, painful, subcutaneous tumors, appearing at any site except the face and head, giving the sensation of a "bag of worms" on palpation. The overlying skin may be ecchymotic. Pubic and axillary hair is sparse. Severe emotional symptoms may be prominent.

Other features that are less constant include decreased sweating, dry skin, epistaxis, and congestive heart failure. There is no evidence that this disease is of endocrine origin [2].

Pathology and Pathophysiology. The subcutaneous nodules are indistinguishable from ordinary lipomas. In addition, there may be areas of necrosis, foreign body granulomas, and fibrosis.

Inheritance. Probably autosomal dominant [3, 4].

Treatment. There is no effective treatment. Surgical excision may sometimes be indicated.

References

1. Dercum, F.X.: Three cases of hitherto unclassified affection resembling in its grosser aspects obesity, but associated with special nervous symptoms – adiposis dolorosa. Amer. J. med. Sci. 104, 521–535 (1892)
2. Steiger, W.A., Litvin, H., Lasché, E.M., Durant, T.M.: Adiposis dolorosa (Dercum's disease). New Engl. J. Med. 247, 393–396 (1952)
3. Lynch, H.T., Harlan, W.L.: Hereditary factors in adiposis dolorosa (Dercum's disease). Amer. J. hum. Genet. 15, 184–190 (1963)
4. Cantu, J.M., Ruiz-Barquin, E., Jimenez, M., Castillo, L., Ruiz-Macotela, E.: Autosomal dominant inheritance in adiposis dolorosa (Dercum's disease). Humangenetik 18, 89–91 (1973)

Leiomyomas

Hereditary Multiple Leiomyomas of Skin

Clinical Presentation. The average age of onset is in the third decade, although in some individuals the lesions may appear during the first year of life [1]. The tumors may be uni- or bilateral and affect predominantly the extensor surfaces of extremities. The trunk and occasionally the face and neck may also be involved (Fig. 12.32). The lesions are multiple, discrete, occasionally coalesced papules and nodules. At times these may be grouped. They are firm, smooth, and fixed to the skin, but not to the underlying tissues. The overlying skin is usually pinkish, and rarely turns whitish when painful [1]. All lesions are painful.

The lesions are slowly progressive in size and number, but there is no malignant transformation [1].

Uterine leiomyomas may be associated with the cutaneous tumors [2]. When this occurs, it is at a younger age.

Pathology and Pathophysiology. The tumors are not encapsulated, are usually in the middermis, but may extend to the upper or lower dermis, and are separated from the overlying epidermis by a narrow zone of normal dermis [1]. There are bundles and masses of smooth muscle cells that make up the

Fig. 12.32. Multiple leiomyomas over the trunk

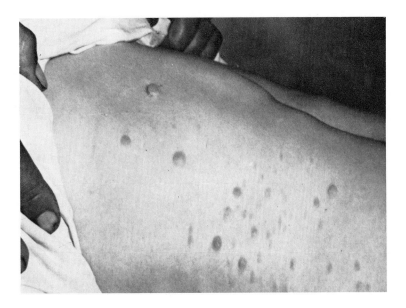

tumors. The origin of these tumors may be the arrectores pilorum muscle [2].

Inheritance. Autosomal dominant.

Treatment. The large and bothersome tumors should be excised.

References

1. Fisher, W.C., Helwig, E.B.: Leiomyomas of the skin. Arch. Derm. *88,* 510–520 (1963)
2. Reed, W.B., Walker, R., Horowitz, R.: Cutaneous leiomyomata with uterine leiomyomata. Acta derm.-venereol. (Stockh.) *53,* 409–416 (1973)

Mast Cell Disease (Urticaria Pigmentosa, Mastocytosis)

Mast cell disease includes a wide spectrum of clinical entities: a solitary cutaneous nodule (mastocytoma); diffuse, cutaneous, multiple hyperpigmented macules or papules (urticaria pigmentosa) with or without systemic involvement; unusual telangiectases of the trunk [telangiectasia macularis eruptiva perstans (TMEP)]; diffuse cutaneous involvement (diffuse mastocytosis); systemic lesions without cutaneous involvement; and, rarely, a malignant mast cell leukemia [1]. Heredity may be operative in some cases which are manifested by any of the clinical spectrum mentioned above [2, 3].

Clinical Presentation. The disease is most common in children, with lesions appearing at birth or within the first few months of life. The typical lesions are hyperpigmented macules or papules symmetrically distributed over the trunk, less so over the neck, scalp, and extremities [1] (Fig. 12.33). Solitary lesions occur exclusively in children and appear as raised brown or tan plaques, 2–5 cm in diameter [1]. Characteristically, all cutaneous lesions urticate on mild trauma (Darier sign): they become erythematous and edematous when rubbed (Fig. 12.34).

Vesiculation of pre-existing lesions is common before the age of two years (Figs. 12.35 and 12.36). In diffuse mastocytosis, a rare variety, the skin is boggy, thickened, and yellowish, with a doughy consistency [3]. Accentuated skin markings, diffuse erythema, and a fine papular eruption may occur. This variety seems to be consistently associated with involvement of internal organs, especially the liver, spleen, gastrointestinal tract, bone marrow, and bone.

In adults, skin lesions usually appear before the age of 18 years [1]. Of the several varieties, TMEP, which is rare, is most often present in adults [1]. The lesions are predominantly on the trunk and are characterized by erythema and telangiectasias. Systemic involvement is more frequent in adults.

Pruritus is the commonest symptom in mast cell disease. Other complaints include flushing, tachycardia, headache, weakness and general malaise, and gastrointestinal complaints [1]. Prognosis and course vary. Isolated mastocytomas regress in a few years. Lesions of urticaria pigmentosa appearing in childhood may regress whereas those appearing in adulthood persist. Diffuse mastocytosis has a poor prognosis.

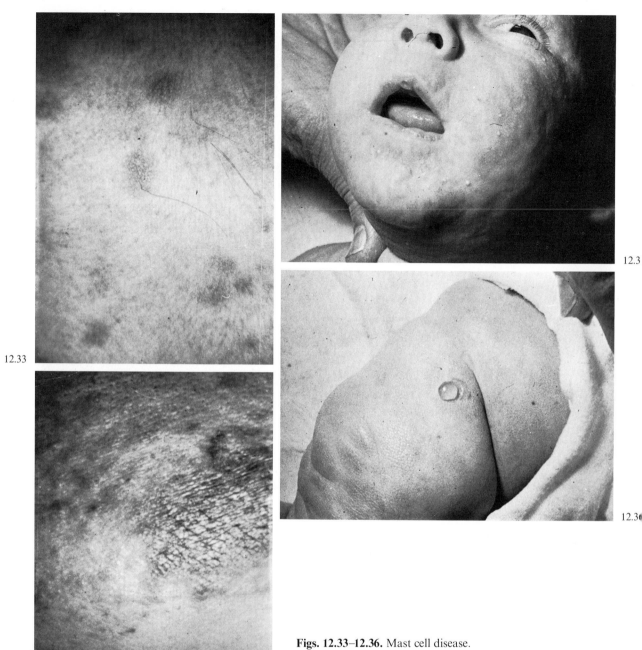

12.33

12.3

12.30

12.34

Figs. 12.33–12.36. Mast cell disease.

Fig. 12.33. Lesions appear as hyperpigmented macules

Fig. 12.34. With rubbing, urtication is evident

Figs. 12.35 and 12.36. Vesiculation is seen

Pathology and Pathophysiology. Characteristically, an infiltrate of mast cells is found in the cutaneous as well as the systemic lesions. Special stains (Giemsa or toluidine blue) may be needed to identify the mast cells. Urinary excretion of histamine may be increased [1].

Inheritance. When familial, inheritance is probably autosomal dominant [2].

Treatment. There is no definitive treatment. Antihistamines may give some symptomatic relief.

References

1. Demis, D.J.: Mast cell disease (urticaria pigmentosa). In: Clinical dermatology. Demis, D.J., Crounse, R.G., Dobson, R.L., McGuire, J. (eds.), Vol. 1, pp. 1–27, Unit 4–11. New York: Harper & Row, Publ. 1974
2. Shaw, J.M.: Genetic aspects of urticaria pigmentosa. Arch. Derm. *97*, 137–138 (1968)
3. Burgoon, C.F., Graham, J.H., McCaffree, D.L.: Mast cell disease. A cutaneous variant with multisystem involvement. Arch. Derm. *98*, 590–605 (1968)

Histiocytic Proliferative Disorders

Histiocytic Dermatoarthritis

Clinical Presentation. The eruption appears in childhood as nodules on the face, ears, dorsa of the hands, feet, and legs, and extensor surfaces of the forearms [1]. The lesions are numerous, 6–30 mm in diameter, and violet to brown in color. Palpation of the extremities reveals multiple, firm, subcutaneous plaques. The skin of the legs and feet is lichenified. There is also severe, symmetric deforming arthritis of the hands, feet, and elbows. Other associated findings are glaucoma, uveitis, polychromatic posterior cataracts, and perceptive deafness [1].

Pathology and Pathophysiology. The nodules are dermal and initially show a granulomatous reaction. Late nodules show chronic inflammation, histiocytic infiltration, and increased fibroblasts and collagen. No multinucleated giant cells are present. Serum protein and lipoprotein electrophoretic patterns are usually normal.

Inheritance. Autosomal dominant [1].

Treatment. There is no definitive treatment.

Reference

1. Zayid, I., Farraj, S.: Familial histiocytic dermatoarthritis. A new syndrome. Amer. J. Med. *54*, 793–800 (1973)

Letterer-Siwe Disease

Letterer-Siwe disease is known, along with Hand-Schüller-Christian disease and eosinophilic granuloma, as one of the three entities classified under the general title of histiocytosis X. Unlike the other two, however, Letterer-Siwe disease or "acute disseminated histiocytosis X" has a familial occurrence.

Clinical Presentation. The disease usually manifests itself during the first year of life and has a rapid progress.

The skin involvement is very frequent and is often the presenting sign. The lesions are usually generalized, maculopapular, pruritic, greasy-appearing, and seborrheic, with a predilection for the hairline, neck, and inguinal regions. Vesicles or pustules may develop and erosions then follow. Hemorrhagic cutaneous involvement may be a terminal manifestation (Figs. 12.37–12.39). In the mouth, there may be gingival hypertrophy, inflammation, necrosis, and retraction, with resultant loss of teeth. Within the span of a few months there may be significant hepatomegaly and splenomegaly, widespread pulmonary infiltration, adenopathy, fever, and intercurrent infections. There may be a diffuse involvement of the medullary cavity with osseous lesions [1, 2].

Roentgenograms of the chest reveal a granular appearance in the pulmonary parenchyma. In some patients osseous lesions may appear on roentgenograms [1, 2].

Death is usually due to marrow failure, asphyxia, or septicemia.

Cutaneous Letterer-Siwe disease with a benign course has also been described [3].

An inbred kindred has been reported [4] in which 12 infants in six sibships died from a disease of the reticuloendothelial system. The disease presented many features of Letterer-Siwe disease, but differed "in the prominence of eosinophils and in the lack of pulmonary infiltration and bone-marrow failure" [4]. Follicular mucinosis may be associated with the cutaneous histiocytosis and eosinophilia.

Pathology and Pathophysiology. The liver and spleen have nodular lesions composed of altered histiocytes or reticulocytes and an associated mononuclear cell. The adrenal glands, bone marrow, and lungs also reveal numerous altered histiocytes [5].

On light microscopy, the cutaneous lesion of Letterer-Siwe disease typically shows infiltration of large, pale histiocytes with homogeneous nuclei and

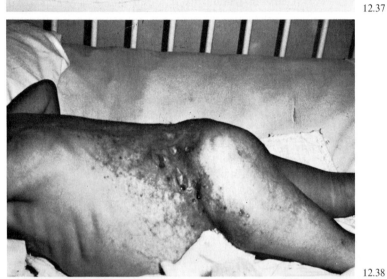

12.37

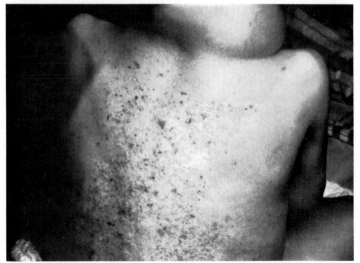

12.38

12.39

clear, slightly granular cytoplasm. Mitotic figures may be present. The nuclei may be pyknotic and assume bizarre shapes. The papular, nodular, petechial, and ulcerative lesions have in common the basic histiocytic proliferation of the skin [6].

On electron microscopy, the large histiocytes contain a greatly indented nucleus with dispersed chromatin and the typical granule or rod-shaped profile (the X-granule). This disclike structure with a central laminar core of 90-Å periodicity was first described in the Langerhans cells of the epidermis. Letterer-Siwe disease is considered to be due to the hyperplasia of such cells [6]. Freeze-fracture replication of X-granules in cells of cutaneous lesions of Letterer-Siwe disease confirms previous reports of variations in overall shape of these granules [7].

Ultrastructural examination of the skin in Letterer-Siwe disease treated with vinblastine reveals that Langerhans granules and other organelles freely scattered in the cytoplasm are trapped within the nuclear membrane during anaphase. Unknown "comma-shaped bodies" are found in the cytoplasm of some macrophages and Langerhans cells [8].

Inheritance. Autosomal recessive, with slightly reduced penetrance [5, 9, 10].

Treatment. Remission of the disease has been produced by the intravenous administration of vinblastine (Velban) [11].

References

1. Christie, A., Batson, R., Shapiro, J., Riley, H.D., Jr., Laughmiller, R., Stahlman, M.: Acute disseminated (nonlipid) reticuloendotheliosis. Acta paediat. *43* (Suppl. 100), 65–76 (1954)
2. Avery, M.E., McAfee, J.G., Guild, H.G.: The course and prognosis of reticuloendotheliosis (eosinophilic granuloma, Schüller-Christian disease and Letterer-Siwe disease). A study of forty cases. Amer. J. Med. *22*, 636–652 (1957)
3. Clark, R.F.: Cutaneous Letterer-Siwe disease: a benign course with conservative management. Cutis *14*, 113–115 (1974)
4. Omenn, G.S.: Familial reticuloendotheliosis with eosinophilia. New Engl. J. Med. *273*, 427–432 (1965)
5. Rogers, D.L., Benson, T.E.: Familial Letterer-Siwe disease. Report of a case. J. Pediat. *60*, 550–554 (1962)
6. Winkelmann, R.K.: The skin in histiocytosis X. Mayo Clin. Proc. *44*, 535–548 (1969)
7. Breathnach, A.S., Gross, M., Basset, F., Nèzelof, C.: Freeze-fracture replication of X-granules in cells of cutaneous lesions of histiocytosis-X (Letterer-Siwe disease). Brit. J. Derm. *89*, 571–585 (1973)
8. Gianotti, F., Caputo. R.: Skin ultrastructure in Letterer-Siwe disease treated with vinblastine. Mode of penetration of Langerhans granules into the nucleus. Brit. J. Derm. *84*, 335–345 (1971)
9. Juberg, R.C., Kloepfer, H.W., Oberman, H.A.: Genetic determination of acute disseminated histiocytosis X (Letterer-Siwe syndrome). Pediatrics *45*, 753–765 (1970)
10. Freundlich, E., Amit, S., Montag, Y., Suprun, H., Nevo, S.: Familial occurrence of Letterer-Siwe disease. Arch. Dis. Child. *47*, 122–125 (1972)
11. Winkelmann, R.K., Burgert, E.O.: Therapy of histiocytosis X. Brit. J. Derm. *82*, 169–175 (1970)

Malignant Lymphomas

Mycosis Fungoides

Mycosis fungoides (MF) is a peculiar type of malignant lymphoma which arises and remains predominantly in the skin. In the later stages of the disease it may disseminate and involve visceral organs. Familial MF seems to be very rare as only a few cases have been reported [1, 2].

Clinical Presentation. MF has a prolonged course, lasting for 20 years or more. Traditionally, the course of the disease has been divided into three stages: the premycotic, mycotic, and tumor stages. In the premycotic stage, the eruption is nonspecific and mimics dermatitis: patchy, erythematous, noninfiltrated, scaly plaques. This phase may last for many years before the mycotic stage becomes evident. Then the plaques are darker in color, scaly, infiltrated, and slightly elevated. These plaques vary in size and shape and gradually extend peripherally (Figs. 12.40 and 12.41). Intense pruritus becomes manifest during this stage, which may last for many years. The tumor stage is characterized by the rather rapid growth of nodules within infiltrated plaques. Some of these tumors are fungating or may ulcerate (Figs. 12.42 and 12.43). Occasionally, at the terminal stage, visceral involvement may occur. Death may be due to the widespread disease, intercurrent complications, secondary infections, or treatment.

In addition to the classic or Alibert form of MF, two rare variants exist: the erythrodermic and *d'emblée* forms. In the former, there is a generalized exfoliative erythroderma that progresses to MF. In the *d'emblée* form, tumors develop on normal skin without the appearance of the erythematous infiltrated plaques.

Pathology and Pathophysiology. The histologic changes in the premycotic stage are not diagnostic. As infiltration in the plaques develops, the histologic changes become suggestive and then diagnostic of MF. The diagnostic features are a polymorphic, bandlike cellular infiltrate in the upper dermis, the presence of large cells with a hyperchromatic,

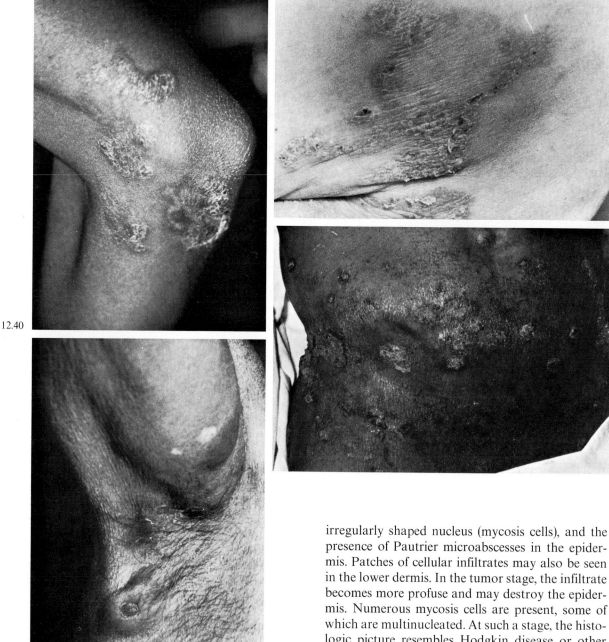

12.40

12.41

12.42

12.43

Figs. 12.40 and 12.41. Mycosis fungoides. Slightly infiltrated, scaly, circinate plaques. (Courtesy of Dr. I. Zeligman)

Figs. 12.42 and 12.43. Mycosis fungoides. Tumefaction and ulceration. (Courtesy of Dr. I. Zeligman)

irregularly shaped nucleus (mycosis cells), and the presence of Pautrier microabscesses in the epidermis. Patches of cellular infiltrates may also be seen in the lower dermis. In the tumor stage, the infiltrate becomes more profuse and may destroy the epidermis. Numerous mycosis cells are present, some of which are multinucleated. At such a stage, the histologic picture resembles Hodgkin disease or other lymphomas.

Inheritance. Inheritance is not definite. The disease has been described in brother and sister and in mother and daughter [1, 2].

Treatment. Treatment depends on the stage. In early stages, topical corticosteroids or UV irradiation may be helpful. In the presence of infiltration, topical nitrogen mustard [3], 8-methoxypsoralen with UVA, fractionated radiotherapy, total body irradiation (electron beam) [4], and cytotoxic drugs (especially cyclophosphamide, 150–200 mg daily,

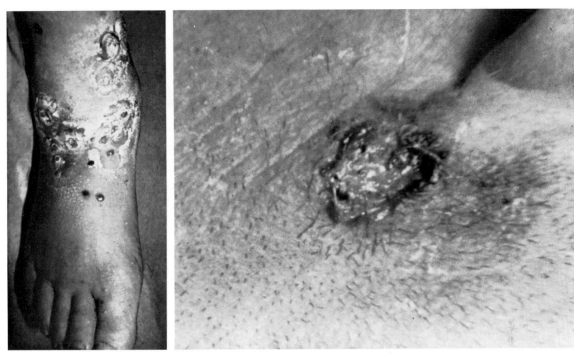

12.44

12.45

Fig. 12.44. Malignant melanoma. Typical satellite nodules

Fig. 12.45. Malignant melanoma. Ulcerated pigmented lesions

with proper monitoring of the blood count) [5] are helpful and may give long remissions.

References

1. Cameron, O.J.: Mycosis fungoides in mother and in daughter. Arch. Derm. Syph. *27*, 232–236 (1933)
2. Sandbank, M., Katzenellenbogen, I.: Mycosis fungoides of prolonged duration in siblings. Arch. Derm. *98*, 620–627 (1968)
3. Van Scott, E.J., Winters, P.L.: Responses of mycosis fungoides to intensive external treatment with nitrogen mustard. Arch. Derm. *102*, 507–514 (1970)
4. Fromer, J.L., Johnston, D.O., Salzman, F.A., Trump, J.G., Wright, K.A.: Management of lymphoma cutis with low megavolt electron beam therapy: nine year follow-up in 200 cases. Southern med. J. *54*, 769–776 (1961)
5. Van Scott, E.J., Auerbach, R., Clendenning, W.E.: Treatment of mycosis fungoides with cyclophosphamide. Arch. Derm. *85*, 499–501 (1962)

Melanocytic Proliferative Disorders

Familial Malignant Melanoma

The occurrence of familial malignant melanoma of the skin was first recorded in 1952 [1]. Since then, numerous additional reports have appeared. Familial patients seem to manifest a younger age

distribution, a significantly earlier average age at first diagnosis, a significantly increased frequency of multiple primary melanomas, and a significantly higher survival rate than nonfamilial patients [2] (Figs. 12.44 and 12.45). There is a tendency for melanomas in familial patients to occur at random over the skin surface with the significant absence of facial lesions [3]. In Australia, people of Scottish, Irish, and Welsh descent are particularly prone to develop familial melanomas [3]. In patients with familial melanoma, the distribution of hair color, eye color, and skin texture as well as reaction to exposure to sunlight does not seem to be different from that of a closely matched control group [3]. Studies of families affected with malignant melanoma indicate a complex genetic mechanism, probably involving several loci [2, 3]. Unknown environmental factors may be responsible for the occurrence of the disease in unrelated individuals in the same household.

References

1. Cawley, E.P.: Genetic aspects of malignant melanoma. Arch. Derm. Syph. *65*, 440–450 (1952)
2. Anderson, D.E.: Clinical characteristics of the genetic variety of cutaneous melanoma in man. Cancer *28*, 721–725 (1971)
3. Wallace, D.C., Beardmore, G.L., Exton, L.A.: Familial malignant melanoma. Ann. Surg. *177*, 15–20 (1973)

Chapter 13   Vascular and Hematologic Disorders

Contents

Anemias and Thrombocytopenias

Congenital Hemolytic Anemias

Congenital hemolytic anemias usually present themselves with nondermatologic manifestations. However, occasionally the presenting sign is an intractable ulcer of the leg. Consequently, the possibility of a blood dyscrasia should be considered in all chronic leg ulcers not due to varicose veins.

Clinical Presentation. The hemolytic anemias responsible for leg ulcers are the following: hereditary spherocytosis, hereditary elliptocytosis, hereditary nonspherocytic hemolytic anemia, thalassemia, and sickle cell anemia [1].

In all of these conditions the onset of anemia is during infancy, except for hereditary spherocytosis, in which the disease manifests itself in childhood or early adult life. In most of these there may be crises characterized by abdominal pain, vomiting, fever, and mild jaundice. Splenomegaly is present in all. Leg ulcers occur in all of these congenital hemolytic anemias with varying incidence (Fig. 13.1). They occur in 6–7% of patients with hereditary spherocytosis and 25–75% of adolescents and adults with sickle cell anemia. The ulcers are unilateral or bilateral, solitary or multiple, irregular, and resistant to conventional therapy. They do not have a distinctive gross appearance and are not pathognomonic of a specific type of anemia. The exact character of the anemia must be determined by appropriate clinical and hematologic studies [2–5]. In sickle cell disease an extra transverse digital crease is found on the palmar surface, just beyond the distal interphalangeal flexion crease [6]. This crease is present at birth and is most frequent on the middle finger. Although it is not a specific and pathognomonic finding, the crease is much more common in children with the disease than in normals.

Pathology and Pathophysiology. The final common pathway of pathologic mechanisms leading to ulcer formation is oxygen deprivation to the cutaneous and subcutaneous tissues overlying the lower portions of the legs, resulting in ischemic necrosis. Histologically, the ulcers show a nonspecific inflammatory process [2–5].

Inheritance. Hereditary spherocytosis, hereditary elliptocytosis, and hereditary nonspherocytic hemolytic anemia have the autosomal dominant pattern of inheritance. In thalassemia and sickle cell anemia, the inheritance follows the autosomal recessive pattern.

Treatment. In hereditary spherocytosis and ellipto-cytosis, splenectomy is usually followed by good results [2–4]. In hereditary nonspherocytic hemo-lytic anemia, splenectomy may or may not be helpful. In thalassemia, the leg ulcers have been treated successfully by streptokinase-strepto-dornase in carboxymethylcellulose jelly [7]. In the treatment of sickle cell ulcers, oral zinc sulfate has been tried with beneficial results in uncontrolled trials [8].

References

1. Smith, C.H.: Blood diseases of infancy and childhood, 3rd ed., pp. 303–311, 317–319, 371–428. Saint Louis: Mosby, C.V. Co. 1972
2. Beinhauer, L.G., Gruhn, J.G.: Dermatologic aspects of congenital spherocytic anemia. Arch. Derm. *75*, 642–646 (1957)
3. Estes, J.E., Farber, E.M., Stickney, J.M.: Ulcers of the leg in Mediterranean disease. Blood *3*, 302–306 (1948)
4. Pascher, F., Keen, R.: Ulcers of the leg in Cooley's anemia. New Engl. J. Med. *256*, 1220–1222 (1957)
5. Gabuzda, T.G.: Sickle cell leg ulcers: current pathophysio-logic concepts. Int. J. Derm. *14*, 322–325 (1975)
6. Zizmor, J.: The extra transverse digital crease: a skin sign found in sickle cell disease. Cutis *11*, 447–449 (1973)
7. Cooper, C.D., Wacker, W.E.C.: The successful therapy with streptokinase-streptodornase of ankle ulcers associated with Mediterranean anemia. Blood *9*, 241–243 (1954)
8. Serjeant, G.R., Galloway, R.E., Gueri, M.C.: Oral zinc sulphate in sickle-cell ulcers. Lancet *1970II*, 891–892

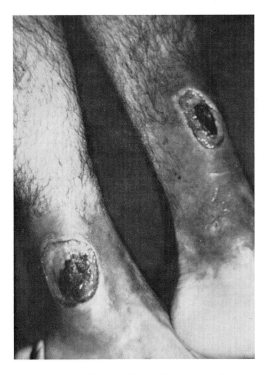

Fig. 13.1. Bilateral, well-defined leg ulcers typically seen in the hereditary anemias. This patient suffers from thalassemia major

Fanconi Anemia (Pancytopenia and Multiple Anomalies)

In 1927 Fanconi [1] described three brothers affect-ed with a disorder characterized by pancytopenia, brown hyperpigmentation, genital hypoplasia, and microcephaly. Since then, more than 150 patients affected with this disorder have been described [2–4].

Clinical Presentation. The most important features of this syndrome are brownish pigmentation of the skin (77%), small stature (56%), small cranium (43%), hypoplasia or aplasia of the thumb and radial bones (78%), and pancytopenia. A small penis, small testes, and cryptorchidism are found in 44% of male patients.

Hyperpigmentation is the most frequent finding [3,4]. The lesions may be of different sizes and have a patchy distribution. The brownish dusky pigmen-tation increases with age. It is most evident in the neck, groin, axilla, trunk, and anogenital areas. Within the hyperpigmented areas there may be depigmented macules and macules of darker pigmentation.

Bleeding, pallor, and recurring infections usually appear between 5 and 10 years of age, although pancytopenia may occur in infancy or as late as the third decade.

Acute leukemia or solid malignant tumors are fatal complications [5] and may occur in family mem-bers lacking the full-blown features of the disorder. It has been reported that male heterozygotes for Fanconi anemia have a risk of malignant neoplasm three to four times that of the general population [6].

A new familial heredodegenerative disorder with pancytopenia, immunologic deficiency, and cu-taneous malignancies has also been reported [7]. Apparently it follows the autosomal recessive pat-tern of inheritance.

Pathology and Pathophysiology. Renal anomalies (unilateral agenesis, hydronephrosis, horseshoe kid-neys) are common. A few patients have presented with congenital heart disease [8,9].

Usually all bone marrow elements are affected with resulting anemia, leukopenia, and thrombo-cytopenia. This pancytopenia develops between 4 and 10 years of age.

The chromosomes (cultured from lymphocytes) of most patients show nonspecific structural abnormalities, such as breaks, gaps, and endoreduplications [8, 10–12]. These are known to exist in patients suffering from acute leukemia or solid malignant tumors. Their presence in Fanconi anemia is of importance, since most of these patients also develop acute leukemia or solid tumors.

Skin fibroblasts from these patients have been shown to be unusually susceptible to transformation by SV40 oncogenic viruses [13].

A deficiency in the ability to excise UV-induced pyrimidine dimers from DNA has been reported in some patients [14]. However, single-strand break production and unscheduled DNA synthesis are intact, thus ruling out the probability of a deficiency of endonuclease, DNA polymerase, or ligase. Therefore it is inferred that the deficiency is that of an exonuclease which specifically recognizes and excises distortions in the tertiary structure of DNA (see also p. 1).

Inheritance. Autosomal recessive [3].

Treatment. Testosterone and corticosteroids may produce temporary improvement in the pancytopenia, but the disease is usually fatal [15]. The use of oxymetholone has recently been advocated [16].

References

1. Fanconi, G.: Familiäre infantile perniziosaartige Anämie (perniziöses Blutbild und Konstitution). Jb. Kinderheilk. *117*, 257–280 (1927)
2. Nilsson, L.R.: Chronic pancytopenia with multiple congenital abnormalities (Fanconi's anaemia). Acta paediat. (Uppsala) *49*, 518–529 (1960)
3. Fanconi, G.: Familial constitutional panmyelocytopathy, Fanconi's anemia (F.A.). I. Clinical aspects. Sem. Hemat. *4*, 233–240 (1967)
4. Gmyrek, D., Syllm-Rapoport, I.: Zur Fanconi-Anämie (FA). Analyse von 129 beschriebenen Fällen. Z. Kinderheilk. *91*, 297–337 (1964)
5. Garriga, S., Crosby, W.H.: The incidence of leukemia in families of patients with hypoplasia of the marrow. Blood *14*, 1008–1014 (1959)
6. Swift, M., Cohen, J., Pinkham, R.: A maximum-likelihood method for estimating the disease predisposition of heterozygotes. Amer. J. hum. Genet. *26*, 304–317 (1974)
7. Abels, D., Reed, W.B.: Fanconi-like syndrome. Arch. Derm. *107*, 419–423 (1973)
8. Bloom, G.E., Warner, S., Gerald, P.S., Diamond, L.K.: Chromosome abnormalities in constitutional aplastic anemia. New Engl. J. Med. *274*, 8–14 (1966)
9. Swift, M., Zimmerman, D., McDonough, E.R.: Squamous cell carcinomas in Fanconi's anemia. J. Amer. med. Ass. *216*, 325–326 (1971)
10. Schroeder, T.M., Anschütz, F., Knopp, A.: Spontane Chromosomenaberrationen bei familiärer Panmyelopathie. Humangenetik *1*, 194–196 (1964)
11. Swift, M.R., Hirschhorn, K.: Fanconi's anemia: inherited susceptibility to chromosome breakage in various tissues. Ann. intern. Med. *65*, 496–503 (1966)
12. Schmid, W.: Familial constitutional panmyelocytopathy. Fanconi's anemia (F.A.). II. A discussion of the cytogenetic findings in Fanconi's anemia. Sem. Hemat. *4*, 241–249 (1967)
13. Todaro, G.J., Green, H., Swift, M.R.: Susceptibility of human diploid fibroblast strains to transformation by SV40 virus. Science *153*, 1252–1254 (1966)
14. Poon, P.K., O'Brien, R.L., Parker, J.W.: Defective DNA repair in Fanconi's anaemia. Nature (London) *250*, 223–225 (1974)
15. Shahidi, N.T., Diamond, L.K.: Testosterone-induced remission in aplastic anemia of both acquired and congenital types. Further observations in 24 cases. New Engl. J. Med. *264*, 953–967 (1961)
16. Allen, D.M., Fine, M.H., Necheles, T.F., Dameshek, W.: Oxymetholone therapy in aplastic anemia. Blood *32*, 83–89 (1968)

Table 13.1. Purpuras, thrombocytopenias, and thrombocytopathies

Name	Inheritance	Clinical presentation and pathophysiology	Ref.
Thrombasthenia of Glanzmann and Naegli (autosomal dominant form)	Autosomal dominant	Petechiae, bleeding from mucous membrane, severe anemia Prolonged bleeding time, abnormal capillary fragility, normal or increased number of platelets, giant platelets, altered concentration of platelet enzymes, absence of surface-localized thrombosthenin in platelets	[1, 2]
Hereditary thrombasthenia-thrombocytopenia	Autosomal dominant	Normal or increased megakaryocytes By electron microscopy vacuoles and abnormal granules in platelets	[3]
Thrombocytopenia (autosomal dominant)	Autosomal dominant	Hemorrhagic diathesis Shortened platelet lifespan	[4]
Hemoglobin Köln hemoglobinopathy	Autosomal dominant	Spontaneous bruising Hemoglobin Köln Hemolytic anemia with thrombocytopenia	[5]
Pigmented purpuric eruption (see also p. 240)	Autosomal dominant	Symmetric pigmented and purpuric eruption beginning early in life	[6]
Purpura simplex	Autosomal dominant (suspected)	Purpura of the extremities, epistaxis, ecchymoses on slight trauma, and menorrhagia	[7, 8]
Thrombasthenia of Glanzmann and Naegeli (autosomal recessive form)	Autosomal recessive	Normal bleeding time, platelet count, coagulation time Deficient clot retraction and abnormal platelet morphology	[1]
Thrombocytopenic purpura (autosomal recessive)	Autosomal recessive (probable)	Thrombocytopenia, easy bruising, epistaxis	[9, 10]
Thrombocytopenic thrombocytopathy	Autosomal recessive	Thrombocytopenia, morphologically abnormal platelets, prolonged bleeding time, low platelet thromboplastin activity, normal clot retraction Phospholipid content of platelets increased	[11]
Thrombocytopenia, aplasia of radius (TAR syndrome)	Autosomal recessive	Aplasia or hypoplasia of radius Thrombocytopenia	[12]
Fanconi anemia (see also p. 237)	Autosomal recessive	Pancytopenia Brownish pigmentation of the skin, small stature, small cranium	[13]
Wiskott-Aldrich syndrome (see also p. 161)	Autosomal recessive	Eczema, thrombocytopenia, immunologic deficiency	[14]
Glycinemia	Autosomal recessive	Episodic vomiting, lethargy, ketosis, neutropenia, periodic thrombocytopenia	[15]
Cystathioninuria	Autosomal recessive	Mental retardation, clubfoot, developmental defects about the ears, convulsions Thrombocytopenia Urinary lithiasis	[16, 17]
Generalized lymphohistiocytic infiltration	Autosomal recessive	High and irregular fever, hepatosplenomegaly, purpura, jaundice, polyneuritis, meningeal reaction, choked disks, moderate anemia, and severe granulocytopenia	[18, 19]
Gaucher disease (see also p. 267)	Autosomal recessive	Splenomegaly, hepatomegaly, anemia, leukopenia, thrombocytopenia, with or without central nervous system damage	[20]
Letterer-Siwe disease (see also p. 231)	Autosomal recessive	Diffuse papular eruption of vesicular nature and scaly petechial dermatitis Hepatomegaly, splenomegaly, thrombocytopenia, marrow failure, pulmonary infiltration, fever, infections	[21]
Thrombocytopenia with elevated serum IgA and renal disease	X-linked recessive (suspected)	Thrombocytopenia due to reduced platelet production Elevated IgA levels in serum Varying degrees of glomerulonephritis	[22]
Thrombocytopenia (X-linked recessive)	X-linked recessive	Thrombocytopenia Mild tendency to infection and eczema	[23, 24]

References

1. Caen, J.P., Castaldi, P.A., Leclerc, J.C., Inceman, S., Larrieu, M.J., Probst, M., Bernard, J.: Congenital bleeding disorders with long bleeding time and normal platelet count. I. Glanzmann's thrombasthenia (report of fifteen patients). Amer. J. Med. *41*, 4–26 (1966)
2. Booyse, F., Kisieleski, D., Seeler, R., Rafelson, M., Jr.: Possible thrombosthenin defect in Glanzmann's thrombasthenia. Blood *39*, 377–381 (1972)
3. Seip, M., Kfaerheim, Å.: A familial platelet disease – hereditary thrombasthenic-thrombopathic thrombocytopenia Scand. J. clin. lab. Invest. *17* (Suppl. 84–86), 159–169 (1965)
4. Murphy, S., Oski, F.A., Gardner, F.H.: Hereditary thrombocytopenia with an intrinsic platelet defect. New Engl. J. Med. *281*, 857–862 (1969)
5. Hutchinson, H.E., Pinkerton, P.H., Waters, P., Douglas, A.S., Lehmann, H., Beale, D.: Hereditary Heinz-body anaemia, thrombocytopenia, and haemoglobinopathy (Hb Köln) in a Glasgow family. Brit. med. J. *1961 II*, 1099–1103
6. Gould, W.M., Farber, E.M.: A familial pigmented purpuric eruption. Dermatologica (Basel) *132*, 400–408 (1966)
7. Davis, E.: Hereditary familial purpura simplex. Review of 27 families. Lancet *1941 I*, 145–146
8. Fisher, B., Zuckerman, G.H., Douglass, R.C.: Combined inheritance of purpura simplex and ptosis in four generations of one family. Blood *9*, 1199–1204 (1954)
9. Roberts, M.H., Smith, M.H.: Thrombopenic purpura. Report of four cases in one family. Amer. J. Dis. Child. *79*, 820–825 (1950)
10. Wilson, S.J., Larsen, W.E., Skillman, R.S., Walters, T.R.: Familial thrombocytopenic purpura. Blood *22* (Abstr.), 827 (1963)
11. Cullum, C., Cooney, D.P., Schrier, S.L.: Familial thrombocytopenic thrombocytopathy. Brit. J. Haemat. *13*, 147–159 (1967)
12. Shaw, S., Oliver, R.A.M.: Congenital hypoplastic thrombocytopenia with skeletal deformities in siblings. Blood *14*, 374–377 (1959)
13. Fanconi, G.: Familial constitutional panmyelopathy, Fanconi's anemia (F.A.). I. Clinical aspects. Sem. Hematol. *4*, 233–240 (1967)
14. Wolff, J.A.: Wiskott-Aldrich syndrome: clinical, immunologic, and pathologic observations. J. Pediat. *70*, 221–232 (1967)
15. Childs, B., Nyhan, W.L., Borden, M., Bard, L., Cooke, R.E.: Idiopathic hyperglycinemia and hyperglycinuria: a new disorder of amino acid metabolism. I. Pediatrics *27*, 522–538 (1961)
16. Harris, H., Penrose, L.S., Thomas, D.H.H.: Cystathioninuria. Ann. hum. Genet. *23*, 442–453 (1959)
17. Shaw, K.N.F., Lieberman, E., Koch, R., Donnell, G.N.: Cystathioninuria. Amer. J. Dis. Child. *113*, 119–128 (1967)
18. Nelson, P., Santamaria, A., Olson, R.L., Nayak, N.C.: Generalized lymphohistiocytic infiltration. A familial disease not previously described and different from Letterer-Siwe disease and Chédiak-Higashi syndrome. Pediatrics *27*, 931–950 (1961)
19. Mozziconacci, P., Nèzelof, C., Attal, C., Girard, F., Pham-Huu-Trung, (NI), Weil, J., Desbuquois, B., Gadot, M.: La lympho-histiocytose familiale. Arch. franç. Pediat. *22*, 385–408 (1965)
20. Brady, R.O., King, F.M.: Gaucher's disease. In: Lysosomes and storage diseases. Hers, H.G., Van Hoof, F. (eds.), pp. 381–394. New York: Academic Press 1973
21. Freundlich, E., Amit, S., Montag, Y., Suprun, H., Nevo, S.: Familial occurrence of Letterer-Siwe disease. Arch. Dis. Child. *47*, 122–125 (1972)
22. Gutenberger, J., Trygstad, C.W., Stiehm, E.R., Opitz, J.M., Thatcher, L.G., Bloodworth, J.M.B., Jr., Setzkorn, J.: Familial thrombocytopenia, elevated serum IgA levels, and renal disease. A report of a kindred. Amer. J. Med. *49*, 729–741 (1970)
23. Vestermark, B.S.: Familial sex-linked thrombocytopenia. Acta paediat. *53*, 365–370 (1964)
24. Ata, M., Fisher, O.D., Holman, C.A.: Inherited thrombocytopenia. Lancet *1965 I*, 119–123

Familial Pigmented Purpuric Eruption

The term "pigmented purpuric eruption" encompasses disorders that have certain morphologic characteristics and possibly share a common pathophysiologic mechanism [1]. These disorders are Schamberg disease (progressive pigmented purpuric dermatosis) [2], pigmented purpuric lichenoid dermatosis of Gougerot and Blum [3], and purpura annularis telangiectodes of Majocchi [4]. Familial occurrence of pigmented purpuric eruptions has rarely been reported [5, 6].

Clinical Presentation. In the familial cases, the eruption primarily involves the legs, but may also affect the thighs and upper extremities. The initial lesion is a red punctum which becomes reddish brown in color – the "cayenne pepper" appearance. The lesions are macular and of various sizes, spreading by peripheral extension. These are asymptomatic and chronic. General health is preserved.

Pathology and Pathophysiology. The main changes are an inflammatory reaction around the upper dermal capillaries, extravasation of erythrocytes, and deposition of hemosiderin.

Inheritance. Autosomal dominant.

Treatment. There is no effective treatment.

References

1. Randall, S.J., Kierland, R.R., Montgomery, H.: Pigmented purpuric eruptions. Arch. Derm. Syph. *64*, 177–191 (1951)
2. Schamberg, J.G.: A peculiar progressive pigmentary disease of the skin. Brit. J. Derm. *13*, 1–5 (1901)
3. Gougerot, H., Blum, P.: Purpura angioscléreux prurigineux avec éléments lichénoïdes. Bull. Soc. franç. Derm. Syph. *32*, 161–163 (1925)
4. Majocchi, D.: Purpura annularis telangiectodes. Arch. Derm. Syph. *43*, 447–468 (1898)
5. Baden, H.P.: Familial Schamberg's disease. Arch. Derm. *90*, 400 (1964)
6. Gould, W.M., Farber, E.M.: A familial pigmented purpuric eruption. Dermatologica (Basel) *132*, 400–408 (1966)

Hemangioma-Thrombocytopenia Syndrome (Kasabach-Merritt Syndrome)

In 1940 Kasabach and Merritt [1] drew attention to the development of thrombycytopenia in patients with large vascular tumors.

Clinical Presentation. The cutaneous lesions are vascular tumors that are usually present at birth or appear within the first months of life. Development in later life is rare [2]. The sites of involvement are the trunk and extremities, less so the face and scalp [2]. The angioma usually undergoes rapid enlargement. Thrombocytopenia and hemorrhages usually appear early in the course. Characteristically, there is ecchymosis around the hemangiomas and internal bleeding is common [2]. Anemia and splenomegaly are frequent and death may ensue. Occasionally, there is regression of the symptoms.

Pathology and Pathophysiology. The vascular tumors are mostly capillary or cavernous hemangiomas, less frequently hemangioendotheliomas, and in one instance an angiosarcoma was observed [2]. There is sequestration of platelets within the hemangiomas. In addition, there are red cell changes of the microangiopathic hemolytic anemia type (compatible with trauma) [3]. Survival time of platelets is markedly shortened [3]. Other unidentified factors may contribute to the bleeding [4].

Inheritance. No evidence of a simple genetic pattern of inheritance has been discovered.

Treatment. Irradiation or surgical excision of the tumor and systemic corticosteroids have been helpful.

References

1. Kasabach, H.H., Merritt, K.K.: Capillary hemangioma with extensive purpura. Amer. J. Dis. Child. *59*, 1063–1070 (1940)
2. Wilson, C.J., Haggard, M.E.: Giant vascular tumors and thrombocytopenia. Arch. Derm. *81*, 432–437 (1960)
3. Propp, R.P., Scharfman, W.B.: Hemangioma-thrombocytopenia syndrome associated with microangiopathic hemolytic anemia. Blood *28*, 623–633 (1966)
4. Rodriguez-Erdmann, F., Murray, J.E., Moloney, W.C.: Consumption-coagulopathy in Kasabach-Merritt syndrome. Trans. Ass. Amer. Phycns. *83*, 168–175 (1970)

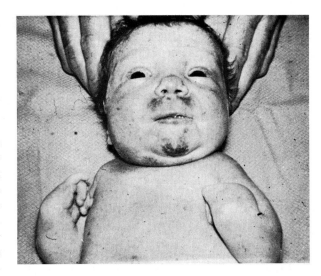

Fig. 13.2. TAR syndrome. Note the ecchymoses on the face and the abnormal upper limbs

Thrombocytopenia and Absent Radius Syndrome (TAR)

In 1956 Gross et al. [1] described this entity in siblings. Shaw and Oliver [2] differentiated this disorder from Fanconi pancytopenia with associated malformations and established it as a separate entity.

Clinical Presentation. The most striking feature of this syndrome is the absence or hypoplasia of the radius. This anomaly is usually bilateral and often associated with defects of the hands, legs, and feet (Fig. 13.2).
Thrombocytopenia, most severe in early infancy, presents with absence or hypoplasia of megakaryocytes. "Leukemoid" granulocytosis occurs in 62% of cases and eosinophilia in 53%. Purpura is almost universal and gastrointestinal hemorrhages occur in nearly half of the cases.
Occasional abnormalities include congenital heart defects (in 25% of cases), small stature, brachycephaly, strabismus, micrognathia, syndactyly, a short humerus, hypoplasia of the shoulder girdle, genu varum, dislocation of the hip, Meckel's diverticulum, and renal anomalies.
In 40% of patients, gastrointestinal and cerebral hemorrhages are the immediate cause of death. After the first year, the prognosis improves.

Pathology and Pathophysiology. The distinguishing feature of the TAR syndrome is the absence or hypoplasia of the erythron. The blood disorder is evident in the first few months of life. Other differences from Fanconi anemia include the absence of both pigmentary abnormalities and chromosomal breaks. Two patients with hypoplastic radius and hypoplastic thrombocytopenia with trisomy 18 have been reported [3, 4]. However, it has not been definitely established that they represent cases of the typical TAR syndrome.

One patient with TAR syndrome developed leukemia. It is of interest that the uncle of another patient died of leukemia. However, unlike Fanconi panmyelopathy, this complication is not very frequent in the TAR syndrome.

Inheritance. Autosomal recessive [2].

Treatment. Treatment is symptomatic, with platelet transfusions in cases of hemorrhage. The skeletal anomalies should have orthopedic care, whenever possible.

References

1. Gross, H., Groh, C., Weippl, G.: Kongenitale hypoplastische Thrombopenie mit Radiusaplasie, ein Syndrom multipler Abartungen. Neue öst. Z. Kinderheilk. *1*, 574 (1956)
2. Shaw, S., Oliver, R.A.M.: Congenital hypoplastic thrombocytopenia with skeletal deformities in siblings. Blood *14*, 374–377 (1956)
3. Rabinowitz, J.S., Moseley, J.E., Mitty, H.A., Hirschhorn, K.: Trisomy 18, esophageal atresia, anomalies of the radius and congenital hypoplastic thrombocytopenia. Radiology *89*, 488–491 (1967)
4. Juif, J.-G., Stoll, C., Korn, R.: Thrombopénie hypoplasique congénitale avec aplasie du radius. Arch. franç. Pédiat. *29*, 513–526 (1972)

Telangiectasias

Hereditary Hemorrhagic Telangiectasia (Osler-Rendu-Weber Disease)

Even though this disease was first discussed by Sutton in 1864 [1], the recognition of its components is credited to Rendu [2], Osler [3], and Weber [4].

Clinical Presentation. The presenting symptom is usually recurrent epistaxis, which appears in childhood, is followed by a period free of hemorrhage, and recurs in the third decade. The cutaneous telangiectases may appear in childhood but usually become prominent in the third decade. The typical skin lesion is punctiform, sometimes depressed, sharply marginated, and covered by a thin skin [5]

(Figs. 13.3–13.5). Very rarely one or more vessels may be connected to the central red area. Nodular lesions, somewhat cyanotic, may be present but these are rare [5]. The lesions involve any part of the body, but the upper part more than the lower. They are frequent on the palmar surfaces, fingernails, lips, ears, face, lower arms, and toes. The trunk is less involved. The mucosal surfaces are always affected, especially in the Kiesselbach area on the nasal septum and the tongue. The conjunctiva, esophagus, bronchial tree, stomach, intestine, vagina, and rectum are also involved [5]. Hemorrhage may occur from any site: gastrointestinal tract, lungs, meninges, brain, retina, sclera, urinary tract, liver, and mesenteric vessels [5]. Pulmonary arteriovenous fistulas become evident as the mucocutaneous lesions become established [5]. When well-developed, polycythemia and clubbing are present, and the lesion can be detected radiologically. Hepatic arteriovenous fistulas with liver fibrosis may also occur [6]. Other sites of aneurysms are splenic and cerebral arteries. Cerebral arteriovenous malformations may be as frequent as pulmonary arteriovenous fistulas [7].

Pathology and Pathophysiology. The lesion is made up of dilated papillary vessels in which there is failure of the muscle and connective tissue to develop properly in the walls [5]. A single layer of endothelial cells may be the only indication of a smaller vessel. The local increase of plasminogen activator in the lesions results in increased fibrinolytic activity and also contributes to the bleeding tendency [8].

Inheritance. Autosomal dominant.

Treatment. The mainstay of treatment is to control hemorrhage and replace the lost blood. Pressure at the site of the bleeding may suffice. Electrocautery of nasal bleeding sites gives temporary relief. Local application of aminocaproic acid is beneficial [8]. When epistaxis is severe, dermoplasty may be useful in replacing the nasal mucosa by a split skin graft. Systemic estrogens may be helpful in enhancing the keratinization of the mucous membrane. In certain cases, extensive surgical intervention in the lungs or intestines may be indicated.

References

1. Sutton, H.G.: Epistaxis as an indication of impaired nutrition and degeneration of the vascular system. Med. Mirror London *1*, 769 (1864)
2. Rendu, H.: Epistaxis répétées chez un sujet porteur de petits angiomes cutanés et muqueux. Bull. Soc. méd. Hosp. Paris *13*, 731–733 (1896)

Figs. 13.3–13.5. Hereditary hemorrhagic telangiectasia. Numerous punctiform telangiectases on the face, tongue, and hands

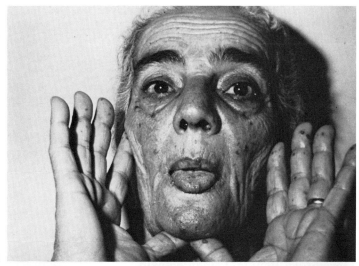

13.3

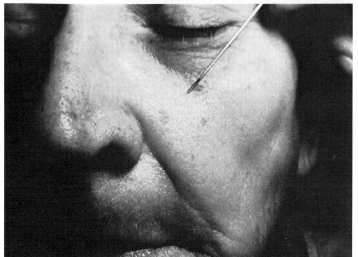

13.4

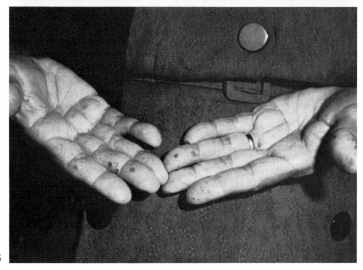

13.5

3. Osler, W.: On a family form of recurring epistaxis, associated with multiple telangiectases of the skin and mucous membranes. Bull. Johns Hopk. Hosp. *12*, 333–337 (1901)
4. Weber, F.P.: Multiple hereditary developmental angiomata (telangiectases) of the skin and mucous membranes associated with recurring haemorrhages. Lancet *1907II*, 160–162
5. Bean, W.B.: Vascular spiders and related lesions of the skin, pp. 132–157. Springfield: Charles C Thomas 1958
6. Zelman, S.: Liver fibrosis in hereditary hemorrhagic telangiectasia. Fibrosis of diffuse insular character. Arch. Path. *74*, 66–72 (1962)
7. Waller, J.D., Greenberg, J.H., Lewis, C.W.: Hereditary hemorrhagic telangiectasia with cerebrovascular malformations. Arch. Derm. *112*, 49–52 (1976)
8. Kwaan, H.C., Silverman, S.: Fibrinolytic activity in lesions of hereditary hemorrhagic telangiectasia. Arch. Derm. *107*, 571–573 (1973)

Hereditary Benign Telangiectasia

Clinical Presentation. In this condition, described in seven kindreds [1], fine telangiectases appear on the face, neck, upper chest, backs of hands, and, in some, the knees and vermilion border of the lip. The lesions are more obvious in exposed areas. The telangiectases become less noticeable with age.

Pathology and Pathophysiology. There is dilatation of the horizontal subpapillary venous plexus with loss of the more superficial capillaries. Microvascular atrophy occurs with increased age. The upper dermis is atrophic.

Inheritance. Autosomal dominant.

Treatment. None is necessary.

Reference

1. Ryan, T.J., Wells, R.S.: Hereditary benign telangiectasia. Trans. St. Johns Hosp. derm. Soc. *57*, 148–156 (1971)

Ataxia Telangiectasia (Louis-Bar Syndrome)

In 1941 Louis-Bar described a patient with telangiectasia of the conjunctiva and skin and cerebellar ataxia [1]. Subsequently, more than 150 patients affected with this syndrome have been reported [2–5].

Clinical Presentation. The main manifestations are telangiectasia, ataxia, and complications due to immune deficiency [2].

The telangiectases become evident at around 3 years of age and are first seen in the bulbar conjunctiva (Fig. 13.6). They eventually spread and involve the eyelids, the bridge of the nose, and the paranasal areas in a "butterfly" pattern. They also involve the pinnae of the ears, the neck (Fig. 13.7), and the antecubital and popliteal areas. Skin areas exposed to the sun are more affected.

A few years after the onset of the skin changes, the subcutaneous fat diminishes. A mottled pattern of hyper- and hypopigmentation occurs with cutaneous atrophy. The skin of the face becomes tense and bound down, assuming a sclerodermatous appearance. Basal cell carcinomas and senile keratoses occur. Seborrheic dermatitis, dry skin, follicular keratosis, and hirsutism of the extremities are common. Nummular eczema, impetigo, and warts may occur (Fig. 13.8). Telangiectasia of the soft and hard palates has also been reported. Occasionally, café-au-lait spots and partial albinism are present [3,4].

Ataxia is the most striking neurologic finding. Choreoathetosis may also occur and even mask the ataxia. As the disease progresses, speech becomes slow and slurred, and mental retardation becomes evident in about one-third of the cases [3].

The immune deficiency is clinically manifested by recurrent infections of the upper and lower respiratory tracts, middle ear, and sinuses. Bronchiectasis is a common complication [3]. The most frequently observed serum immunoglobulin abnormalities are diminished levels of IgA and IgE [5].

Occasional features of the disease include the following: growth deficiency (with variable age of onset), malignancies (leukemia, sarcoma, Hodgkin disease, cutaneous malignancies), and sexual immaturity.

Pulmonary disease, debilitation, and malignancies are the most common causes of death, which usually occurs by the age of 25 years.

Pathology and Pathophysiology. The histopathologic study of the skin reveals flattening of the epidermis. In the upper dermis there is fibrosis and the vessels are congested and dilated [4]. All of these changes resemble those seen with actinic damage. The cutaneous telangiectatic vessels branch from the subpapillary venous plexuses. Likewise, the ocular vascularity arises primarily from the dilated connecting venules of the conjunctival vessels [4].

Neuropathologic findings include atrophy of the cerebellar cortex, demyelination of the posterior columns of the spinal cord, and degeneration of neurons in the spinal ganglia [6].

In addition to reduced levels of serum IgA and IgE, the immune deficiency is manifested by inadequate

Figs. 13.6–13.8. Ataxia telangiectasia

Fig. 13.6. Involvement of the bulbar conjunctiva

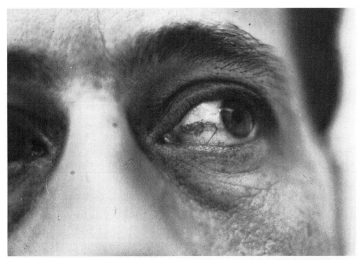

Fig. 13.7. Telangiectases on the side of the neck

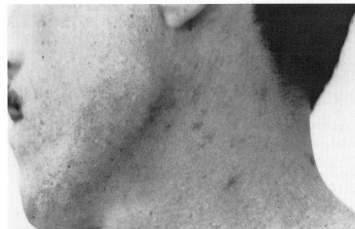

Fig. 13.8. Multiple viral warts on the hands, due to the immune deficiency. (Courtesy of Dr. V. A. McKusick)

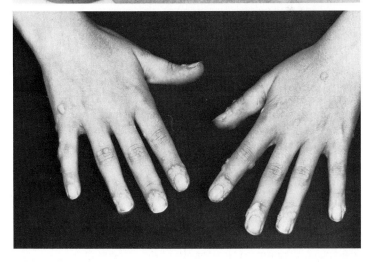

cellular immunity with a deficient delayed type of hypersensitivity, thymic hypoplasia, hypoplasia of the tonsils and adenoids, and lymphopenia [7] (see also p. 156).

Many patients have been reported with antibodies to thyroid and to smooth and striated muscle cells, suggesting the presence of autoimmune phenomena [8].

A high incidence of leukemia, lymphosarcoma, and basal cell carcinoma is noted [3, 5].

Raised levels of α-fetoprotein have been consistently reported in the blood of patients affected with ataxia telangiectasia [9]. This finding is suggestive of immaturity of the liver. It favors the hypothesis that the primary defect in this disease is in tissue differentiation, resulting from faulty mesoderm-entoderm interaction.

Abnormalities of the amino acid content of collagen have also been reported [10]. They consist of moderately diminished hydroxylysine and elevated proline and alanine in the collagen.

Cultured lymphocytes reveal chromosomal breaks [11, 12] and impaired responsiveness to phytohemagglutinin. Postradiation colony-forming assays have recently been used in the study of ataxia telangiectasia (AT). Cells from patients with AT were found to have decreased post-γ-ray colony-forming ability [13]. This may be a consequence of faulty DNA repair of γ-ray-induced DNA damage [14]. Chemical mutagens, especially actinomycin D, have been shown to have similar effects [15].

There are certain common features among Fanconi anemia, Bloom syndrome, and ataxia telangiectasia: (a) generalized growth deficiency; (b) skin disorders; (c) propensity to develop lymphoreticular malignancy; and (d) high frequency of chromosomal breakage in cultured lymphocytes [16].

Thus, in its homozygous state, the gene causing this disease has a severe pleiotropic effect, since it causes growth retardation, immune deficiency, and deterioration of the central nervous system, skin, and respiratory tract. However, no specific cellular metabolic defect has yet been detected.

Inheritance. Autosomal recessive [2].

Treatment. Treatment is symptomatic, especially focusing on the recurrent infections. Transplantation of the neonate thymus-sternum complex has been attempted [17].

References

1. Louis-Bar, D.: Sur un syndrôme progressif comprenant des télangiectasies capillaires cutanées et conjonctivales symétriques, à disposition naevoïde et des troubles cérébelleux. Confin. neurol. (Basel) *4*, 32–34 (1941)
2. McFarlin, D.E., Strober, W., Waldmann, T.A.: Ataxia-telangiectasia. Med. (Baltimore) *51*, 281–314 (1972)
3. Boder, E., Sedgwick, R.P.: Ataxia-telangiectasia. A review of 101 cases. In: Little club clinics in developmental medicine. Walsh, G. (ed.), No. 8, pp. 110–118. London: The National Spastics Society and Heinemann Medical Books Ltd. 1963
4. Reed, W.B., Epstein, W.L., Boder, E., Sedgwick, R.: Cutaneous manifestations of ataxia-telangiectasia. J. Amer. med. Ass. *195*, 746–753 (1966)
5. Ammann, A.J., Cain, W.A., Ishizaka, K., Hong, R., Good, R.A.: Immunoglobulin E deficiency in ataxia-telangiectasia. New Engl. J. Med. *281*, 469–472 (1969)
6. Aguilar, M.J., Kamoshita, S., Landing, B.H., Boder, E., Sedgwick, R.P.: Pathological observations in ataxia-telangiectasia. A report on five cases. J. Neuropath. exp. Neurol. *27*, 659–676 (1968)
7. Peterson, R.D.A., Kelly, W.D., Good, R.A.: Ataxia-telangiectasia. Its association with a defective thymus, immunological-deficiency disease, and malignancy. Lancet *1964 I*, 1189–1193
8. Ammann, A.J., Hong, R.: Autoimmune phenomena in ataxia-telangiectasia. J. Pediat. *78*, 821–826 (1971)
9. Waldmann, T.A., McIntire, K.R.: Serum-alpha-fetoprotein levels in patients with ataxia-telangiectasia. Lancet *1972 II*, 1112–1115
10. McReynolds, E.W., Dabbous, M.K., Hanissian, A.S., Duenas, D., Kimbrell, R.: Abnormal collagen in ataxia telangiectasia. Amer. J. Dis. Child. *130*, 305–307 (1976)
11. Hecht, F., Koler, R.D., Rigas, D.A., Dahnke, G.S., Case, M.P., Tisdale, V., Miller, R.W.: Leukemia and lymphocytes in ataxia-telangiectasia. Lancet *1966 II*, 1193
12. Lisker, R., Cobo, A.: Chromosome breakage in ataxia-telangiectasia. Lancet *1970 I*, 618
13. Taylor, A.M.R., Harnden, D.G., Arlett, C.F., Harcourt, S.A., Lehmann, A.R., Stevens, S., Bridges, B.A.: Ataxia telangiectasia: a human mutation with abnormal radiation sensitivity. Nature (Lond.) *258*, 427–429 (1975)
14. Paterson, M.C., Smith, B.P., Lohman, P.H.M., Anderson, A.K., Fishman, L.: Defective excision repair of γ-ray-damaged DNA in human (ataxia telangiectasia) fibroblasts. Nature (Lond.) *260*, 444–447 (1976)
15. Hoar, D.I., Sargent, P.: Chemical mutagen hypersensitivity in ataxia telangiectasia. Nature (Lond.) *261*, 590–592 (1976)
16. German, J.: Genetic disorders associated with chromosomal instability and cancer. J. invest. Derm. *60*, 427–434 (1973)
17. Lopukhin, Y., Morosov, Y., Petrov, R.: Transplantation of neonate thymus-sternum complex in ataxia-telangiectasia. Transplant. Proc. *5*, 823–827 (1973)

Familial Multiple Nevi Flammei

The presenting symptoms are multiple "birthmarks." These appear as asymptomatic, dark red, sharply circumscribed, angular macules, 0.1–0.7 × 3.5–8 cm (Fig. 13.9). There is some blanching on pressure, leaving a residual brownish color [1]. The lesions are distributed over the hands, upper and lower extremities, and trunk. Histologically, there are increased numbers of capillaries [1]. Inheritance is autosomal dominant.

Reference

1. Shelley, W.B., Livingood, C.S.: Familial multiple nevi flammei. Arch. Derm. Syph. *59*, 343–345 (1949)

Telangiectatic Nevus of Nape (Nevus Flammeus of Nape)

This is a rather common condition in which a nevus flammeus or a "salmon patch" appears on the nape of the neck. The lesion is apparent at birth as a pale pink macule with fine telangiectasia. Many persist into adulthood and are asymptomatic.

Inheritance. Autosomal dominant [1].

Treatment. None is usually needed.

Reference

1. Zumkeller, R.: A propos de la fréquence et de l'hérédité du naevus vasculosus nuchae (Unna). J. Génét. hum. *6*, 1–12 (1957)

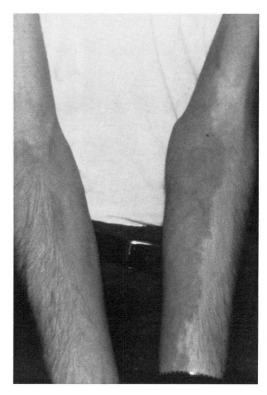

Fig. 13.9. Familial multiple nevus flammeus

Lymphedemas

Hereditary Lymphedema

Edema resulting from inadequate lymphatic drainage is referred to as lymphedema. Hereditary lymphedema due to failure of development, in varying degrees, of the lymphatic vessels in embryonic life [1] can be classified as to the age of onset.
Early-onset type (Nonne-Milroy)
Late-onset type
   Hereditary lymphedema (onset about puberty)
   Hereditary lymphedema associated with yellow nails
   Hereditary lymphedema associated with distichiasis
   Hereditary lymphedema associated with ptosis

Early-Onset Type (Nonne-Milroy)

This type of congenital lymphedema was described by Nonne in 1891 [2] and Milroy in 1892 [3].

Clinical Presentation. Edema is present at birth and is usually confined to the lower extremities. Genital involvement in males is not uncommon. The edema is firm, pitting, and permanent [1]. The overlying skin appears normal. There are no constitutional symptoms and general health is usually unaffected. Chylous ascites with loss of protein into the intestinal tract was observed in one patient [4] and bilateral pleural effusion in two other patients [5].

Inheritance. Autosomal dominant.

Treatment. There is no treatment.

Late-Onset Type

Hereditary Lymphedema with Onset about Puberty (Meige Disease, Lymphedema Praecox)

Meige, in 1898 [6], described this type of lymphedema.

Clinical Presentation. Characteristically, the edema develops around puberty. There is insidious development of painless edema of the lower extremities

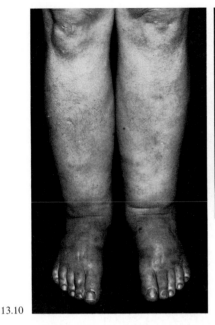

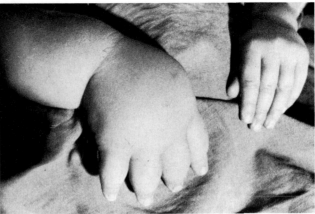

13.11

13.10

Fig. 13.10. Lymphedema of late onset (associated with distichiasis). (See p. 194)

Fig. 13.11. Lymphedema of late onset. Affection of the upper extremity. (Courtesy of Dr. F. C. Fraser)

[7]. There may be accompanying signs of acute inflammation. The edema is firm with minimal pitting. Histologic examination of the skin shows edema and mild chronic inflammation of the dermis [7].

Inheritance. Probably autosomal dominant.

Treatment. There is no treatment.

Hereditary Lymphedema with Yellow Nails

A characteristic nail change is often associated with lymphedema of late onset.
The initial manifestation is a marked decrease in the growth rate of the fingernails (less than 0.2 mm per week compared to the normal 0.5–1.2 mm) [8]. The nails remain smooth but are curved from side to side and the cuticle is lost. The nail plate becomes pale yellow or greenish with a darker color on the edges. Onycholysis may also be present and some of the partially separated nails may show a distinct hump [8].
The edema usually follows the nail changes and affects the legs, less often the face and hands, or may be generalized. Pleural effusion [9] and bronchiectasis [10] may also be present. The edema has been attributed to hypoplasia of lymphatic vessels [8]. Other reports, however, cast doubt on the invariable association of lymphedema with yellow nails [11]. The familial occurrence of lymphedema with yellow nails [12] strongly suggests an autosomal dominant mode of inheritance. No specific treatment is available.

Hereditary Lymphedema with Distichiasis

The association of distichiasis with lymphedema of late onset is a constant feature of this syndrome [13, 14] (Figs. 13.10 and 13.11). Webbed neck [14], lower lid ectropion [14], and vertebral changes with or without extradural cysts [13] may be present.
There is hypoplasia of the lymphatics demonstrable by lymphangiograms [13]. Inheritance is autosomal dominant (see p. 194).

Hereditary Lymphedema with Ptosis

Ptosis of the eyelids may be associated with hereditary lymphedema of the legs [14, 15]. This rare combination is probably inherited as autosomal dominant.

References

1. Esterly, J.R.: Congenital hereditary lymphoedema. J. med. Genet. 2, 93–98 (1965)
2. Nonne, M.: Vier Fälle von Elephantiasis congenita hereditaria. Virchows Arch. path. Anat. 125, 189 (1891)
3. Milroy, W.F.: An undescribed variety of hereditary oedema. N.Y. State J. Med. 56, 505 (1892)
4. Rosen, F.S., Smith, D.H., Earle, R., Jr., Janeway, C.A., Giltlin, D.: The etiology of hypoproteinemia in a patient with congenital chylous ascites. Pediatrics 30, 696–706 (1962)
5. Hurwitz, P.A., Pinals, D.J.: Pleural effusion in chronic hereditary lymphedema (Nonne, Milroy, Meige's disease). Report of two cases. Radiology 82, 246–248 (1964)
6. Meige, H.: Dystrophie œdémateuse héréditaire. Presse méd. 6, 341–343 (1898)
7. Goodman, R.M.: Familial lymphedema of the Meige's type. Amer. J. Med. 32, 651–656 (1962)

Fig. 13.12. Raynaud disease. Blanching and bluish coloration of the fingers

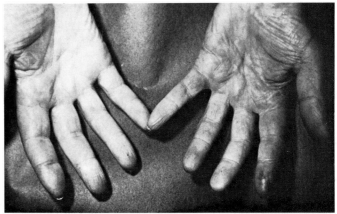

Fig. 13.13. Chronic Raynaud disease with ulceration of the fingertips

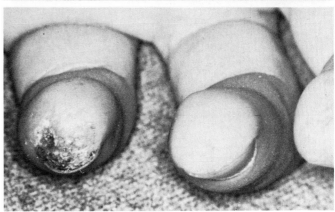

8. Samman, P.D., White, W.F.: The "yellow nail" syndrome. Brit. J. Derm. *76*, 153–157 (1964)
9. Emerson, P.A.: Yellow nails, lymphoedema, and pleural effusions. Thorax *21*, 247–253 (1966)
10. Zerfas, A.Z.: Yellow nail syndrome with bilateral bronchiectasis. Proc. roy. Soc. Med. *59*, 448 (1966)
11. Marks, R., Ellis, J.P.: Yellow nails. A report of six cases. Arch. Derm. *102*, 619–623 (1970)
12. Wells, G.C.: Yellow nail syndrome: with familial primary hypoplasia of lymphatics, manifest late in life. Proc. roy. Soc. Med. *59*, 447 (1966)
13. Robinow, M., Johnson, G.F., Verhagen, A.D.: Distichiasis – lymphedema. A hereditary syndrome of multiple congenital defects. Amer. J. Dis. Child. *119*, 343–347 (1970)
14. Falls, H.F., Kertesz, E.D.: A new syndrome combining pterygium colli with developmental anomalies of the eyelids and lymphatics of the lower extremities. Trans. Amer. ophthal. Soc. *62*, 248–275 (1964)
15. Bloom, D.: Hereditary lymphedema (Nonne-Milroy-Meige). Report of a family with hereditary lymphedema associated with ptsosis of the eyelids in several generations. N.Y. State J. Med. *41*, 856–863 (1941)

Raynaud Disease

The Raynaud phenomenon, in which there is intermittent paroxysmal decrease of blood flow to the extremities, is associated with several pathologic conditions. Raynaud disease describes those cases in which no other disease is found.

Clinical Presentation. The disease is commoner in women (5:1), and the age of onset is usually under 40 years. Cooling or emotional stress brings about a typical attack. One or more fingers become white or pale blue in color with numbness of the finger to touch and occasionally to pain [1]. Only the tip of the finger may be involved or the whole palm may be affected (Figs. 13.12 and 13.13). Recovery is usually in a few minutes and is manifested by erythema or cyanosis. Usually the affection is symmetric and the fingers are more often involved than the toes. The disease is generally progressive. Secondary changes may occur in the skin which becomes atrophic and sclerotic. The nails also become thin, longitudinally ridged, and brittle [2]. Koilonychia and partial onycholysis may appear [2].

Pathology and Pathophysiology. In the early stages, there is no structural abnormality. Intimal thickening may be seen in later stages. The pathogenesis of this disease is uncertain. An abnormal sympathetic nerve supply has been postulated. Other postulates incriminate the small arterioles [1], increased blood viscosity [3], or increased circulating epinephrine and norepinephrine [4].

Inheritance, Most cases are sporadic. When familial, inheritance is autosomal dominant.

Treatment. Patients are instructed to avoid exposure to cold. Vasodilators may be tried, although these are not usually helpful. Sympathectomy may be resorted to, if other measures fail.

References

1. Lewis, T., Pickering, G.W.: Observations upon maladies in which the blood supply to digits ceases intermittently or permanently and upon bilateral gangrene of digits; observations relevant to so-called "Raynaud's disease". Clin. Sci. *1*, 327–366 (1933–1934)
2. Samman, P.D.: The nails in disease, 2nd ed., pp. 96–97. London: William Heinemann Medical Books 1972
3. Pringle, R., Walder, D.N., Weaver, J.P.A.: Blood viscosity and Raynaud's disease. Lancet *1965 I*, 1086–1088
4. Peacock, J.H.: Peripheral venous blood concentrations of epinephrine and norepinephrine in primary Raynaud's disease. Circulat. Res. *7*, 821–827 (1959)

Cold Hypersensitivity (Familial Cold Urticaria)

Clinical Presentation. The symptoms appear soon after birth and persist indefinitely. On exposure to a cold environment, and after a latency period of several hours, symptoms appear. There is a diffuse erythema especially over the extremities, followed by the appearance of papules [1, 2]. The papules coalesce, flatten out, and appear purpuric [1]. Itching is rare, but there may be pain, tenderness, and a burning sensation [1, 2]. Other manifestations include fever, chills, nausea, arthralgia, and muscle pain [1, 2]. Leukocytosis is a constant feature [1]. The symptoms last for about a day and then subside. Skin tests with ice cubes and passive transfer tests with serum are negative [2]. In one family, systemic amyloidosis was associated with the cold hypersensitivity [3].·

Pathology and Pathophysiology. The skin lesions show dilated dermal vessels and, characteristically, an intense inflammatory infiltrate [1]. Initially the infiltrate is predominantly neutrophilic, then lymphocytes appear. Leukocytoclasis is also evident [1].

The syndrome of cold hypersensitivity seems to be mediated by a humoral factor other than histamine,

catecholamines, adrenocortical steroids, or etiocholanolone [1]. Intravenous administration of *Pseudomonas* polysaccharide complex prevents the generalized reaction by an as yet unidentified mechanism [1].

Inheritance. Autosomal dominant [1, 2].

Treatment. Desensitization by gradual exposure may be helpful. Warming and induction of sweating give symptomatic relief.

References

1. Tindall, J.P., Beeker, S.K., Rosse, W.F.: Familial cold urticaria. A generalized reaction involving leukocytosis. Arch. intern. Med. *124*, 129–134 (1969)
2. Doeglas, H.M.G.: Familial cold urticaria. Arch. Derm. *107*, 136–137 (1973)
3. Shepard, M.K.: Cold hypersensitivity. In: The clinical delineation of birth defects. Bergsma, D. (ed.), Vol. VII, No. 8, pt. XII, p. 352. Baltimore: Williams & Wilkins Co. 1971

Palmar Erythema (Erythema Palmare Hereditarium)

This rare disorder is characterized by asymptomatic redness of the palms. The bright red color is limited to the palms and terminates abruptly at the junction of the palmar skin with that of the wrist and sides of the hand [1]. The palmar surface of the fingers may be involved, as well as the backs of the tips of the terminal phalanges. There are no telangiectases and no other skin abnormalities. Inheritance is autosomal dominant.

Reference

1. Lane, J.E.: Erythema palmare hereditarium (red palms). Arch. Derm. Syph. *20*, 445–448 (1929)

Other Disorders

Familial Localized Heat Urticaria

This unique syndrome has been described in three generations of a family [1]. The symptoms appear in childhood and persist. Wheals, localized and sharply marginated, appear at sites of exposure to heat. Characteristically, the wheals do not appear immediately but 11/2–2 h after the heat exposure and may persist for 12–14 h [1]. Pretreatment with a local anesthetic and compound 48/80 completely inhibits the reaction. Repeated heat challenges, oral antihistamines, and locally injected atropine diminish the whealing.

Histologic examination of the wheal shows an inflammatory reaction in the dermis which is more pronounced than in cases of acute urticaria. A high percentage of the circulating basophils of affected individuals are degranulated [1]. The mechanism for the delayed whealing is unknown, but mediators other than histamine may be involved in this reaction [1]. Inheritance is probably autosomal dominant. Antihistamines are advised for symptomatic relief.

Reference

1. Michaëlsson, G., Ros, A.-M.: Familial localized heat urticaria of delayed type. Acta derm.-venereol. (Stockh.) *51*, 279–283 (1971)

Hereditary Inflammatory Vasculitis with Persistent Nodules

Several members of three generations in a family have been described with this disorder [1]. The main feature is the appearance of recurring nodules in the skin and subcutaneous tissue from early childhood or birth. The nodules are of two types. In one type, they appear on the arms, legs, and buttocks and are multiple, small to medium-sized, persistent, and nonulcerating. In the other type, the nodules occur over bony prominences and are multiple, larger, firm, and erythematous [1]. The condition is aggravated by sunlight.

Rheumatoid factor, antinuclear factor, and chronic discoid lupus erythematosus may be present in some members of the affected family. It is possible that this type of vasculitis may be a particular familial form of lupus erythematosus.

Histologic examination shows a marked perivascular lymphocytic infiltrate and edema throughout the dermis, especially in the lower dermis near the sweat coils and extending to the fat [1]. The vessels are essentially intact and no granulomatous reaction or fat necrosis is found. Mucinous edema separates the collagen bundles. Inheritance is probably autosomal dominant. Treatment with chloroquine (250 mg daily) results in rapid resolution of the lesions.

Reference

1. Reed, W.B., Bergeron, R.F., Tuffanelli, D., Wilson Jones, E.: Hereditary inflammatory vasculitis with persistent nodules. A genetically-determined new entity probably related to lupus erythematosus. Brit. J. Derm. *87*, 299–307 (1972)

Chapter 14   Neurocutaneous Syndromes

Contents

Familial Dysautonomia (Riley-Day Syndrome)

In 1949 Riley et al. [1] described this syndrome for the first time. Since then, over 200 affected families have been identified, almost all of whom are Ashkenazi Jews [2].

Clinical Presentation. The most striking and characteristic features of this disease are absence of overflow tears (alacrimia), corneal anesthesia, relative indifference to pain, and a peculiar reaction to anxiety manifested by hypotension, excessive sweating, drooling, and blotchy skin. Whenever these patients are anxious or excited, they develop erythematous blotches over any part of their bodies, except the palms and soles. These start as small red macules and then increase in number, size, and intensity to become confluent and dark red within a few seconds [2–4].

Other common findings are myopia, exotropia, corneal hyposthesia with ulcerations and opacities, anisocoria, tortuous retinal vessels, absence of the fungiform and vallate papillae of the tongue (Fig. 14.1), kyphoscoliosis, and short stature. Some patients develop neuropathic arthropathy of the knees, shoulders, or elbows.

The most common neurologic abnormalities are patchy and variable insensitivity to pain, impaired coordination, and dysesthesia (an abnormal re-

action to touch stimuli). The intellect is unimpaired [2–4].

The intradermal injection of histamine produces little pain or erythema [5]. The ratio of homovanillic acid to vanillylmandelic acid in the urine is elevated [6]. The concentrations of epinephrine and norepinephrine in the adrenal glands of three affected children were higher than normal [7].

Congenital insensitivity to pain with anhidrosis has also been reported [8]. This condition should be differentiated from hereditary insensitivity to pain (inherited as autosomal recessive), in which the skin presents no anatomic abnormalities in the nerve endings, nerve trunks, or central nervous system. Cuts, burns, or bruises are frequent and may heal poorly, leaving prominent scars.

Pathology and Pathophysiology. A 1-year-old child with no taste buds had extreme paucity of subcutaneous sensory nerves and reduced neuron populations in sensory and autonomic ganglia [9]. Demyelination of the posterior columns of the spinal cord was also observed [10].

A decrease in synthesis of noradrenaline [11] and decreased dopamine-β-hydroxylase (DBH), the enzyme that converts dopamine to norepinephrine, have been found [12].

Inheritance. Autosomal recessive [4].

Treatment. No specific treatment is available. The treatment is aimed at complications such as aspiration pneumonia.

References

1. Riley, C.M., Day, R.L., Greeley, D.M., Langford, W.S.: Central autonomic dysfunction with defective lacrimation. I. Report of five cases. Pediatrics 3, 468–478 (1949)
2. McKusick, V.A., Norum, R.A., Farkas, H.J., Brunt, P.W., Mahloudji, M.: The Riley-Day syndrome – observations on genetics and survivorship. An interim report. Israel J. med. Sci. 3, 372–379 (1967)
3. Moses, S.W., Rotem, Y., Jagoda, N., Talmor, N., Eichhorn, F., Levin, S.: A clinical, genetic and biochemical study of familial dysautonomia in Israel. Israel J. med. Sci. 3, 358–371 (1967)

4. Brunt, P.W., McKusick, V.A.: Familial dysautonomia. A report of genetic and clinical studies, with a review of the literature. Med. (Baltimore) *49*, 343–374 (1970)

5. Smith, A.A., Dancis, J.: Response to intradermal histamine in familial dysautonomia – a diagnostic test. J. Pediat. *63*, 889–894 (1963)

6. Smith, A.A., Taylor, T., Wortis, S.B.: Abnormal catecholamine metabolism in familial dysautonomia. New Engl. J. Med. *268*, 705–707 (1963)

7. Smith, A.A., Dancis, J.: Catecholamine release in familial dysautonomia. New Engl. J. Med. *277*, 61–64 (1967)

8. Swanson, A.G., Buchan, G.C., Alvord, E.C., Jr.: Anatomic changes in congenital insensitivity to pain. Absence of small primary sensory neurons in ganglia, roots, and Lissauer's tract. Arch. Neurol. *12*, 12–18 (1965)

9. Pearson, J., Finegold, M.J., Budzilovich, G.: The tongue and taste in familial dysautonomia. Pediatrics *45*, 739–745 (1970)

10. Fogelson, M.H., Rorke, L.B., Kaye, R.: Spinal cord changes in familial dysautonomia. Arch. Neurol. *17*, 103–108 (1967)

11. Goodall, M., Gitlow, S.E., Alton, H.: Decreased noradrenaline (norepinephrine) synthesis in familial dysautonomia. J. clin. Invest. *50*, 2734–2740 (1971)

12. Weinshilboum, R.M., Axelrod, J.: Reduced plasma dopamine-β-hydroxylase activity in familial dysautonomia. New Engl. J. Med. *285*, 938–942 (1971)

Tuberous Sclerosis
(Epiloia, Bourneville Disease)

This disorder affects about 1 per 100,000 individuals in the USA and Western Europe. It is worldwide in distribution and involves both sexes.

Clinical Presentation. The disease has protean manifestations and affects every organ, even though the classic features are mental deficiency, epilepsy, and adenoma sebaceum. Four types of skin lesions are pathognomonic:

1. *Adenoma sebaceum (Pringle)* (Figs. 14.2 and 14.3) is rarely present at birth but usually appears around the age of 5 or 6 years. The lesions increase in size and number until puberty and remain stationary thereafter. They are pink to red nodules with a smooth, glistening surface [1], symmetrically distributed in the nasolabial folds, cheeks, and nose in a butterfly pattern. The upper lip is notably spared [1]. The chin, ears, forehead, and eyelids may be involved. The lesions are usually discrete, but occasionally they may coalesce. Fibromatous plaques, flesh-colored or brownish, may appear on the forehead or cheek.

2. *Periungual fibromas (Könen tumors)* (Fig. 14.4) are present in about 50% of affected individuals. These tumors appear as smooth buds at the base of the nail or subungually and may reach a size sufficient to disrupt the nail bed [1]. They are flesh-colored, usually multiple, and may affect fingers and toes.

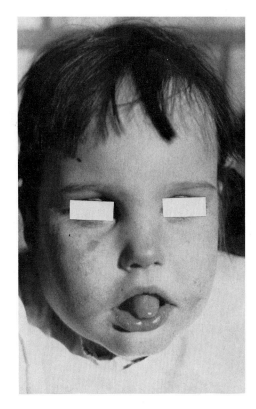

Fig. 14.1. Familial dysautonomia. Note the smooth tongue with absence of papillae. (Courtesy of Dr. F.C. Fraser)

3. *Shagreen patch (peau chagrinée)* (Fig. 14.5) is an irregularly shaped plaque of thickened skin, slightly elevated, with a *peau d'orange* surface. Characteristically, the patch is in the lumbosacral region. Occasionally, a central patch may have smaller satellite lesions around it [1].

4. *Leaf-shaped white macules* (Figs. 14.6 and 14.7) are usually present at birth and are of great diagnostic importance [2]. In fair-skinned individuals, Wood's light helps in their detection [2]. These macules may be the only cutaneous sign of tuberous sclerosis.

Other less pathognomonic lesions are multiple skin tags of the neck and axillae, café-au-lait spots, poliosis, port-wine hemangiomas, and mucosal fibromas.

Neurologic manifestations are prominent. Mental retardation becomes evident in early childhood and affects 70% of patients. Epilepsy affects all individuals with mental deficiency and many of those with normal intelligence. The seizures are local at first but change pattern. A variety of motor peculiarities and behavioral deviations may appear. There is correlation between the severity of skin lesions and the neurologic manifestations. Radiologic examination of the skull reveals cal-

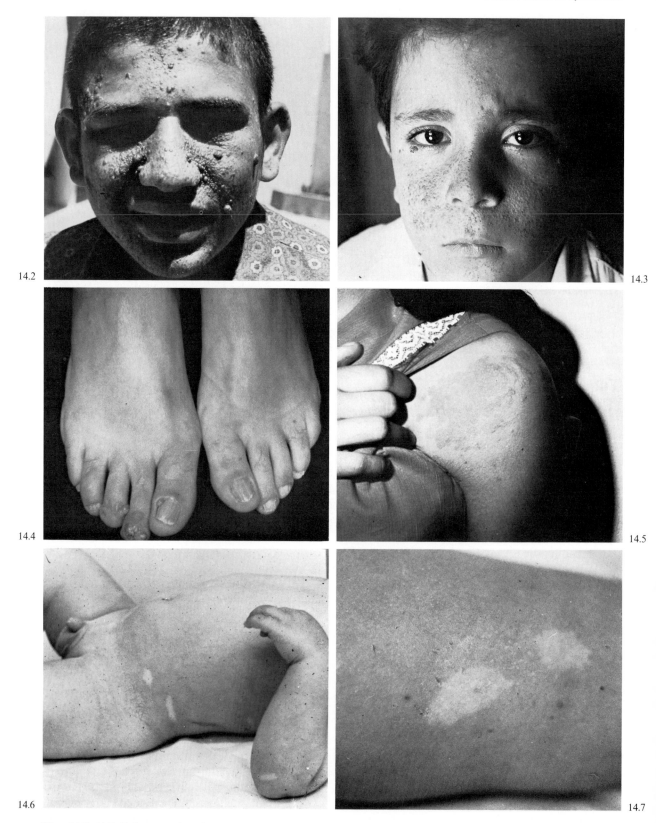

14.2

14.3

14.4

14.5

14.6

14.7

Figs. 14.2–14.7. Tuberous sclerosis

Figs. 14.2 and 14.3. Adenoma sebaceum

Fig. 14.4. Periungual fibromas. (Courtesy of Dr. I. Zeligman)

Fig. 14.5. Shagreen patch

Figs. 14.6 and 14.7. Leaf-shaped depigmented macules

cified nodules especially in the region of the basal ganglia.

Other organs are also involved. Retinal phakoma is the most frequent ocular sign and appears as a whitish plaque in more than half of the cases [3]. Rarer eye manifestations are congenital blindness, congenital cataract, chorioretinitis, optic atrophy, and areas of depigmentation [3]. Renal hamartomas appear in about half the cases of tuberous sclerosis and are usually bilateral and multiple [3]. Rhabdomyomas of the heart may be the cause of death in childhood. Pulmonary involvement is uncommon and its symptoms include dyspnea, hemoptysis, and recurrent spontaneous pneumothorax [3]. Over 80% of patients with tuberous sclerosis have radiologic evidence of bone involvement, pseudocysts in the phalanges, and irregular cortical thickening especially in the metatarsal and metacarpal bones [3].

Pathology and Pathophysiology. The skin lesions are basically hamartomas of vascular and connective tissues. In lesions of adenoma sebaceum (the latter term is obviously a misnomer), there is an angiofibromatous proliferation; in the fibromas and shagreen patch, a predominantly fibrous tissue proliferation has been noted [1]. In the leaflike white macules, the melanocytes contain decreased tyrosinase activity and reduced melanin deposition in the melanosomes [2].

The brain lesions are made up of glial tissue in which are scattered large glial and nerve cells of bizarre patterns [3]. These masses may be calcified.

Inheritance. Autosomal dominant.

Treatment. For cosmetic purposes, lesions of adenoma sebaceum can be excised or curetted. Anticonvulsant therapy may be helpful. Surgical intervention may be resorted to in certain cases.

References

1. Nickel, W.R., Reed, W.B.: Tuberous sclerosis. Special reference to the microscopic alterations in the cutaneous hamartomas. Arch. Derm. *85*, 209–226 (1962)
2. Fitzpatrick, T.B., Szabó, G., Hori, Y., Simone, A.A., Reed, W.B., Greenberg, M.H.: White leaf-shaped macules. Earliest visible sign of tuberous sclerosis. Arch. Derm. *98*, 1–6 (1968)
3. Reed, W.B., Nickel, W.R., Campion, G.: Internal manifestations of tuberous sclerosis. Arch. Derm. *87*, 715–728 (1963)

Neurofibromatosis (Von Recklinghausen Disease)

This disease affects 30–40 individuals per 100,000 [1]. It is worldwide in distribution.

Clinical Presentation. The pathognomonic skin findings are hyperpigmentation and multiple tumors. Pigmentation, present in practically all cases, appears in infancy as brown macules, the café-au-lait spots. These spots increase in number and size during childhood, and can involve any part of the skin surface. They vary in size from a few millimeters to several centimeters (Fig. 14.8). It is postulated that any individual with six or more café-au-lait spots greater than 1.5 cm in diameter may be considered as having the disease [1]. The presence of frecklelike pigmentation in the axillae and perineum is pathognomonic of the disease [2]. Leukodermic macules may also be present.

The cutaneous and subcutaneous tumors vary in size and consistency (Figs. 14.9 and 14.10). The cutaneous tumors (molluscum fibrosum) are soft or firm, a few millimeters to several centimeters in diameter, and appear on any part of the skin, but are most numerous on the trunk. Their number varies from a few to several hundred. They are pinkish or flesh-colored and may be pedunculated or sessile. Characteristically, when pressed, these tumors invaginate through a dermal defect ("button-holing") [1]. The subcutaneous tumors are also multiple and arise in relation to nerve trunks. "Plexiform neuroma" designates such discrete nodular tumors, usually along the cranial or cervical nerves. Accompanied by excessive overgrowth of subcutaneous tissue and skin, these tumors may reach enormous size and are grotesque and disfiguring. Such growths, referred to as elephantiasis neuromatosa or *tumeur royale*, are like a bag of worms and evolve rapidly [3].

Tumors of the oral mucosa are infrequent. Scoliosis, kyphosis, bone cysts, and pathologic fractures are not uncommon. Neurologic manifestations include oligophrenia (frequent), cranial nerve tumors (especially optic and acoustic), and peripheral nerve tumors. Endocrine involvement is manifested by acromegaly, Addison disease, hyper- and hypothyroidism, sexual precocity, and cretinism. There is a fairly common association of neurofibromatosis with pheochromocytoma [4]. Involvement of the gastrointestinal tract gives rise to hemorrhage or obstruction. Malignant change in the tumors of neurofibromatosis may occur especially in the deeper lesions with an incidence of 3–4% [1, 5].

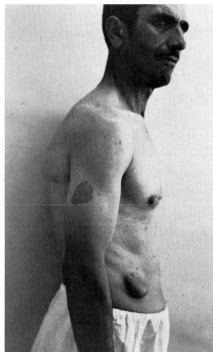

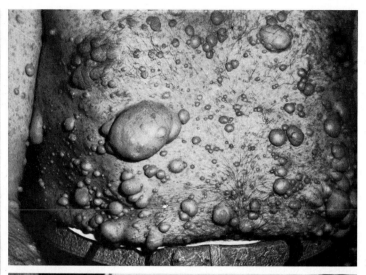

14.9

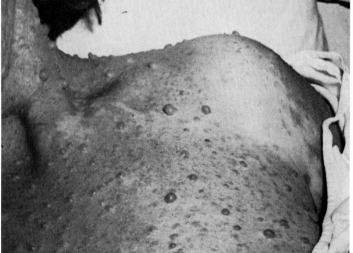

14.8

14.10

Fig. 14.8. Neurofibromatosis. Café-au-lait spot with a cutaneous tumor

Figs. 14.9 and 14.10. Neurofibromatosis. Numerous cutaneous and subcutaneous tumors interspersed with hyperpigmented macules

Such sarcomas appear later in life. There also seems to be a higher incidence of other cutaneous neoplasms in patients with neurofibromatosis [6].

Pathology and Pathophysiology. The cutaneous neurofibromas are not encapsulated although they are usually well-circumscribed. Three basic features comprise these tumors: fibrils, cellular proliferation, and degenerative phenomena [7]. The fibrils are usually wavy, thin, and eosinophilic. The cells have oval or spindle-shaped nuclei and occasionally tend to be palisaded as in Verocay bodies, although the latter are not well-developed. Many mast cells are present [1, 7] and special stains reveal nonspecific cholinesterase [7] and nerve fibers. Mucoid degeneration of the stroma may occur as a homogeneous ground substance in which the cells are embedded.

The café-au-lait spots show increased melanin in the melanocytes and keratinocytes as well as giant melanin granules [8]. Ultrastructurally, these characteristic giant melanin granules are shown to be giant melanosomes or "macromelanosomes" rather than phagolysosomes [9].

Inheritance. Autosomal dominant with high penetrance and wide variability in expression. About 50% of patients have a fresh mutation.

Treatment. Management is mainly palliative and symptomatic. If malignant change is suspected, surgery is indicated.

References

1. Crowe, F.W., Schull, W.J., Neel, J.V.: Clinical, pathological, and genetic study of multiple neurofibromatosis. Springfield: Charles C Thomas 1956
2. Crowe, F.W.: Axillary freckling as a diagnostic aid in neurofibromatosis. Ann. intern. Med. *61*, 1142–1143 (1964)

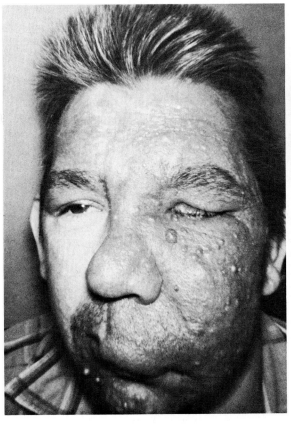

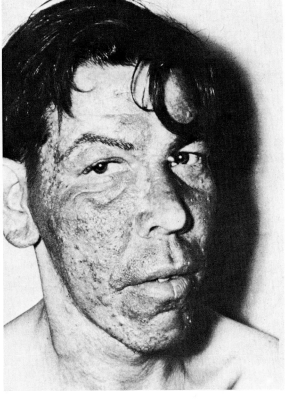

Fig. 14.11. Sturge-Weber syndrome. Unilateral cutaneous angioma with involvement of the eye. (Courtesy of Dr. I. Zeligman)

Fig. 14.12. Sturge-Weber syndrome. Hemangioma involving the whole face. (Courtesy of Dr. I. Zeligman)

3. Basset, A., Collomb, H., Quéré, N.A., Sicard, D., Faye, I.: Quelques aspects de la maladie de Recklinghausen en Afrique de l'Ouest. A propos de 35 cas observés à Dakar de 1959 à 1964. Ann. Derm. Syph. (Paris) *93*, 43–51 (1966)
4. Healey, F.H., Jr., Mekelatos, C.J.: Pheochromocytoma and neurofibromatosis. New Engl. J. Med. *258*, 540–543 (1958)
5. D'Agostino, A.N., Soule, E.H., Miller, R.H.: Sarcomas of the peripheral nerves and somatic soft tissues associated with multiple neurofibromatosis (von Recklinghausen's disease). Cancer *16*, 1015–1027 (1963)
6. Knight, W.A., III, Murphy, W.K., Gottlieb, J.A.: Neurofibromatosis associated with malignant neurofibromas. Arch. Derm. *107*, 747–750 (1973)
7. Winkelmann, R.K., Johnson, L.A.: Cholinesterases in neurofibromas. Arch. Derm. *85*, 106–114 (1962)
8. Benedict, P.H., Szabo, G., Fitzpatrick, T.B., Sinesi, S.J.: Melanotic macules in Albright's syndrome and in neurofibromatosis. J. Amer. med. Ass. *205*, 618–626 (1968)
9. Jimbow, K., Szabo, G., Fitzpatrick, T.B.: Ultrastructure of giant pigment granules (macromelanosomes) in the cutaneous pigmented macules of neurofibromatosis. J. invest. Derm. *61*, 300–309 (1973)

Angiomatoses

Sturge-Weber Syndrome (Encephalotrigeminal Angiomatosis)

Clinical Presentation. This syndrome comprises hemangiomas involving the skin, eye, and cerebral meninges [1, 2]. The cutaneous angioma is usually present at birth and involves one side of the face in the distribution of the trigeminal nerve (mainly the ophthalmic division) (Fig. 14.11). Occasionally, it spreads beyond the midline and may involve the head, neck, and trunk (Fig. 14.12). The lesion is usually of the port-wine nevus flammeus type, although nodular thickenings may be present within it.

The eye may be involved and congenital glaucoma (buphthalmos) may develop. Other eye changes are megalocornea and angiomatosis of the conjunctiva, iris, and choroid.

Epilepsy is the main manifestation of intracranial involvement. This usually appears in early infancy or childhood. Occasionally, seizures may not appear in spite of meningeal involvement [1]. Hemiplegia and mental retardation develop in many cases. The association of facial angioma and brain involvement is not always present. When the facial lesion affects the region below the eyelids and nose (below the ophthalmic division of the trigeminal nerve), cerebral involvement is usually absent.

Occasionally Sturge-Weber and Klippel-Trénaunay syndromes coexist [3].

Pathology and Pathophysiology. The cutaneous lesion is the capillary hemangioma type (nevus flammeus). The intracranial lesion is an angiomatosis of the leptomeninges with secondary calcifications [4]. The underlying brain tissue exhibits pressure atrophy.

Inheritance. Suspected autosomal dominant, although there is no clear evidence of heredity. Trisomy of chromosome 22 has been found associated with the syndrome [5].

Treatment. Neurosurgical intervention may be helpful. Similarly, the eye condition may be helped by control of the glaucoma. For the nevus flammeus, many modalities are available although none is satisfactory. These modalities include the use of a camouflaging cosmetic material, ionizing irradiation, carbon dioxide snow, tattooing with insoluble pigments, and, at times, surgical excision.

References

1. Chao, D.H.-C.: Congenital neurocutaneous syndromes of childhood. III. Sturge-Weber disease. J. Pediat. 55, 635–649 (1959)
2. Royale, H.E.: The Sturge-Weber syndrome. Oral Surg. 22, 490–497 (1966)
3. Furukawa, T., Igata, A., Toyokura, Y., Ikeda, S.: Sturge-Weber and Klippel-Trénaunay syndrome with nevus of Ota and Íto. Arch. Derm. 102, 640–645 (1970)
4. Morgan, G.: Pathology of the Sturge-Weber syndrome. Proc. roy. Soc. Med. 56, 422–423 (1963)
5. Hayward, M.D., Bower, B.D.: Chromosomal trisomy associated with the Sturge-Weber syndrome. Lancet 1960 II, 844–846

von Hippel-Lindau Syndrome (Hemangioblastoma of Cerebellum and Retina)

This rare syndrome is characterized by angiomatosis of cerebellum or medulla, retinal angiomas (in 20% of cases), and occasional cutaneous angio-

mas, especially of the occipitocervical region [1]. Associated findings are hypernephromas [2], pheochromocytomas [3], polycystic disease of the pancreas and kidneys, and hemangiomas of the spinal cord, adrenals, lungs, and liver.

The presence of hypertension with the vascular cerebellar lesion leads to subarachnoid hemorrhage. Polycythemia may be present and could be due to the cerebellar hemangioblastoma [4] or the hypernephroma.

Inheritance. Autosomal dominant.

Treatment. Only symptomatic treatment is available.

References

1. Christoferson, L.A., Gustafson, M.B., Petersen, A.G.: Von Hippel-Lindau's disease. J. Amer. med. Ass. 178, 280–282 (1961)
2. Kaplan, C., Sayre, G.P., Greene, L.F.: Bilateral nephrogenic carcinomas in Lindau-von Hippel disease. J. Urol. 86, 36–42 (1961)
3. Sharp, W.V., Platt, R.L.: Familial pheochromocytoma. Association with von Hippel-Lindau's disease. Angiology 22, 141–146 (1971)
4. Hennessy, T.G., Stern, W.E., Herrick, S.E.: Cerebellar hemangioblastoma: erythropoietic activity by radioiron assay. J. nucl. Med. 8, 601–606 (1967)

Diffuse Corticomeningeal Angiomatosis of Divry and Van Bogaert

The cutaneous features in this syndrome are congenital cutis marmorata (marble skin) affecting mainly the back and spreading to the flanks, buttocks, and legs; acrocyanosis affecting mainly the hands, forearms, elbows, and knees; and patches of hyperpigmentation on the trunk. The neurologic manifestations include epileptic seizures, progressive dementia, visual field defects, and pyramidal and extrapyramidal signs [1, 2].

There is a noncalcifying corticomeningeal angiomatosis and diffuse degeneration of the white matter. Inheritance is autosomal recessive. There is no treatment for this condition.

References

1. Divry, P., Van Bogaert, L.: Une maladie familiale caractérisée par une angiomatose diffuse cortico-méningée non calcifiante et une démyélinisation progressive de la substance blanche. J. Neurol. Neurosurg. Psychiat. 9, 41–54 (1946)
2. Martin, J.J., Navarro, C., Roussel, J.M., Michielssen, P.: Familial capillaro-venous leptomeningeal angiomatosis. Europ. Neurol. 9, 202–215 (1973)

Chapter 15 Metabolic Disorders

Contents

Aminoacidemias and Aminoacidurias

Alkaptonuria

In 1859 Bödeker [1] made the diagnosis of this condition with certainty for the first time. Virchow [2], in 1866, described a peculiar type of generalized pigmentation in the connective tissues of a 67-year-old man. He named the condition ochronosis because the pigment was brownish yellow (ochre) microscopically. In 1902 Albrecht [3] demonstrated the connection between ochronosis and alkaptonuria. In 1908, partly as a result of his studies on alkaptonuria, Sir Archibald Garrod [4] developed his whole concept of heritable metabolic diseases.

Clinical Presentation. The most important features of alkaptonuria are (a) the signs due to the presence of homogentisic acid in the urine, (b) pigmentation of cartilage and other connective tissues (Fig. 15.1), and (c) arthritis in later years [5].
The earliest physical findings in this disease are slight pigmentation of the sclerae or the ears, usually noticeable after the age of 20 or 30 years. The eye pigmentation is usually found about midway between the cornea and outer and inner canthi, at the site of the insertions of the recti muscles. A more diffuse pigmentation may involve the conjunctiva and cornea (Figs. 15.2 and 15.3). The ear pinna is slate-blue or gray and feels irregular and thickened. Sometimes a dusky discoloration, corresponding to the tendons, may be seen through the skin over the hands. Since the pigment may appear in perspiration, clothing near the axillary regions

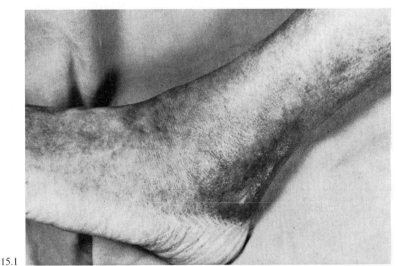

Fig. 15.1. Alkaptonuria. Dusky discoloration over the Achilles tendon. (Courtesy of Dr. I. Zeligman)

15.1

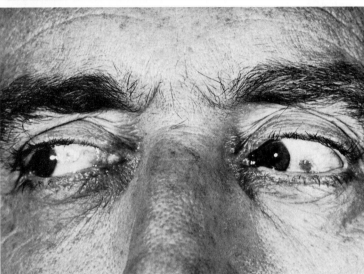

Figs. 15.2 and 15.3. Alkaptonuria. Pigmentation in the sclera. (Fig. 2 – courtesy of Dr. B. N. La Du, Jr., from Bunim, J. J., et al.: Ann. intern. Med. *47*, 1210–1224, 1957)

15.2

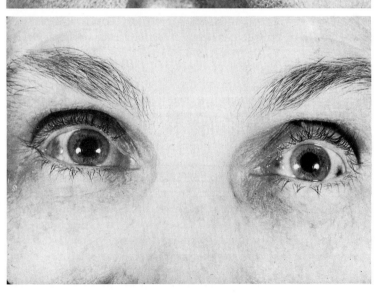

15.3

Fig. 15.4. Metabolic pathways. Block at ① produces one type of oculocutaneous albinism. Block at ② produces phenylketonuria. Block at ③ produces alkaptonuria

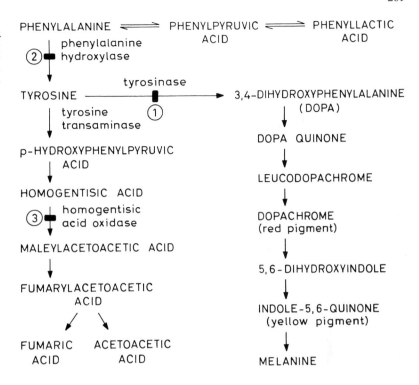

may be stained and the skin may have a brownish discoloration in the axillary and genital areas [6].

Long-standing alkaptonuria may lead to "ochronotic arthritis." The earliest symptoms are usually some degree of limitation of motion of the hip and knee joints or the shoulders. The arthritic complications are often severe and painful and may lead to a completely bedridden existence later in life [6].

Most patients give a history of urine which turns dark on standing. This is due to the presence of an abnormal constituent, homogentisic acid. The darkening is greatly accelerated by alkali. Homogentisic acid can be identified more specifically after precipitation as the lead salt [7] or by paper chromatography [8].

Pathology and Pathophysiology. The metabolic defect in alkaptonuria is a failure to synthesize active homogentisic acid oxidase in the liver and kidneys [9] (see Fig. 15.4 for metabolic pathways and site of defect). This results in the accumulation of homogentisic acid in tissues, leading to an abnormal pigmentation that involves the cartilage in many regions (costal, laryngeal, tracheal). Pigmentation is also present throughout the body in fibrous tissues, tendons, and ligaments. It may be found in the endocardium, intima of the larger vessels, kidneys, lungs, and epidermis as well [6].

Inheritance. Autosomal recessive [10].

Treatment. Large amounts of ascorbic acid may prevent the deposition of ochronotic pigment in the different tissues [11].

References

1. Bödeker, C.: Über das Alkapton; ein neuer Beitrag zur Frage: welche Stoffe des Harns können Kupferreduktion bewirken? Z. Rat. Med. 7, 130 (1859)
2. Virchow, R.: Ein Fall von allgemeiner Ochronose der Knorpel und knorpelähnlichen Teile. Virchows Arch. path. Anat. 37, 212 (1866)
3. Albrecht, H.: Über Ochronose. Z. Heilk. 23, 366 (1902)
4. Garrod, A.E.: The Croonian lectures on inborn errors of metabolism. Lecture II. Alkaptonuria. Lancet 1908 II, 73–79
5. O'Brien, W.M., La Du, B.N., Bunim, J.J.: Biochemical, pathologic and clinical aspects of alcaptonuria, ochronosis, and ochronotic arthropathy. Review of world literature (1584–1962). Amer. J. Med. 34, 813–838 (1963)
6. La Du, B.N.: Alcaptonuria. In: The metabolic basis of inherited disease. Stanbury, J.B., Wyngaarden, J.B., Fredrickson, D.S. (eds.), 4th ed., pp. 268–282. New York: McGraw-Hill Book Co. 1978
7. Medes, G.: Modification of Garrod's method for preparation of homogentisic acid from urine. Proc. Soc. exp. Biol. (N.Y.) 30, 751 (1932–1933)
8. Knox, W.E., Le May-Knox, M.: The oxidation in liver of L-tyrosine to acetoacetate through p-hydroxyphenylpyruvate and homogentisic acid. Biochem. J. 49, 686–693 (1951)
9. La Du, B.N., Zannoni, V.G., Laster, L., Seegmiller, J.E.: The nature of the defect in tyrosine metabolism in alcaptonuria. J. biol. Chem. 230, 251–260 (1958)
10. Khachadurian, A., Abu Feisal, K.: Alkaptonuria. Report of a family with seven cases appearing in four successive generations with metabolic studies in one patient. J. chron. Dis. 7, 455–465 (1958)
11. Sealock, R.R., Galdston, M., Steele, J.M.: Administration of ascorbic acid to an alkaptonuric patient. Proc. Soc. exp. Biol. (N.Y.) 44, 580–583 (1940)

Argininosuccinic Aciduria

In 1958 Allan et al. [1] described two severely mentally retarded siblings with a grossly increased excretion of a urinary amino acid. In 1959 Dent [2] identified this amino acid as argininosuccinic acid (ASA). The disease is very rare; less than 50 cases have been reported to date.

Clinical Presentation. Patients can be divided clinically into two groups:
1. *Late-onset type* – with mental retardation, seizures, intermittent ataxia, and vomiting, apparent in the second year of life.
2. *Early-onset (malignant) type* – with failure to thrive, recurrent vomiting, hepatomegaly, seizures, and coma in the early months of life, death sometimes occurring in the first few days of life from massive pulmonary hemorrhage [3].
Argininosuccinic acid is excreted in massive amounts in the urine and is found in elevated levels in the blood and CSF. The diagnosis can be made easily by two-dimensional chromatoelectrophoresis. The hair abnormality is trichorrhexis nodosa. It has been observed in approximately half of the patients with argininosuccinic aciduria. The hair is "dry," fracturing at the ends, especially over the occipital region. There is irregular growth, giving a tufted, matted appearance. Patches of dry skin and brittle nails may be present.

Pathology and Pathophysiology. The basic biochemical defect is the absence of argininosuccinase (ASase) in human red blood cells [4] as well as in the liver, brain, and kidneys [3].
Prenatal diagnosis is possible by means of amniocentesis and the demonstration of absent ASase in amniotic fluid cells [5].
The hairs show nodose swellings and constrictions as well as longitudinal splitting along the shaft. Transverse fractures may result at the nodes. On exposure to acridine orange, an abnormal red fluorescence appears. The cause of the hair abnormality is not clear. It has been postulated that the keratin is abnormal because of arginine deficiency secondary to the absence of ASase.
The general pathologic status of various organs is nonspecific.

Inheritance. Autosomal recessive [3].

Treatment. A low-protein diet in combination with arginine supplement started at 6 weeks of age seems promising [6].

References

1. Allan, J.D., Cusworth, D.C., Dent, C.E., Wilson, V.K.: A disease, probably hereditary, characterised by severe mental deficiency and a constant gross abnormality of aminoacid metabolism. Lancet *1958 I*, 182–187
2. Dent, C.E.: Argininosuccinic aciduria. A new form of mental deficiency due to metabolic causes. Proc. roy. Soc. Med. *52*, 885 (1959)
3. Shih, V.E.: Urea cycle disorders. In: The metabolic basis of inherited disease and other congenital hyperammonemic syndromes. Stanbury, J.B., Wyngaarden, J.B., Fredrickson, D.S. (eds.), 4th ed., pp. 362–386. New York: McGraw-Hill Book Co. 1978
4. Tomlinson, S., Westall, R.G.: Argininosuccinic aciduria. Argininosuccinase and arginase in human blood cells. Clin. Sci. *26*, 261–269 (1964)
5. Shih, V.E., Littlefield, J.W.: Argininosuccinase activity in amniotic-fluid cells. Lancet *1970 II*, 45
6. Shih, V.E.: Early dietary management in an infant with argininosuccinase deficiency: preliminary report. J. Pediat. *80*, 645–648 (1972)

Tyrosinemia II
(Richner-Hanhart Syndrome)

A deficiency of hepatic tyrosine aminotransferase in humans is responsible for a syndrome of keratitis, palmar and plantar erosions, hyperkeratosis, and mental retardation. Serum tyrosine increases due to the enzymatic deficiency lead to the deposition of tyrosine crystals in the eye and especially the cornea. This deposition and possible lysosomal activation leads to inflammation in the cornea and the skin. The inheritance follows the autosomal recessive pattern [1]. (See Disseminate Palmoplantar Keratodermia with Corneal Dystrophy, p. 44).

Reference

1. Goldsmith, L.A.: Molecular biology and molecular pathology of a newly described molecular disease – Tyrosinemia II (The Richner-Hanhart syndrome). Exp. Cell Biol. *46*, 96–113 (1978)

Aspartylglycosaminuria

In 1967 Jenner and Pollitt described two mentally retarded adult patients with this condition [1]. More recently, 34 patients with this disorder have been recognized in Finland in the course of a systematic investigation in institutions for the mentally retarded [2].

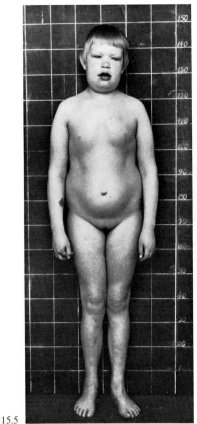

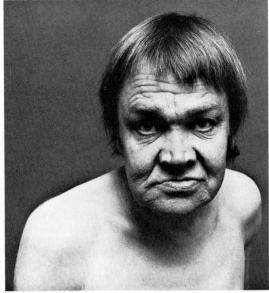

15.6

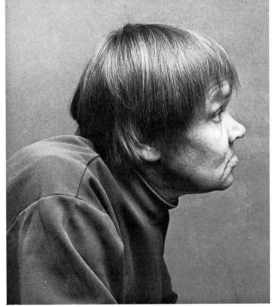

15.5

Figs. 15.5–15.7. Aspartylglycosaminuria. Coarse features with deep sagging cheeks, broad nose and face, and short neck. Note acneiform lesions on the face in Fig. 6. (Courtesy of Dr. J. Palo)

15.7

Clinical Presentation. All patients exhibit mental retardation, bone or connective tissue abnormalities, and coarse features, including deep sagging cheeks, broad nose and face, and short neck (Figs. 15.5–15.7). Cranial asymmetry and thoracic or lumbar scoliosis are frequent findings. About half the patients have cutaneous manifestations, including large nevi, acne, and photosensitive pigmentation. Aggressive behavior is frequent. The IQ varies from 10–40. Lymphocyte vacuolization is a constant hematologic finding. Most patients develop slowly and suffer from recurrent infections of the skin or the upper respiratory tract. The ages of the diagnosed patients vary from 13–37 years [3].

Pathology and Pathophysiology. Normally, aspartylglycosylamine is split to aspartate, ammonia, and N-acetylglucosylamine by aspartylglycosylamine amidase, a lysosomal enzyme. No activity of this enzyme is detected in the plasma or seminal fluid of these patients [4]. In the brain and liver the activity of the enzyme is decreased to about 16–20% of the normal mean value. In these tissues the activity of α-fucosidase is also decreased to about one-third the normal, whereas N-acetyl-β-glucosaminidase is five to eight times more active than normally [5]. Electron microscopically, numerous large lysosomes containing electron-dense membranous material are seen in the glial cells and neurons. The hepatocytes reveal large, clear vacuoles containing a pale, flocculent material [5].

Inheritance. Autosomal recessive [3].

Treatment. No specific treatment is known.

References

1. Jenner, F.A., Pollitt, R.J.: Large quantities of 2-acetamido-1-(β-L-aspartamido)-1,2-dideoxyglucose in the urine of mentally retarded siblings. Biochem. J. *103*, 48P–49P (1967)
2. Palo, J., Savolainen, H.: Thin-layer chromatographic demonstration of aspartylglycosylamine and a novel acidic carbohydrate in human tissues. J. Chromatog. *65*, 447–450 (1972)
3. Palo, J., Mattsson, K.: Eleven new cases of aspartylglucosaminuria. J. ment. Defic. Res. *14*, 168–173 (1970)
4. Pollitt, R.J., Jenner, F.A., Merskey, H.: Aspartylglycosaminuria. An inborn error of metabolism associated with mental defect. Lancet *1968II*, 253–255
5. Palo, J., Riekkinen, P., Arstila, A., Autio, S.: Biochemical and fine structural studies on brain and liver biopsies in aspartylglucosaminuria. Neurology (Minneap.) *21*, 1198–1204 (1971)

Citrullinuria

Citrullinuria (citrullinemia) was first reported by McMurray in 1962 [1, 2].

Clinical Presentation. This is an extremely rare metabolic disorder (less than 20 cases reported to date) characterized by mental retardation, marked accumulation of citrulline in the blood, CSF, and urine, and elevation of the blood ammonia concentration in the postabsorptive state. The condition is heterogeneous. The neonatal type is characterized by irritability, lethargy, and convulsions, followed by coma and death [3].
The hair is fragile and has an atrophic bulb. On microscopic examination, it is banded and hence is referred to as "bamboo hair."

Pathology and Pathophysiology. The primary biochemical defect in citrullinemia is the deficiency of hepatic argininosuccinic acid (ASA) synthetase activity, an enzyme involved in the synthesis of ASA.

Inheritance. Autosomal recessive.

Treatment. No specific treatment is available.

References

1. McMurray, W.C., Mohyuddin, F., Rossiter, R.J., Rathbun, J.C., Valentine, G.H., Koegler, S.J., Zarfas, D.E.: Citrullinuria: a new aminoaciduria associated with mental retardation. Lancet *1962I*, 138
2. McMurray, W.C., Rathbun, J.C., Mohyuddin, F., Koegler, S.J.: Citrullinuria. Pediatrics *32*, 347–357 (1963)
3. Shih, V.E.: Urea cycle disorders and other congenital hyperammonemic syndromes. In: The metabolic basis of inherited disease. Stanbury, J.B., Wyngaarden, J.B., Fredrickson, D.S. (eds.), 4th ed., pp. 362–386. New York: McGraw-Hill Book Co. 1978

Phenylketonuria

In 1934 Følling [1] described ten patients who excreted phenylpyruvic acid and were mentally deficient. Later, in 1939, Jervis [2] showed that the condition was inherited through an autosomal recessive gene and that these patients exhibited a high level of phenylalanine accumulation.

Clinical Presentation. The infant with phenylketonuria (PKU) is not clinically abnormal at birth. During the first year, the usual developmental milestones are often delayed and convulsions may supervene. A characteristic "mousy" odor is usually present. The incidence of PKU is 1 per 10,000 in the general population.
The physical findings involve mainly two systems: the skin and the nervous system.
Characteristically, affected individuals have fair skin, blond or light brown hair (Fig. 15.8), and blue eyes [3]. Eczematous dermatitis and/or atopic dermatitis (affecting 5–50% of PKU cases) usually begin in infancy and may persist to adolescence or adulthood. A dry or rough skin is often noted. Papuloerythematous eruptions may appear over the forearms.
Untreated patients are moderately to severely mentally retarded and may have abnormal neurologic manifestations, e.g., agitated behavior, EEG abnormalities, muscular hypertonicity, microcephaly, hyperactive reflexes, inability to talk, hyperkinesis, incontinence, tremors, and seizures.
An easy and helpful screening method consists of adding a few drops of a fresh 10% ferric chloride solution to a few milliliters of acidified urine. A bluish green color appears in a few seconds when the disease is present. The same test can be performed by adding the ferric chloride to a diaper wet with urine. The more reliable and diagnostic method is determination of the level of phenylalanine in plasma. The diagnosis of PKU is made if the level is 20 mg/100 ml or above (normal 2–4 mg/100 ml) along with a normal tyrosine level.

Pathology and Pathophysiology. The basic biochemical defect is the hereditary inactivity of

Fig. 15.8. Hair from phenylketonurics, with or without dietary treatment. (Courtesy of the Department of Medical Illustration, Institute of Child Health and Hospital for Sick Children, London, England, through Dr. L.I. Woolf)

HAIR FROM PHENYLKETONURICS

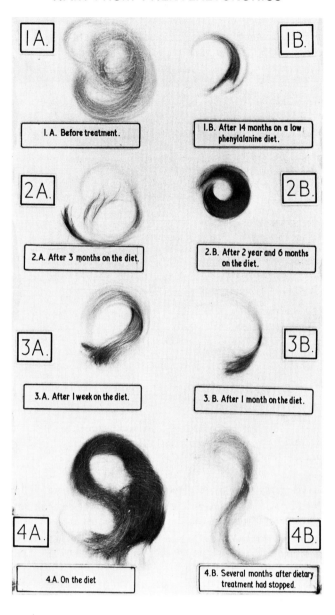

I.A. Before treatment.

I.B. After 14 months on a low phenylalanine diet.

2.A. After 3 months on the diet.

2.B. After 2 year and 6 months on the diet.

3.A. After I week on the diet.

3.B. After I month on the diet.

4.A. On the diet

4.B. Several months after dietary treatment had stopped.

phenylalanine hydroxylase, a liver enzyme. Normally, the liver enzyme oxidizes L-phenylalanine to tyrosine, which is involved in melanin synthesis. The deficiency of phenylalanine hydroxylase results in the accumulation of phenylalanine and the formation, through other pathways, of phenylpyruvic, phenyllactic, phenylacetic, and δ-hydroxyphenyllactic acids. These, in turn, compete for the tyrosinase necessary to convert tyrosine to melanin, resulting in fair hair and blue eyes (see Fig. 15.4 for these metabolic pathways and the block in PKU). At least three enzymes are known to be involved in the hydroxylation of phenylalanine. Mutation can affect two of these [4].

The pathologic changes of the nervous system are due to defective myelination. Phenylpyruvic acid inhibits pyruvate decarboxylase in the brain, but not the liver. This may account for the defect in formation of myelin and mental retardation in this disease [5].

One form of hyperphenylalaninemia with levels of >20 mg/100 ml is manifested by myoclonus, uncontrolled movements, tetraplegia, greasy skin, and recurrent hyperthermia. It is associated with a functional abnormality of dihydropteridine reductase [3].

Inheritance. Autosomal recessive [3, 4].

Treatment. A low phenylalanine diet should be administered. If this is started during the first 4 weeks of life, normal physical, neurologic, and mental development is expected. Overtreatment may result in an acute, weeping eczematous dermatitis.

References

1. Følling, A.: Über Ausscheidung von Phenylbrenztrauben- säure in den Harn als Stoffwechselanomalie in Verbindung mit Imbezillität. Z. physiol. Chem. *227*, 169–176 (1934)
2. Jervis, G.A.: The genetics of phenylpyruvic oligophrenia. J. ment. Sci. *85*, 719 (1939)
3. Tourian, A.Y., Sidbury, J.B.: Phenylketonuria. In: The metabolic basis of inherited disease. Stanbury, J.B., Wyngaarden, J.B., Fredrickson, D.S. (eds.), 4th ed., pp. 240–255. New York: McGraw-Hill Book Co. 1978
4. McKusick, V.A.: Mendelian inheritance in man, 4th ed., pp. 538–540. Baltimore: Johns Hopkins University Press 1975
5. Bowden, J.A., McArthur, C.L., III: Possible biochemical model for phenylketonuria. Nature (Lond.) *235*, 230 (1972)

Endocrinopathies

Testicular Feminization Syndrome

This condition was brought to the attention of geneticists by Pettersson and Bonnier in 1937 [1].

Clinical Presentation. Affected individuals are always considered to be female and are reared accordingly. At adolescence they feminize very well with good breast development and feminine features, voice, and habitus. The vagina is blind and estrinized, the uterus is absent, and abdominal or inguinal testes are present [2].

Most of them lack pubic and axillary hair ("hairless pseudofemale") (Fig. 15.9). The hair of the scalp is abundant, without temporal balding.

The syndrome may have three main presentations [3]: (a) complete testicular feminization; (b) incomplete testicular feminization with ambiguous genitalia and an enlarged clitoris; and (c) testicular feminization with hypospadias.

The karyotype is usually 46,XY. Female carriers may show almost no secondary sex hair, but have normal menstruation, conception, and pregnancies.

Pathology and Pathophysiology. The affected males exhibit normal, fetal testicular development and regression of the Müllerian ducts. In children the testes are histologically normal, whereas in adults they show pathognomonic histologic changes which develop after gonadotropic stimulation [3].

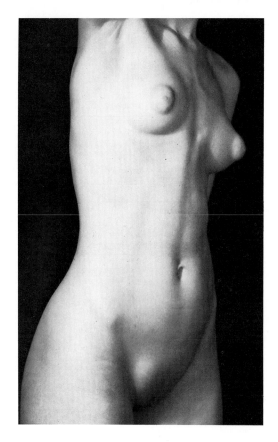

Fig. 15.9. Testicular feminization syndrome. Note absence of axillary hair and very scanty pubic hair. (Courtesy of Dr. L. Pinsky)

The hair follicles of the axillary and pubic areas are anatomically normal but unresponsive to local or parenteral administration of androgens. The beard, voice, and clitoris are also unresponsive. These patients have normal testosterone levels [4].

A receptor protein specific for 5α-androstan-17β-ol-3-one [dihydrotestosterone (DHT)] was found in cells from males and females of all ages [5, 6]. The binding activity was observed in dermal fibroblasts from neck, abdomen, buttocks, foreskin, and wrist. The locus for the receptor protein was found to be on the X chromosome and to lyonize [7]. Lyonization may be responsible for the wide spectrum of phenotypes in heterozygote females.

Inheritance. X-linked recessive [7].

Treatment. The treatment consists of orchidectomy and maintenance on estrogen.

References

1. Pettersson, G., Bonnier, G.: Inherited sex-mosaic in man. Hereditas 23, 49–69 (1937)
2. Wilkins, L.: The diagnosis and treatment of endocrine disorders in childhood and adolescence, 3rd ed., pp. 320–330. Springfield: Charles C Thomas 1965
3. Jirásek, J.A.: Androgen-insensitive male pseudohermaphroditism. In: The clinical delineation of birth defects. Bergsma, D. (ed.), Vol. VII, No. 6, pt. X, pp. 179–184. Baltimore: Williams & Wilkins Co. 1971
4. Southren, A.L., Saito, A.: The syndrome of testicular feminization. A report of three cases with chromatographic analysis of the urinary neutral 17-ketosteroids. Ann. intern. Med. 55, 925–931 (1961)
5. Keenan, B.S., Meyer, W.J., III, Hadjian, A.J., Migeon, C.J.: Androgen receptor in human skin fibroblasts: characterization of specific 17β-hydroxy-5α-androstan-3-one-protein complex in cell sonicates and nuclei. Steroids 25, 535–552 (1975)
6. Keenan, B.S., Meyer, W.J., III, Hadjian, A.J., Jones, H.W., Migeon, C.J.: Syndrome of androgen insensitivity in man: absence of 5α-dihydrotestosterone binding protein in skin fibroblasts. J. clin. Endocr. 38, 1143–1146 (1974)
7. Meyer, W.J., III, Migeon, B.R., Migeon, C.J.: Locus on human X chromosome for dihydrotestosterone receptor and androgen insensitivity. Proc. nat. Acad. Sci. (Wash.) 72, 1469–1472 (1975)

Storage Diseases

Gaucher Disease

In 1882 Gaucher [1] published the first clinical description of this disease which was ultimately named after him.

Clinical Presentation. The most important clinical features of Gaucher disease are splenomegaly, hepatomegaly, erosion of the cortices of the long bones and the head of the femur, hypochromic anemia, leukopenia, and thrombocytopenia. The skin may have a brownish yellow pigmentation, mainly on the face, body, or legs, darker in areas exposed to light. Hemorrhagic folliculitis and furuncles occur on the thighs, legs, and forearms [2]. The skin coloration may be associated with wedge-shaped pigmentation and thickening of the conjuctiva (pingueculae). These skin changes are part of only the chronic form of Gaucher disease.

The wide variation in the clinical forms suggests that Gaucher disease is genetically heterogeneous. Three main clinical categories are distinguished: (a) infantile form – most rapidly progressing, with extensive damage to the central nervous system and death occurring during infancy; (b) juvenile form – with rapidly progressing organomegaly and bone involvement, but without nervous system difficul-

ties; and (c) adult form – with late onset of splenomegaly and varying degrees of clinical severity [2]. The diagnosis is usually made by detecting Gaucher cells in the bone marrow or spleen. Prenatal detection of Gaucher disease is presently possible by amniocentesis, fetal cell culture, and enzymatic determination [2].

Pathology and Pathophysiology. The disease is characterized by deposition of glucocerebroside in histiocytes, forming the Gaucher cells. The rate of formation of this substance is normal. The accumulation of glucocerebroside is due to a deficiency of the catabolic enzyme glucocerebrosidase, required for the hydrolysis of the β-glucosidic bond of glucocerebroside [3]. Since the highest glucocerebroside activity in normal individuals is found in lysosomes [4], Gaucher disease can be considered a lysosomal disease.

Inheritance. Autosomal recessive [2].

Treatment. Treatment is symptomatic, but unsatisfactory. Splenectomy is indicated when hypersplenism is evident in the adult form. Recently, infusion of purified glucocerebrosidase has been reported, with promising results [5].

References

1. Gaucher, C.P.E.: Thesis, University of Paris 1882
2. Brady, R.O., King, F.M.: Gaucher's disease. In: Lysosomes and storage diseases. Hers, H.G., Van Hoof, F. (eds.), pp. 381–394. New York: Academic Press 1973
3. Brady, R.O., Kanfer, J.N., Shapiro, D.: Metabolism of glucocerebrosides. II. Evidence of an enzymatic deficiency in Gaucher's disease. Biochem. biophys. Res. Commun. 18, 221–225 (1965)
4. Weinreb, N.J., Brady, R.O., Tappel, A.E.: The lysosomal localization of sphingolipid hydrolases. Biochim. biophys. Acta (Amst.) 159, 141–146 (1968)
5. Brady, R.O.: The lipid storage diseases: new concepts and control. Ann. intern. Med. 82, 257–261 (1975)

Niemann-Pick Disease

In 1914 Niemann described this condition for the first time in an 18-month-old female infant [1]. Pick later delineated the entity more clearly and called it lipoid cell hepatosplenomegaly [2, 3].

Clinical Presentation. At least five different phenotypes are defined clinically [4–6]. Some, but not all, types are associated with deficient activity of the enzyme sphingomyelinase [5]. This suggests heterogeneity in the underlying genetic abnormalities.

Type A: acute neuronopathic form. The characteristic findings are progressive hypotonia, listlessness, hepatosplenomegaly, and petechiae. About half of the patients have generalized lymph node enlargement. Late in the illness a cherry-red spot is present in the macula. Xanthomas of the skin may be present. They occur as yellow, orange, or pink papules with a predilection for the face, hands, extremities, and shoulders. The skin has a yellowish brown appearance, especially on the exposed parts. The children are normal at birth; the disease manifests itself in the early months of life and is rapidly progressive, with death occurring before 2–3 years of age [6].

It is hard to diagnose Niemann-Pick disease definitively with routine laboratory tests. Sphingomyelinase assay is diagnostic for type A, since the enzyme is absent in the spleen, white blood cells, and skin fibroblasts of affected individuals. It is also helpful in differentiating the other forms of the disease in which the percentage of sphingomyelinase activity varies. Prenatal diagnosis by amniocentesis is possible [7].

Type B: chronic form without central nervous system involvement. Splenic enlargement occurs between 2 and 6 years of age as the first sign of illness. The activity of sphingomyelinase in the spleen and cultured fibroblasts is 1–5% of normal [5].

Type C: subacute form with central nervous system involvement. The clinical features include spasticity, seizures, and the presence of a cherry-red spot in the fundus. The activity of sphingomyelinase is normal.

Type D: Nova Scotia variant. All patients in this group are from Nova Scotia. Neonatal jaundice may be present and persists until 6 months of age. The neurologic symptoms are prominent. The activity of sphingomyelinase is normal.

Type E: adult, non-neuronopathic form. A small number of adults without neurologic difficulties, but with moderate hepatosplenomegaly and foam cells in the marrow, have been reported as having a variant form of Niemann-Pick disease on the basis of some increase in the quantity of sphingomyelin in the liver and spleen [6].

Pathology and Pathophysiology. Niemann-Pick disease is characterized by deposition of sphingomyelin in various tissues forming the typical Niemann-Pick foam cells. Concerning the enzymatic defect, the following was observed. Two major isoenzymes of sphingomyelinase were found (I and II) in normal liver. Cultured fibroblasts in type A demonstrated a virtual absence of both isoenzymes. In type B, there was a marked decrease in the activity of both isoenzymes. Liver tissue

from a patient with type C contained only isoenzyme I. As to the Nova Scotia variant, it may be due to a primary disturbance of cholesterol metabolism, accompanied by an ancillary accumulation of sphingomyelin [8].

Inheritance. Autosomal recessive [6].

Treatment. There is no specific treatment.

References

1. Niemann, A.: Ein unbekanntes Krankheitsbild. Jb. Kinderheilk. *29*, 1–10 (1914)
2. Pick, L.: Über die lipoidzellige Splenohepatomegalie Typus Niemann-Pick als Stoffwechselerkrankung. Med. Klin. *23*, 1483–1488 (1927)
3. Pick, L.: II. Niemann-Pick's disease and other forms of so-called xanthomatosis. Amer. J. med. Sci. *185*, 601–616 (1933)
4. Crocker, A.C.: The cerebral defect in Tay-Sachs disease and Niemann-Pick disease. J. Neurochem. 7, 69–80 (1961)
5. Schneider, P.B., Kennedy, E.P.: Sphingomyelinase in normal human spleens and in spleens from subjects with Niemann-Pick disease. J. Lipid Res. *8*, 202–209 (1967)
6. Brady, R.O.: Sphingomyelin lipidosis: Niemann-Pick disease. In: The metabolic basis of inherited disease. Stanbury, J.B., Wyngaarden, J.B., Fredrickson, D.S. (eds.), 4th ed., pp. 718–730. New York: McGraw-Hill Book Co. 1978
7. Epstein, C.J., Brady, R.O., Schneider, E.L., Brady, R.M., Shapiro, E.: In utero diagnosis of Niemann-Pick disease. Amer. J. hum. Genet. *23*, 533–535 (1971)
8. Brady, R.O., King, F.M.: Niemann-Pick's disease. In: Lysosomes and storage diseases. Hers, H.G., Van Hoof, F., pp. 439–452. New York: Academic Press 1973

Farber Lipogranulomatosis

In 1947, in a Mayo Foundation lecture, Farber described a 14-month-old girl with what appeared to be a lipid metabolic disorder with granulomatous components [1]. In 1952, at the meeting of the American Pediatric Society, he presented clinical and pathologic data on her and two other children with similar findings [1]. Finally, in 1957, Farber et al. [2] described the three patients who died in infancy with an illness characterized by progressive development of swollen joints, a hoarse cry, and progressive neurologic deterioration. Since then, around ten patients have been described with this disease.

Clinical Presentation. Soon after birth, tender, swollen joints and a hoarse, weak cry develop. Joint involvement becomes increasingly severe and generalized and multiple subcutaneous and periarticular nodules appear (Fig. 15.10). Subcutaneous nodules may also develop over pressure points, along with slight to moderate enlargement of

Fig. 15.10. Farber lipogranulomatosis. Periarticular nodules. (From Moser, H.W., et al.: Amer. J. Med. *47*, 869–890, 1969)

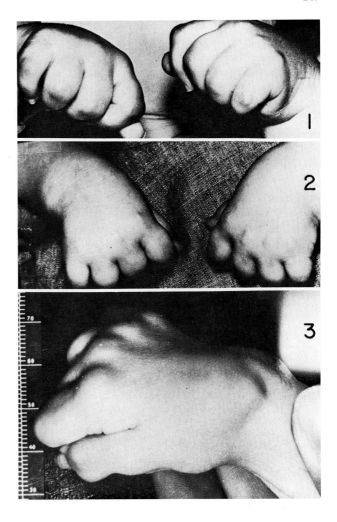

lymph nodes. The liver is of normal size or slightly enlarged. The spleen is not enlarged. There are frequent episodes of fever and dyspnea associated with pulmonary infiltrates. Some patients have neurologic abnormalities. Most of them have a loss of the deep tendon reflexes and mental deterioration in the terminal phase of their illness. The CSF protein level is elevated in many patients [3].

X-rays show a nodular swelling around the peripheral joints associated with muscle atrophy and juxta-articular bone erosion. The lungs show finely nodular parenchymal and interstitial infiltrations [4].

The disease leads progressively to debilitation and finally death, which occurs between the ages of 7 and 22 months [3]. A patient with late onset and long survival has been reported [5].

Pathology and Pathophysiology. Pathologic examination of the subcutaneous nodules reveals that the dermis and subcutaneous tissue are replaced by a pleomorphic, focally necrotic infiltrate of foam cells, histiocytes, lymphocytes, and plasma cells. Soft tissue nodules are present in the larynx and are composed of dense collagen bundles interspersed with foam cells, histiocytes, and mesenchymal cells. Foam cells are also present in some bronchi and alveoli, the red pulp of the spleen, lymph nodes, and bone marrow. Histochemical staining of the foam cells is positive for both carbohydrate and lipid.

There is also ballooning of large neurons in the central and autonomic nervous systems, particularly the anterior horn cells, medulla, pons, and cerebellum. The distension of the neurons is due to PAS-positive cytoplasmic material [3].

The lymph nodes, liver, kidneys, lungs, and subcutaneous nodules reveal a 10- to 60-fold increase in free ceramide and a 5- to 10-fold increase in ganglioside [3]. No ceramidase activity was detected in the kidneys or cerebellum of a patient with Farber disease. The demonstrated accumulation of ceramide along with the deficiency of ceramidase suggests that a genetically determined defect in ceramide degradation forms the biochemical basis of this disorder [6]. Fibroblasts from patients with this disease reveal severe deficiency in acid ceramidase (around 5% of normal values) [7]. The ceramidase level in heterozygotes is also decreased (around 50%) [7].

Inheritance. Autosomal recessive.

Treatment. All modes of therapy have failed. Chlorambucil was helpful in a mildly affected patient with moderate involvement of the joints and subcutaneous tissues [6].

References

1. Farber, S.: A lipid metabolic disorder – "disseminated lipogranulomatosis" – a syndrome with similarity to and important difference from Niemann-Pick and Hand-Schüller-Christian diseases. Amer. J. Dis. Child. *84*, 499–500 (1952)
2. Farber, S., Cohen, J., Uzman, L.L.: Lipogranulomatosis. A new lipo-glyco-protein "storage" disease. J. Mt. Sinai Hosp. *24*, 816–837 (1957)
3. Moser, H.W., Prensky, A.L., Wolfe, H.J., Rosman, N.P.: Farber's lipogranulomatosis. Report of a case and demonstration of an excess of free ceramide and ganglioside. Amer. J. Med. *47*, 869–890 (1969)
4. Schanche, A.F., Bierman, S.M., Sopher, R.L., O'Loughlin, B.J.: Disseminated lipogranulomatosis: early roentgenographic changes. Radiology *82*, 675–678 (1964)
5. Sugita, M., Dulaney, J.T., Moser, H.W.: Ceramidase deficiency in Farber's disease (lipogranulomatosis). Science *178*, 1100–1102 (1972)
6. Crocker, A.C., Cohen, J., Farber, S.: The "lipogranulomatosis" syndrome; review with report of patient showing milder involvement. In: Inborn disorders of sphingolipid metabolism. Aronson, S.M., Volk, B.W. (eds.), pp. 485–503. New York: Pergamon Press 1966
7. Dulaney, J.T., Milunsky, A., Sidbury, J.B., Hobolth, N., Moser, H.W.: Diagnosis of lipogranulomatosis (Farber's disease) by use of cultured fibroblasts. J. Pediat. *89*, 59–61 (1976)

Fucosidosis

In 1966 Durand et al. [1] described two siblings with the clinical picture of severe progressive cerebral degeneration. In 1968 Van Hoof and Hers [2] found a deficiency in α-fucosidase activity in the liver of these patients, hence the appellation of the disease. Less than ten cases have been described [3]. In 1972 Patel et al. [4] described a different phenotype with angiokeratoma of the skin as well as α-L-fucosidase deficiency. Our discussion will concentrate on this latter type since, unlike the previously reported types of fucosidosis, it presents with important dermatologic manifestations.

Clinical Presentation. The patient was a young adult with severe mental and motor retardation apparent since the age of 14 months. He had anhidrosis and consequently was unable to control his body temperature. At the age of 4 years he developed blue-brown, pinhead-sized, raised skin lesions on the abdomen, back, and extremities. These were diagnosed as angiokeratoma corporis diffusum, as in Fabry disease. However, unlike patients with Fabry disease, he was severely retarded and had normal renal function. At the age of 16 years he developed severe kyphoscoliosis with a pigeon chest. He did not have any organomegaly. Leukocytic and urinary α-fucosidase activity was less than 10% of normal controls [4].

Pathology and Pathophysiology. The histology of the skin lesions reveals multiple telangiectases [4]. Electron microscopy of the skin shows massive alterations in all endothelial cells and most fibrocytes. There is cytoplasmic distension by tertiary lysosomes in the form of small vacuoles, but without lamellated membranous bodies as in Fabry disease.

The disease is presumably due to α-L-fucosidase deficiency. Fucosidosis is considered an inborn lysosomal disorder because α-L-fucosidase is a lysosomal enzyme.

If human α-L-fucosidase has the same tetrameric structure as that found in the rat [5], there is the possibility of at least two nonallelic varieties of fucosidosis.

Inheritance. Autosomal recessive. Heterogeneity in fucosidosis has been emphasized [6]. It may represent an example of allelism with the production of quite a different clinical picture, as in the case of the Hurler and Scheie syndromes.

In the variety reported with important dermatologic manifestations [4], heterozygotes have intermediate levels of α-L-fucosidase activity and no overlap with normals.

Treatment. No treatment is known.

References

1. Durand, P., Borrone, C., Della Cella, G.: A new mucopolysaccharide lipid-storage disease? Lancet *1966II*, 1313–1314
2. Van Hoof, F., Hers, H.G.: Mucopolysaccharidosis by absence of α-fucosidase. Lancet *1968I*, 1198
3. Van Hoof, F.: Fucosidosis. In: Lysosomes and storage diseases. Hers, H.G., Van Hoof, F. (eds.), pp. 277–290. New York: Academic Press 1973

4. Patel, V., Watanabe, I., Zeman, W.: Deficiency of α-L-fucosidase. Science *176*, 426–427 (1972)
5. Carlsen, R.B., Pierce, J.G.: Purification and properties of an α-L-fucosidase from rat epididymis. J. biol. Chem. *247*, 23–32 (1972)
6. Gatti, R., Borrone, C., Trias, X., Durand, P.: Genetic heterogeneity in fucosidosis. Lancet *1973 II*, 1024

Anderson-Fabry Disease
(Angiokeratoma Corporis Diffusum, Glycosphingolipid Lipidosis)

In 1898 Anderson [1] in England and Fabry [2] in Germany independently described this disease. Although the trend is to avoid eponyms, the designation Anderson-Fabry disease (AFD) seems to be the most suitable at present and will be used until a better one is introduced and generally accepted. Over 265 cases have been reported to date, most of them since 1961 [3–5].

Clinical Presentation. The characteristic features of the disease involve predominantly the skin, eyes, kidneys, and nervous system.

The patients have a characteristic skin lesion described as *angiokeratoma corporis diffusum universale*. Although telangiectases may be one of the earliest manifestations and may lead to diagnosis in childhood, the eruption is seldom conspicuous before the late teens. With age, the cutaneous vascular lesions progressively increase. They consist of superficial, blood-filled cavities, which may project above the surface as roughly hemispherical, violaceous papules, varying between a pinhead and a few millimeters in size (Fig. 15.11). They do not blanch with pressure. The clusters of lesions are more dense between the umbilicus and the knees and involve the hips, back, thighs, buttocks, penis, and scrotum (Figs. 15.12–15.14). Involvement of the oral mucosa and conjunctiva is common, but the tongue, face, scalp, ears, and nail beds are usually spared [3, 4]. Since angiokeratoma corporis can also occur in one type of fucosidosis, confusion with Anderson-Fabry disease can be avoided by enzymatic analysis (see also p. 270).

The eye lesions consist of corneal opacities, posterior capsular cataracts, aneurysmal dilatation of thin-walled venules of the conjunctiva and retina, and edema of the eyelids [3,4].

Renal dysfunction is manifested by peripheral edema, proteinuria, and, terminally, azotemia [3,4].

Cerebral manifestations include seizures, hemiplegia, hemianesthesia, aphasia, labyrinthine disorders, and clinical evidence of cerebral hemorrhage or thrombosis.

The clinical course of the disease comprises episodes of fever and a very severe burning pain felt deep in the skin of the extremities, sometimes leading to drug addiction or suicide. The pain may be severe even in childhood and the patient may give the impression of exaggerating or simulating. Prolonged attacks of pain, often accompanied by fever, malaise, and an elevated erythrocyte sedimentation rate, have led, on several occasions, to the erroneous diagnosis of acute rheumatic fever or polyarteritis nodosa. Diminished sweating and heat intolerance are noted in many patients.

Death usually occurs in adult life from renal failure or cardiac and cerebral complications. Few patients live beyond the fourth decade.

Pathology and Pathophysiology. The disease is due to a mutation of the gene coding for the lysosomal enzyme α-galactosidase A [3]. The gene is X-linked and lyonizes [6]. α-Galactosidase A is absent in the tissues and plasma of affected individuals [3]. Consequently, the defect is mainly in the catabolism of ceramide trihexoside and partly in that of digalactosyl ceramide, both of which accumulate in most tissues. The determination of ceramide levels in plasma, urinary sediment, and cultured skin fibroblasts affords a biochemical means for the diagnosis of hemizygotes and heterozygotes before the clinical onset of the disease [3]. The enzymatic determination in plasma is easy and provides a definitive diagnosis [3].

Prenatal diagnosis by amniocentesis has been achieved [7].

Skin pathology reveals lesions in the upper dermis, where they may produce elevation and flattening of the epithelium. There may be slight to moderate keratosis. Capillaries, venules, and arterioles contain pathologic lipid stores in the endothelium, perithelium, or smooth muscle. Atrophic or scarce sweat and sebaceous glands have been reported [3].

Vascular involvement is prominent in almost all organs. Glycosphingolipid deposits are present in different parts of the eye and heart.

The characteristic corneal dystrophy and lipid deposits are almost invariably found in skin biopsies from childhood onward and afford the simplest method of diagnosis [4].

Inheritance. X-linked. The gene is highly penetrant in hemizygous males who present the typical features of the disease. Heterozygous females may

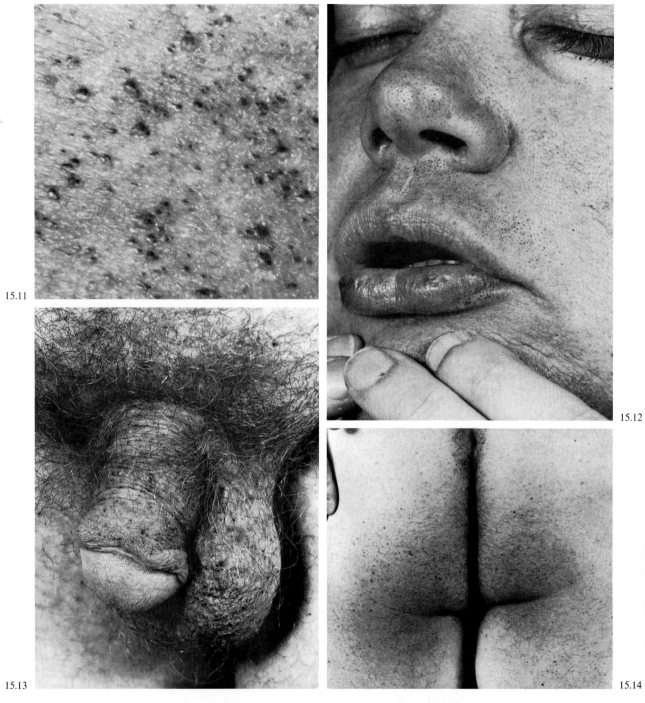

15.11

15.12

15.13

15.14

Fig. 15.11. Anderson-Fabry disease. Closer view showing the small blood-filled cavities. (Courtesy of Dr. V.A. Mc-Kusick, from Hussels, I.E.: In: The clinical delineation of birth defects. Bergsma, D. (ed.), Vol. VII, No. 8, pt. XII, pp. 318–321. Baltimore: Williams & Wilkins Co. 1971

Figs. 15.12–15.14. Anderson-Fabry disease. Angiomatous lesions typically involving the genitalia, buttocks, lips, and perioral area. (Courtesy of Dr. V.A. McKusick, from Hussels, I.E.: In: The clinical delineation of birth defects. Bergsma, D. (ed.), Vol. VII, No. 8, pt. XII, pp. 318–321. Baltimore: Williams & Wilkins Co. 1971

exhibit variable expressivity of the disease explained by the "lyonization" of the gene [6].

Treatment. Bodily exertion and changes in temperature should be avoided. Enzyme replacement by infusion of purified enzyme (ceramidetrihexosidase) has been attempted [8] with promising results. Striking improvement was obtained when diphenylhydantoin was used to relieve the crises [9]. Although renal allograft was effective in the treatment of the renal insufficiency of a heterozygous woman and seemed to correct the primary defect, further confirmation is needed [10].

References

1. Anderson, W.: A case of angeio-keratoma. Brit. J. Derm. *10*, 113 (1898)
2. Fabry, J.: Ein Beitrag zur Kenntnis der Purpura haemorrhagica nodularis (purpura papulosa haemorrhagica Hebrae). Arch. Derm. Syph. (Berl.) *43*, 187 (1898)
3. Desnick, R.J., Klionsky, B., Sweeley, C.C.: Fabry's disease (α-galactosidase A deficiency). In: The metabolic basis of inherited disease. Stanbury, J.B., Wyngaarden, J.B., Fredrickson, D.S. (eds.), 4th ed., pp. 810–840. New York: McGraw-Hill Book Co. 1978
4. Wallace, H.J.: Anderson-Fabry disease. Brit. J. Derm. *88*, 1–23 (1973)
5. Kint, J.A., Carton, D.: Fabry's disease. In: Lysosomes and storage diseases. Hers, H.G., Van Hoof, F. (eds.), pp. 357–380. New York: Academic Press 1973
6. Romeo, G., Migeon, B.R.: Genetic inactivation of the α-galactosidase locus in carriers of Fabry's disease. Science *170*, 180–181 (1970)
7. Brady, R.O., Uhlendorf, B.W., Jacobson, C.B.: Fabry's disease: antenatal detection. Science *172*, 174–175 (1971)
8. Brady, R.O.: The lipid storage diseases: new concepts and control. Ann. intern. Med. *82*, 257–261 (1975)
9. Lockman, L.A., Krivit, W., Desnick, R.J.: Relief of the painful crises of Fabry's disease by diphenylhydantoin. Neurology (Minneap.) *21*, 423 (1971)
10. Desnick, R.J., Allen, K.Y., Simmons, R.L., Najarian, J.S., Krivit, W.: Treatment of Fabry's disease: correction of the enzymatic deficiency by renal transplantation. J. Lab. clin. Med. *78*, 989–990 (1971)

Amyloidosis

Amyloidosis denotes a group of varied disorders in which there is extracellular deposition of "amyloid" in one or more organs. Amyloid is an amorphous, glassy, hyaline substance, primarily proteinaceous [1]. Under the electron microscope amyloid consists of fine, rigid, nonbranching fibrils that are made up of filaments of about 75 Å in diameter. Amyloid is identified by a variety of staining reactions, the most popular of which are a pinkish color with hematoxylin and eosin, metachromasia with crystal violet and methyl violet, birefringence with Congo red in polarized light, and fluorescence with thioflavin T or S [1].

Amyloidosis may be secondary to chronic inflammatory disease or tumors, it may be found without evidence of another underlying disease, or it may be hereditary. Hereditary amyloidosis occurs in a number of syndromes which can be classified as follows:
Amyloidosis I (Andrade or Portuguese type)
Amyloidosis II (Indiana or Rukavina type)
Amyloidosis III (cardiac form)
Amyloidosis IV (Iowa or Van Allen type)
Amyloidosis V (Finland or Meretoja type)
Amyloidosis, cerebral arterial
Amyloidosis, familial visceral
Amyloidosis, primary cutaneous (familial lichen amyloidosus)
Amyloidosis, cutaneous bullous
Amyloidosis with urticaria and deafness
Amyloidosis with cold hypersensitivity
Amyloidosis with familial Mediterranean fever
Amyloidosis with pheochromocytoma and medullary thyroid carcinoma (Sipple syndrome)
The cutaneous lesions in systemic amyloidosis are varied and include translucent, waxy, yellow papules and nodules, especially on the eyelids, perioral area, nasolabial folds, neck, and chest. Occasionally, the amyloid deposits produce indurated plaques that could involve the face, trunk, or extremities (Figs. 15.15–15.17). Purpura may be prominent and appears when the skin is rubbed. In general, however, cutaneous involvement in the hereditofamilial types of amyloidosis is less common than in primary systemic amyloidosis.

Amyloidosis I (Andrade or Portuguese Type) (Familial Amyloid Polyneuropathy)

Clinical Presentation. The disease affects young adults with progressive fatal peripheral neuropathy [2]. The lower limbs are especially involved ("foot disease"), together with alimentary and sexual dysfunction [1, 2]. There is painful paresthesia of the lower extremities with muscular atrophy, absent deep tendon reflexes, loss of heat sensation, trophic lesions, and steppage gait. Affected individuals complain of constipation with bouts of diarrhea, weight loss, sexual impotence, and sphincteric disorders [2]. There may be vitreous opacities that lead to amaurosis [1]. Electromyography shows peripheral neurogenic atrophy with impaired motor conduction [2]. Death occurs in 7–10 years [1]. The disease is endemic in Portugal and has been reported in other parts of the world as well.

Pathology and Pathophysiology. There is amyloidosis of the blood vessels in all tissues [1]. Amyloid deposits are commonly seen in the interstitial tissue of the endoneurium and less frequently in the peri- and epineurium and around blood vessels. The amyloid fibrils are separated from the nerve parenchyma by collagen except in areas of marked nerve degeneration where the amyloid invades the Schwann cell cytoplasm [2]. The nerve fiber changes probably precede the interstitial amyloid deposition [3].

Inheritance. Autosomal dominant.

Treatment. There is no definitive treatment.

Amyloidosis II
(Indiana or Rukavina Type)

Clinical Presentation. This is characterized, in order of descending frequency, by peripheral neuropathy (especially in the upper limbs), skin changes, hepatic enlargement and dysfunction, cardiovascular insufficiency, eye changes, gastrointestinal symptoms, and splenomegaly [4]. The carpal tunnel syndrome is a prominent finding in this disorder [4]. The skin changes are mainly a parchmentlike erythematous skin of the hands [4]. In the eyes there are amyloid deposits around the retinal vessels [4]. An atypical peak between β- and α-globulin has been identified with serum electrophoresis [4].

Pathology and Pathophysiology. There are amyloid deposits in most of the tissues studied.

Inheritance. Autosomal dominant.

Treatment. There is no definitive treatment.

Amyloidosis III (Cardiac Form)

The disease presents with dyspnea on exertion, appearing in the age range 37–46 years [5]. The dyspnea is rapidly progressive and in a few months the patients are incapacitated [5]. Signs of right heart failure appear and general deterioration sets in, leading to protracted cachexia and anasarca [5]. There are no neurologic manifestations nor vitreous opacities [5].
The electrocardiographic changes are either those of right bundle branch block with left axis deviation or left ventricular hypertrophy and strain with left axis deviation or low voltage [5]. In some,

there may be persistent atrial standstill [6]. Hemodynamic studies show elevation of right atrial and pulmonary wedge pressures. The right ventricle systolic pressure is increased and recordings show dip-plateau configurations [5].

Pathology and Pathophysiology. There are extensive amyloid deposits in the myocardium and endocardium, and smaller deposits in other organs [5]. In particular, small vessels, adipose tissue, and skin are generally involved [5].

Inheritance. Autosomal dominant.

Treatment. There is no definitive treatment.

Amyloidosis IV
(Iowa or Van Allen Type)

Onset of symptoms is in the third or fourth decade. Chronic progressive sensorimotor neuropathy, more severe in the lower extremities, appears at the onset [7]. Duodenal ulcer is present at some time in most of the affected individuals. Terminally, there is nephropathy leading to renal failure [7]. The average life span is 17 years [7]. Bilateral deafness is present in most of the patients. Cataracts appear early in life in a few. None has vitreous opacities.

Pathology and Pathophysiology. There are deposits of amyloid in the heart, liver, spleen, gastrointestinal tract, adrenals, kidneys, testes, aorta, peripheral nerves, sympathetic ganglia, and nerve roots [7].

Inheritance. Autosomal dominant.

Treatment. There is no definitive treatment.

Amyloidosis V
(Finland or Meretoja Type)

This variety of systemic amyloidosis is characterized by corneal lattice dystrophy and cranial neuropathy [8]. Inheritance is autosomal dominant.

Cerebral Arterial Amyloidosis

The main feature is cerebral hemorrhage at a young age [9]. Amyloidosis seems to be limited to the cerebral arteries [9]. Inheritance is autosomal dominant.

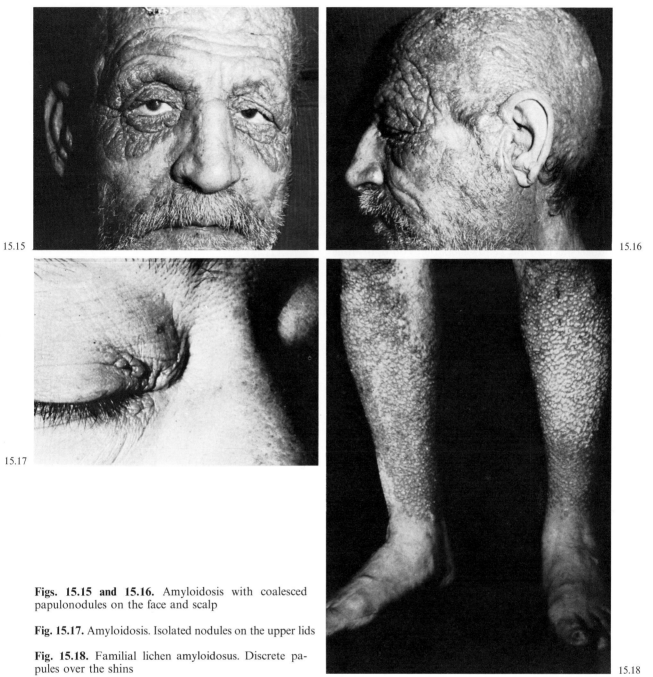

15.15

15.16

15.17

15.18

Figs. 15.15 and 15.16. Amyloidosis with coalesced papulonodules on the face and scalp

Fig. 15.17. Amyloidosis. Isolated nodules on the upper lids

Fig. 15.18. Familial lichen amyloidosus. Discrete papules over the shins

Familial Visceral Amyloidosis

The main feature is involvement of visceral organs, especially the kidneys, with manifestations of nephropathy [10]. Inheritance is autosomal dominant.

Primary Cutaneous Amyloidosis (Familial Lichen Amyloidosus)

Clinical Presentation. Amyloidosis localized in the skin is the main feature of this variety. The familial type of cutaneous amyloidosis is indistinguishable from the nonfamilial type. In familial lichen amyloidosus, the characteristic lesions appear around puberty as discrete, yellowish papules on both shins [11] (Fig. 15.18). The eruption is pruritic, gradually progressive, and may involve the thighs and forearms. When fully developed, the papules are brownish yellow and hyperkeratotic, 1–3 mm in diameter [11]. Another morphologic variant of cutaneous amyloidosis is the so-called "macular amyloidosis," in which the lesions appear predominantly over the back as hyperpigmented macular plaques with a reticulated lacy pattern and scattered, primarily perifollicular, hypopigmented spots [12]. In some, fine pinpoint papules are present [12]. The plaques may be pruritic [13].

Pathology and Pathophysiology. There are discrete deposits of amyloid in the dermal papillae with varying changes in the overlying epidermis. Incontinence of pigment is prominent in the macular type. No amyloid is found in any other tissue.

Inheritance. Autosomal dominant.

Treatment. Intralesional corticosteroids may relieve the pruritus; otherwise treatment is not helpful.

Cutaneous Bullous Amyloidosis

Bullous lesions, especially around the joints, characterize this variety of cutaneous amyloidosis reported in four sibs [14]. Inheritance is probably autosomal recessive.

Amyloidosis with Urticaria and Deafness

This is characterized by urticaria and chills and fever which appear in adolescence, followed in a few years by progressive perceptive deafness and eventually nephropathy [15]. Other findings are loss of libido, skin-thickening, glaucoma, pes cavus, and elevated erythrocyte sedimentation rate [15]. Limb pains are present in other affected kindreds [16]. No specific cause for the urticaria can be elicited. The deafness is not due to infiltration by amyloid, but to absence of the organ of Corti and atrophy of the cochlear nerve [15]. Amyloid deposits are found in most organs, especially the kidneys. Inheritance is autosomal dominant.

Amyloidosis with Cold Hypersensitivity (see p. 250)

Amyloidosis with Familial Mediterranean Fever (see p. 317)

Amyloidosis with Pheochromocytoma and Medullary Thyroid Carcinoma (Sipple Syndrome)

This autosomal dominantly inherited syndrome is characterized by pheochromocytoma and medullary thyroid carcinoma in which the tumor produces amyloid deposited locally or even in distant organs [17].

See also Mucosal Neuromas with Endocrine Tumors, p. 206.

References

1. Cohen, A.S.: Amyloidosis. New Engl. J. Med. *277*, 522–530; 574–583; 628–638 (1967)
2. Coimbra, A., Andrade, C.: Familial amyloid polyneuropathy: an electron microscope study of the peripheral nerve in five cases. I. Interstitial changes. Brain *94*, 199–206 (1971)
3. Coimbra, A., Andrade, C.: Familial amyloid polyneuropathy: an electron microscope study of the peripheral nerve in five cases. II. Nerve fibre changes. Brain *94*, 207–212 (1971)
4. Rukavina, J.G., Block, W.D., Jackson, C.E., Falls, H.F., Carey, J.H., Curtis, A.C.: Primary systemic amyloidosis: a review and an experimental, genetic, and clinical study of 29 cases with particular emphasis on the familial form. Med. (Baltimore) *35*, 239–334 (1956)
5. Frederiksen, T., Gøtzsche, H., Harboe, N., Kiær, W., Mellemgaard, K.: Familial primary amyloidosis with severe amyloid heart disease. Amer. J. Med. *33*, 328–348 (1962)
6. Allensworth, D.C., Rice, G.J., Lowe, G.W.: Persistent atrial standstill in a family with myocardial disease. Amer. J. Med. *47*, 775–784 (1969)
7. Van Allen, M.W., Frohlich, J.R., Davis, J.R.: Inherited predisposition to generalized amyloidosis. Clinical and pathological study of a family with neuropathy, nephropathy, and peptic ulcer. Neurology (Minneap.) *19*, 10–25 (1969)
8. Meretoja, J.: Genetic aspects of familial amyloidosis with corneal lattice dystrophy and cranial neuropathy. Clin. Genet. *4*, 173–185 (1973)
9. Gudmundsson, G., Hallgrímsson, J., Jónasson, T.Á., Bjarnason, Ó.: Hereditary cerebral haemorrhage with amyloidosis. Brain *95*, 387–404 (1972)

10. Weiss, S.W., Page, D.L.: Amyloid nephropathy of Ostertag: report of a kindred. In: The clinical delineation of birth defects. Bergsma, D. (ed.), Vol. X, No. 4, pt. XVI, pp. 67–68. Baltimore: Williams & Wilkins Co. 1974

11. Rajagopalan, K., Tay, C.H.: Familial lichen amyloidosis. Report of 19 cases in 4 generations of a Chinese family in Malaysia. Brit. J. Derm. 87, 123–129 (1972)

12. Kurban, A.K., Malak, J.A., Afifi, A.K., Mire, J.: Primary localized macular cutaneous amyloidosis: histochemistry and electron microscopy. Brit. J. Derm. 85, 52–60 (1971)

13. Sagher, F., Shanon, J.: Amyloidosis cutis. Familial occurrence in three generations. Arch. Derm. 87, 171–175 (1963)

14. De Souza, A.R.: Amiloidose cutanea bolbosa familial. Observacao de 4 casos. Rev. Hosp. Clin. Fac. Med. Sao Paulo 18, 413–417 (1963)

15. Muckle, T.J., Wells, M.: Urticaria, deafness and amyloidosis: a new heredo-familial syndrome. Quart. J. Med. 31, 235–248 (1962)

16. Black, J.T.: Amyloidosis, deafness, urticaria, and limb pains: a hereditary syndrome. Ann. intern. Med. 70, 989–994 (1969)

17. Schimke, R.N., Hartmann, W.H.: Familial amyloid-producing medullary thyroid carcinoma and pheochromocytoma. A distinct genetic entity. Ann. intern. Med. 63, 1027–1039 (1965)

Lipoid Proteinosis
(Hyalinosis Cutis et Mucosae, Urbach-Weithe Syndrome)

Siebenmann, in 1908, described the first patient with this condition [1]. Up to 1969 some 170 cases had been reported, 20% of which were from South Africa [2].

Clinical Presentation. The onset of symptoms is usually at birth or in early infancy. The first manifestation is hoarseness followed by cutaneous and mucosal lesions [3]. The initial skin lesions are regarded as impetigo that heals with atrophic scars [2] (Fig. 15.19). These are commonly seen on the face and proximal parts of the extremities. As the patient grows older, the skin assumes a pasty, waxy appearance, especially in the exposed parts of the body (Fig. 15.20). Often, pearly, beadlike papules appear on the margins of the eyelids. Larger plaques and papules, having a yellowish tinge, appear over the neck and upper trunk. Yellowish brown verrucous plaques may appear on the elbows, hands, and knees (Fig. 15.21). Similar coarse nodularities appear on the scrotum or vulva, perineum, and perianal area. In nonwhites, varied pigmentary changes are seen. The nails are not involved. The teeth may be lost early [4] and there is patchy hair loss [2].

Similar nodularities and diffuse irregular thickening are present in the lips, frenulum of the tongue, buccal mucosa, epiglottis, tonsils, uvula, vocal cords [2, 3], vaginal vestibule [3], and rectum [5].

Intracranial calcification has frequently been described. When present, the calcification is symmetric and bilateral in the hippocampal gyri of the temporal lobes and could result in epileptic seizures. This roentgenographic sign is considered pathognomonic of lipoid proteinosis [2]. Mental abnormalities have been noted in some patients [6]. Other complications include upper respiratory tract obstruction and suffocation in infancy [6], salivary and nasolacrimal gland obstruction [2], and carpal tunnel syndrome [2]. The lifespan is normal.

Pathology and Pathophysiology. The disease is due to the deposition of a glycolipoprotein. This is easily demonstrable as a hyaline material, which is periodic acid-Schiff (PAS)-positive, in the dermis, submucosa, and around the vessels and appendages, especially the sweat glands [3, 7]. In the upper dermis, the PAS-positive material appears as vertically oriented bands. Similar material is deposited in and around blood vessels in the kidneys, muscle, lungs, and jejunum [5].

The initial change is hyaline material deposition in the capillary wall beneath the basement membrane [7]. The deposition gradually increases, pushing aside the connective tissue and eventually incorporating it. This hyaline material is predominantly a neutral mucopolysaccharide and a tryptophan-containing moiety, as well as neutral fat and cholesterol [7]. Electron microscopic studies show islands of hyaline substance separated by fibroblasts exhibiting active fibrilogenesis [8]. It is postulated that the hyaline material is produced locally by abnormal fibroblasts [8] or is at least partially derived from blood plasma [7]. One study using fibroblast cultures from the skin of a patient with this disorder failed to demonstrate an increase in lipid content of the fibroblasts [9]. It was concluded that the hyaline material is principally a glycoprotein and the lipids adhere secondarily.

Inheritance. Autosomal recessive [2].

Treatment. Cosmetic improvement can be achieved by dermabrasion [10]. Dermabrasion of the mucous membranes of the mouth and pharynx may be helpful [11].

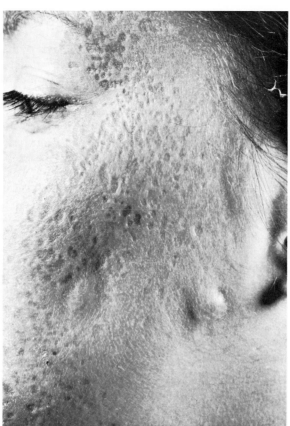

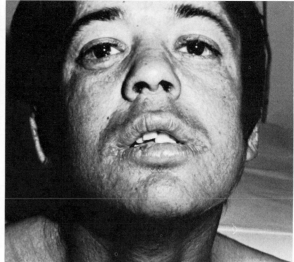

15.20

15.19

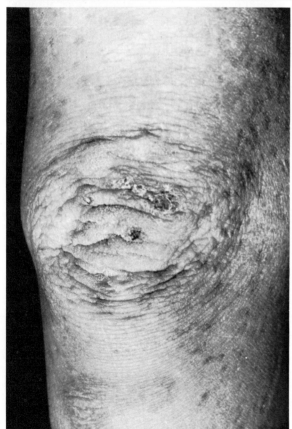

15.21

Figs. 15.19–15.21. Lipoid proteinosis

Fig. 15.19. Atrophic scars on the face. (Courtesy of Dr. G.W. Hambrick, Jr.)

Fig. 15.20. Waxy appearance of the facial skin

Fig. 15.21. Yellowish verrucous plaques of the elbow. (From Ward, W.Q., et al. In: The clinical delineation of birth defects. Bergsma, D. (ed.), Vol. VII, No. 8, pt. XII, pp. 288–291. Baltimore: Williams & Wilkins Co. 1971

References

1. Siebenmann, F.: Über Mitbeteiligung der Schleimhaut bei allgemeiner Hyperkeratose der Haut. Arch. Laryng. Rhin. (Berl.) *20*, 101 (1908)
2. Gordon, H., Gordon, W., Botha, V., Edelstein, I.: Lipoid proteinosis. In: The clinical delineation of birth defects. Bergsma, D. (ed.), Vol. VII, No. 8, pt. XII, pp. 164–177. Baltimore: Williams & Wilkins Co. 1971
3. Zaynoun, S.T., Kurban, A.K.: Lipoid proteinosis. Leb. med. J. *27*, 91–97 (1974)
4. Hofer, P.-Å., Berbenholtz, A.: Oral manifestations in Urbach-Weithe disease (lipoglycoproteinosis; lipoid proteinosis; hyalinosis cutis et mucosae). Odontol. Rev. *26*, 39 (1975)
5. Caplan, R.M.: Visceral involvement in lipoid proteinosis. Arch. Derm. *95*, 149–155 (1967)
6. Grosfeld, J.C.M., Spaas, J., van de Staak, W.J.B.M., Stadhouders, A.M.: Hyalinosis cutis et mucosae (lipoidproteinosis Urbach-Weithe). Dermatologica (Basel) *130*, 239–266 (1965)
7. van der Walt, J.J., Heyl, T.: Lipoid proteinosis and erythropoietic protoporphyria. A histological and histochemical study. Arch. Derm. *104*, 501–507 (1971)
8. Hashimoto, K., Klingmüller, G., Rodermund, O.-E.: Hyalinosis cutis et mucosae. An electron microscopic study. Acta derm.-venereol. (Stockh.) *52*, 179–195 (1972)
9. Shore, R.N., Howard, B.V., Howard, W.J., Shelley, W.B.: Lipoid proteinosis. Demonstration of normal lipid metabolism in cultured cells. Arch. Derm. *110*, 591–594 (1974)
10. Buchan, N.G., Kemble, J.V.H.: Successful surgical treatment of lipoid proteinosis. Brit. J. Derm. *90*, 561–566 (1974)
11. Vukas, A.: Hyalinosis cutis et mucosae. Regenerative properties of tissues involved in chronic pathology. Dermatologica (Basel) *144*, 168–175 (1972)

Wolman Disease
(Primary Familial Xanthomatosis)

This entity was first described by Abramov et al. in 1956 [1]. The identification of this disease as a separate entity was made by Wolman et al. in 1961 [2].

Clinical Presentation. The clinical onset is marked by vomiting and diarrhea in the early weeks of life, with poor weight gain, a protuberant abdomen, irritability, and pallor. The patients also show hepatosplenomegaly, signs of wasting, anemia, vacuolated lymphocytes in the blood smear, foam cells in the marrow, and, by X-ray, striking calcification within enlarged adrenal glands.

The skin is always pale, with a slightly yellow discoloration. A vesiculo-papulo-pustular rash may be noted over the face, neck, shoulders, and chest. Lungs and fundi show no abnormalities and there are no special signs of serious neurologic involvement [3].

A new form of Wolman disease with hypolipoproteinemia and acanthocytosis was described in a Japanese infant [4].

Pathology and Pathophysiology. There is xanthomatous transformation in the adrenals, spleen, liver, lymph nodes, bone marrow, small intestine, lungs, and thymus. Slight involvement is noted in the skin, vascular endothelia of various organs, retina, and central nervous system. The xanthomatous change is caused by deposition of triglycerides and cholesterol, mixed in some organs with phospholipids. The affected organs have foam cells in which the lipid is stored [2]. In the adrenals and some other tissues, crystallization of the lipids may occur, with a foreign body reaction as well as secondary widespread calcification [2].

Abnormal accumulations of triglycerides and cholesterol esters are found in vacuolated and enlarged liver cells. Enlarged Kupffer cells and collections of macrophages in the portal areas contain cholesterollike crystals. E600-resistant acid esterase activity is deficient in liver cells. Electron microscopy shows the lipid droplets to be enclosed by a limiting membrane associated with acid phosphatase activity. All of these findings suggest that Wolman disease is a lysosomal disease [5].

The clinical diagnosis of Wolman disease can be confirmed by histochemical staining of blood films. Acid esterase activity is normally found in lymphocytes, but in this disease only a very low level of activity can be detected. An intermediate level of activity is demonstrated in heterozygotes. The method may be applicable in prenatal diagnosis [6].

Inheritance. Autosomal recessive [3].

Treatment. No specific treatment is available.

References

1. Abramov, A., Schorr, S., Wolman, M.: Generalized xanthomatosis with calcified adrenals. Amer. J. Dis. Child. *91*, 282–286 (1956)
2. Wolman, M., Sterk, V.V., Gatt, S., Frenkel, M.: Primary familial xanthomatosis with involvement and calcification of the adrenals. Report of two more cases in siblings of a previously described infant. Pediatrics *28*, 742–757 (1961)
3. Crocker, A.C., Vawter, G.F., Neuhauser, E.B.D., Rosowsky, A.: Wolman's disease: three new patients with a recently described lipidosis. Pediatrics *35*, 627–640 (1965)
4. Eto, Y., Kitagawa, T.: Wolman's disease with hypolipoproteinemia and acanthocytosis: clinical and biochemical observations. J. Pediat. *77*, 862–867 (1970)
5. Lake, B.D., Patrick, A.D.: Wolman's disease: deficiency of E600-resistant acid esterase activity with storage of lipids in lysosomes. J. Pediat. *76*, 262–266 (1970)
6. Lake, B.D.: Histochemical detection of the enzyme deficiency in blood films in Wolman's disease. J. clin. Path. *24*, 617–620 (1971)

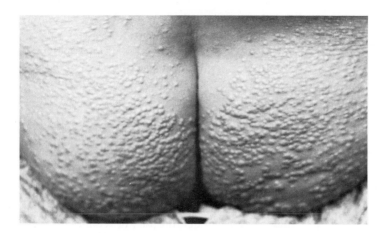

Fig. 15.22. Type I hyperlipoproteinemia. Eruptive lesions over the buttocks. (Courtesy of Drs. A. Khachadurian and S. Uthman)

Familial Hyperlipoproteinemias

Familial hyperlipoproteinemia was initially discovered through the presence of xanthomatoses. The study of a large number of such cases revealed significant heterogeneity. The present classification of hyperlipidemia and hyperlipoproteinemia was recommended by the World Health Organization in 1970 [1], with the addition of a sixth type described since then [2].

Type I: Familial lipoprotein lipase-deficient hyperchylomicronemia

Type II: Familial hyperbetalipoproteinemia

Type III: Familial "broad beta" disease

Type IV: Familial hyperprebetalipoproteinemia

Type V: Familial hyperbetalipoproteinemia and hyperchylomicronemia

Type VI: Familial combined hyperlipidemia

Even though there is at present a tendency to abandon this classification, a new one has not been generally accepted.

Type I: Familial Lipoprotein Lipase-Deficient Hyperchylomicronemia

In 1932 Bürger and Grütz [3] reported the first patient suffering from this very rare disease. To date, less than 50 cases have been reported.

Clinical Presentation. Both sexes are affected. Seventy percent of the cases are detected in childhood. Xanthomas occur in 45–50% of the cases and hepatosplenomegaly, in 75%. One of the striking features of the disease is the occurrence of attacks of diffuse abdominal pain (75% of cases) lasting 1–3 days, usually related to a recent dietary intake of fat and, occasionally, preceded by the appearance of eruptive xanthomas (Fig. 15.22). Spasm, rigidity,

rebound tenderness, leukocytosis, and fever may be present. The pain is relieved by narcotics. Pancreatitis may occur in 40% of patients. Lipemia retinalis may also be present [4].

The high-density lipoprotein (HDL) and low-density lipoprotein (LDL) concentrations are markedly decreased. The very low-density lipoprotein (VLDL) is normal or slightly increased. Plasma free fatty acid (FFA) concentrations are very low, even after fat ingestion. Chylomicrons are markedly increased. Postheparin lipolytic activity (PHLA) is decreased [4].

Pathology and Pathophysiology. In severe cases foam cells may be found in the bone marrow, spleen, and liver. The changes in the blood vessels are not remarkable and there is no evidence of myocardial infarction.

Lipoprotein lipase activity is deficient. The metabolic defect is in the hydrolysis of the initial ester bond in triglycerides [4].

Inheritance. Autosomal recessive [4]. Heterozygotes may show slight hyperlipemia, reduced PHLA, and intermediate levels of lipoprotein lipase.

Treatment. The aim is to reduce chylomicronemia to a minimum. It can be achieved by low fat diets [4].

Type II: Familial Hyperbetalipoproteinemia

Familial type II is the commonest single disorder characterized by an abnormality in plasma lipoprotein concentrations [5].

Clinical Presentation. The homozygous and heterozygous forms of hyperbetalipoproteinemia differ in their clinical presentations [6].

In the homozygote, multiple, large tendon xanthomas and tuberous xanthomas appear over the elbows (Fig. 15.23), dorsal aspects of the hands, buttocks (Fig. 15.24), and soles, usually by the age of 4 years. Arcus corneae may appear before the age of 10 years. Angina may develop in adolescence and significant coronary artery disease may be obvious during young adulthood. The xanthomas progress even on a low cholesterol diet. The patients usually succumb to myocardial infarction before the age of 30 years [4].

In the heterozygote, tendon and tuberous xanthomas appear in young adulthood (Fig. 15.25). Angina pectoris may appear around the age of 30 years, frequently with myocardial infarction. Superficial skin lesions are rare, but xanthelasmas (Fig. 15.26) are common [4].

Both heterozygotes and homozygotes have recurrent attacks of "polyarthritis" involving the ankles, knees, or hands. The attacks last a few days and are most common in young adults [4].

Type II hyperlipoproteinemia is characterized by an increase in LDL (β). The mean LDL concentration in homozygotes is roughly double that of heterozygotes. An LDL cholesterol level of 150 mg/100 ml provides a reasonable screen for the detection of all possible abnormal levels in individuals below 30 years of age [4]. Two subtypes of type II can be distinguished. In both there is an increase in LDL (β). In type IIa, VLD (pre-β) is normal, whereas it is elevated in type IIb. The mean trigylcerides and VLDL of type IIb heterozygotes are almost twice those in normal subjects. The total concentration of phospholipids is also usually increased in type II [4].

Pathology and Pathophysiology. The xanthomas represent accumulation of lipids in the dermis in large macrophages or free in the interstitial spaces. The lipids in tendinous and tuberous lesions include phospholipids, cholesterol, cholesterol esters, and triglycerides.

The pathologic picture of the coronary and cerebral vessels in heterozygotes is similar to that of the general population. However, the homozygotes have a remarkable degree of atheroma formation leading to extensive pathology of the coronaries and aorta. Cultured skin fibroblasts from persons homozygous for the gene of this disorder reveal a 40–60-fold higher level of activity of 3-hydroxy-3-methyl-glutaryl coenzyme A reductase (HMG CoA reductase), the rate-controlling enzyme in cholesterol synthesis. The fibroblasts of heterozygotes have an intermediate level of the enzyme. The enhanced enzyme results from complete absence of normal feedback suppression by LDL [7]. It has been demonstrated that a cell surface receptor for LDL is defective or missing; thus, the degradation of LDL and the inhibition of HMG CoA reductase are impaired [8].

Inheritance. Autosomal dominant [6, 9]. However, families with suspected polygenic inheritance have also been described [2].

Treatment. Treatment involving a special diet has been effective in lowering the plasma cholesterol and LDL concentrations in heterozygotes. Instructions for this special diet are available from various sources [10]. Combined with diet, the use of cholestyramine and nicotinic acid gives satisfactory results with relatively low toxicity [11].

Type III: Familial "Broad Beta" Disease

Familial type III hyperlipoproteinemia is characterized by the presence of detectable amounts of plasma VLDL with an abnormal composition.

Clinical Presentation. The disease manifests itself during young adulthood with the appearance of xanthomas on the elbows, buttocks, and creases of the palms. During the third and fourth decades intermittent claudication begins, frequently associated with myocardial infarctions. Forty percent of the patients have a diabetic type of glucose tolerance test. The mean age of detection of the disease is 34 years for men and 49 years for women. The incidence of premature vascular disease is high and is indicated by decreased pulses in the femoral, popliteal, or smaller leg arteries. Plasma cholesterol and phospholipids are elevated. The glycerides may also be elevated.

The disease should be suspected in the presence of the following manifestations: (a) hypercholesterolemia and hypertriglyceridemia responsive to changes in body weight; (b) a ratio of plasma cholesterol to triglyceride varying from 0.3–1.5; (c) plantar xanthomas; and (d) peripheral vascular disease with hyperglyceridemia and diabetes. The diagnosis can be confirmed by lipoprotein analysis. There is a lack of β-migrating lipoproteins on polyacrylamide gel electrophoresis and presence of a "broad beta band" on paper, agarose, or cellulose acetate electrophoresis. However, the absolute diagnostic test is provided by preparative ultracentrifugation of plasma.

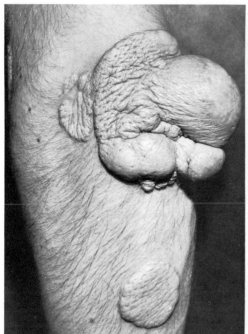

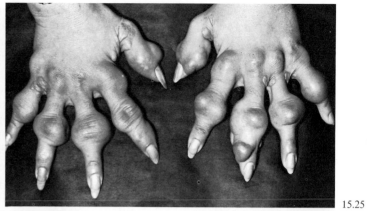

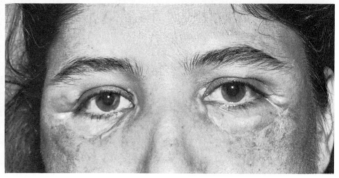

15.23

15.25

15.26

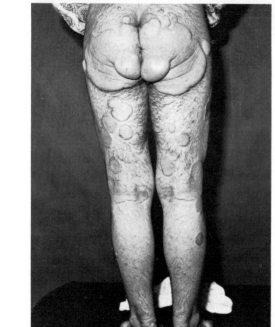

15.24

Figs. 15.23–15.26. Type II hyperlipoproteinemia

Fig. 15.23. Tuberous xanthomas over the elbow. (Courtesy of Drs. A. Khachadurian and S. Uthman)

Fig. 15.24. Tuberous xanthomas over the buttocks. (Courtesy of Drs. A. Khachadurian and S. Uthman)

Fig. 15.25. Tuberous xanthomas with deformities at the joints. (Courtesy of Drs. A. Khachadurian and S. Uthman)

Fig. 15.26. Xanthelasmas. (Courtesy of Drs. A. Khachadurian and S. Uthman)

Pathology and Pathophysiology. The lipid composition of the xanthomas is not different from that in type II. The basic defect remains unknown.

Inheritance. Not clear, probably autosomal dominant [12].

Treatment. Treatment is very rewarding and involves diet control and drugs, aiming at the maintenance of plasma cholesterol and triglyceride concentrations within normal limits. The drugs used are clofibrate (2.0 g per day), nicotinic acid (3.0 g per day), or D-thyroxine (4–8 mg per day) [4].

Type IV: Familial Hyperprebetalipoproteinemia

Type IV hyperlipoproteinemia is characterized by increased VLDL or prebetalipoproteins without chylomicronemia.

Clinical Presentation. Common features of the disease are mild labile hypertension, gout, abnormal glucose tolerance test, atheroeruptive xanthomas, and, in some patients, myocardial infarction. The association of rheumatic manifestations has been emphasized [13]. There is a slight elevation of the plasma cholesterol, with striking elevations of the VLDL and triglycerides [4].

Pathology and Pathophysiology. The condition is considered endogenous hyperglyceridemia because the increased amounts of glycerides are synthesized in the liver and intestine from fatty acids that have not come directly from the diet. It is called "carbohydrate-induced hyperlipemia" because there is an exaggerated response to the usual carbohydrate content of the diet.
The exact basic metabolic defect is still unknown.

Inheritance. Probably autosomal dominant [12].

Treatment. After reducing to ideal body weight, a maintenance diet with low carbohydrate and alcohol content is instituted. Drugs such as clofibrate or nicotinic acid may be helpful.

Type V: Familial Hyperbetalipoproteinemia and Hyperchylomicronemia

The type V pattern is a combination of exogenous hyperglyceridemia (postabsorptive chylomicronemia) and endogenous hyperglyceridemia (increased VLDL).

Clinical Presentation. The most striking feature of this disease is abdominal pain that occurs in bouts, associated with lethargy, nausea, and vomiting. These episodes occur several times a year, last a few hours or days, and are precipitated by fatty foods. The patients have prebetalipoproteinemia with high plasma cholesterol and triglycerides. Obesity and eruptive xanthomas are frequent physical findings. Xanthomas do not occur on the palms. Other common manifestations are pancreatitis, hepatomegaly, and hyperuricemia. There is no evidence of accelerated vascular disease [4].

Pathology and Pathophysiology. The exact basic metabolic defect is still unknown.

Inheritance. Although type V patients are genotypically different from type IV patients, their mode of inheritance is still not clearly understood [4].

Treatment. Ideal weight should be maintained with special diets high in protein and limited in fat or carbohydrate. Drugs such as nicotinic acid or norethindrone acetate may be helpful.

Type VI: Familial Combined Hyperlipidemia

Clinical Presentation. This type is characterized clinically by an increased frequency of myocardial infarctions and xanthomas. Affected individuals manifest any one of four lipoprotein phenotypes: type IIa, type IIb, type IV, or type V patterns. In the individual family with combined hyperlipidemia, the pedigree is often confusing because of this variability in phenotypes [2].

Pathology and Pathophysiology. The primary biochemical abnormality in this disorder may involve triglyceride metabolism with secondary effects on cholesterol metabolism. Additional evidence supporting this hypothesis is the fact that triglyceride levels in relatives appear to segregate into two distributions, whereas their cholesterol levels show a less clear-cut bimodality [2].

Inheritance. Probably autosomal dominant, with variable expression [2].

Treatment. Ideal weight should be maintained with special diets high in protein and limited in fat and carbohydrate. The drug therapy should be decided according to the lipoprotein types, until more information on the treatment of this relatively newly discovered type is available.

References

1. Beaumont, J.L., Carlson, L.A., Cooper, G.R., Fejfar, Z., Fredrickson, D.S., Strasser, T.: Classification of hyperlipidaemias and hyperlipoproteinaemias. Bull. W.H.O. *43*, 891–915 (1970)
2. Goldstein, J.L., Schrott, H.G., Hazzard, W.R., Bierman, E.L., Motulsky, A.G.: Hyperlipidemia in coronary heart disease. II. Genetic analysis of lipid levels in 176 families and delineation of a new inherited disorder, combined hyperlipidemia. J. clin. Invest. *52*, 1544–1568 (1973)
3. Bürger, M., Grütz, O.: Über hepatosplenomegale Lipoidose mit xanthomatösen Veränderungen in Haut und Schleimhaut. Arch. Derm. Syph. (Berl.) *166*, 542 (1932)
4. Fredrickson, D.S., Goldstein, J.L., Brown, M.S.: The familial hyperlipoproteinemias. In: The metabolic basis of inherited disease. Stanbury, J.B., Wyngaarden, J.B., Fredrickson, D.S. (eds.), 4th ed., pp. 604–655. New York: McGraw-Hill Book Co. 1978
5. Lever, W.F., Smith, P.A.J., Hurley, N.A.: Idiopathic hyperlipemic and primary hypercholesteremic xanthomatosis. I. Clinical data and analysis of the plasma lipids. J. invest. Derm. *22*, 33–51 (1954)
6. Khachadurian, A.K.: The inheritance of essential familial hypercholesterolemia. Amer. J. Med. *37*, 402–407 (1964)
7. Goldstein, J.L., Brown, M.S.: Familial hypercholesterolemia: identification of a defect in the regulation of 3-hydroxy-3-methylglutaryl coenzyme A reductase activity associated with overproduction of cholesterol. Proc. nat. Acad. Sci. (Wash.) *70*, 2804–2808 (1973)
8. Brown, M.S., Goldstein, J.L.: Receptor-mediated control of cholesterol metabolism. Science *191*, 150–154 (1976)
9. Schrott, H.G., Goldstein, J.L., Hazzard, W.R., McGoodwin, M.M., Motulsky, A.G.: Familial hypercholesterolemia in a large kindred. Evidence for a monogenic mechanism. Ann. intern. Med. *76*, 711–720 (1972)
10. Fredrickson, D.S., Levy, R.I., Jones, E., Bonell, M., Ernst, N.: The dietary management of hyperlipoproteinemia: a handbook for physicians. Washington, D.C.: U.S. Dept. of Health, Education, and Welfare, Public Health Service 1970
11. Levy, R.I., Fredrickson, D.S.: The current status of hypolipidemic drugs. Postgrad. Med. *47*, 130–136 (1970)
12. McKusick, V.A.: Mendelian inheritance in man, 5th ed., p. 214. Baltimore: Johns Hopkins University Press 1978
13. Goldman, J.A., Glueck, C.J., Abrams, N.R., Steiner, P., Herman, J.: Musculoskeletal disorders associated with type-IV hyperlipoproteinaemia. Lancet *1972 II*, 449–452

β-Sitosterolemia

In 1973 and 1974 Bhattacharyya and Connor [1, 2] described two patients with this disease.

Clinical Presentation. Tendon xanthomas are noted in childhood. They gradually involve the extensor tendons of both hands and the patellar, plantar, and Achilles tendons. Tuberous xanthomas involve the elbows.

There is elevation of β-sitosterol and two other plant sterols (campesterol and stigmasterol) in the blood.

Pathology and Pathophysiology. The tendon xanthomas and adipose tissue contain plant sterols. Despite the high concentration of β-sitosterol in the xanthomas, the increase in xanthoma cholesterol is quantitatively more important, because cholesterol is the predominant sterol.

The proposed pathogenetic mechanism is the intestinal absorption of abnormally large amounts of β-sitosterol.

Inheritance. Autosomal recessive.

Treatment. No special treatment is presently available.

References

1. Bhattacharyya, A.K., Connor, W.E.: β-Sitosterol and xanthomatosis: a newly described lipid storage disease in two sisters. J. clin. Invest. *52* (Abstr.), 9a (1973)
2. Bhattacharyya, A.K., Connor, W.E.: β-Sitosterolemia and xanthomatosis. A newly described lipid storage disease in two sisters. J. clin. Invest. *53*, 1033–1043 (1974)

Cerebral Cholesterinosis (Cerebrotendinous Xanthomatosis)

In 1937 Van Bogaert et al. [1] described this disease with cholesterinosis involving the tendons, lungs, and central nervous system.

Clinical Presentation. The patients demonstrate cerebellopyramidal signs, myoclonus of the soft palate, mental debility, cataracts, xanthelasmas, and tendon xanthomas. The lungs may also be involved.

The disease is characterized by three stages. The initial stage begins in childhood with dementia and is followed by an adolescent phase of progressive ataxia, spasticity, and cataracts. Finally, the third stage is characterized by prominent tendon tumefactions (especially in the Achilles tendons), a severe spastic ataxic syndrome, and a bulbar phase leading to death [2].

The serum cholesterol levels are within normal limits. Serum cholestanol concentrations are elevated. Premature atherosclerosis may occur [3].

The diagnosis can be made by demonstrating cholestanol in abnormal amounts in the serum and tendons of persons suspected of being affected.

Pathology and Pathophysiology. Light microscopy of Achilles tendon sections reveals a dense accumulation of narrow crystalline clefts within granulomatous lesions that contain many large mononuclear cells with foamy cytoplasm and multinucleated giant cells. Sections of lung show granulomatous lesions containing large, foamy mononuclear cells, multinucleated giant cells, and needle-shaped clefts.

The brain stem and cerebellum are the two most affected parts within the nervous system. Microscopic examination reveals myelin destruction, a variable degree of atheromas, and xanthoma cells. Massive deposits of cholesterol crystals are observed in the white matter, suggesting a derangement in cholesterol metabolism [4].

Fifteen tissues obtained post mortem contained 10–400 times more cholestanol and 30% more cholesterol [3].

Bile acid production in cerebrotendinous xanthomatosis is subnormal, yet the activity of cholesterol 7α-hydroxylase, the rate-determining enzyme of bile acid synthesis, is elevated. It is suggested that decreased bile acid synthesis in cerebrotendinous xanthomatosis results from impaired oxidation of the cholesterol side chain [5].

Inheritance. Autosomal recessive [2].

Treatment. There is no specific treatment.

References

1. Van Bogaert, L., Scherer, H.J., Froehlich, A., Epstein, E.: Une deuxième observation de cholestérinose tendineuse symétrique avec symptômes cérébraux. Ann. Méd. *42*, 69–101 (1937)
2. Schimschock, J.R., Alvord, E.C.,Jr., Swanson, P.D.: Cerebrotendinous xanthomatosis. Clinical and pathological studies. Arch. Neurol. *18*, 688–698 (1968)
3. Salen, G.: Cholestanol deposition in cerebrotendinous xanthomatosis. A possible mechanism. Ann. intern. Med. *75*, 843–851 (1971)
4. Menkes, J.H., Schimschock, J.R., Swanson, P.D.: Cerebrotendinous xanthomatosis. The storage of cholestanol within the nervous system. Arch. Neurol. *19*, 47–53 (1968)
5. Setoguchi, T., Salen, G., Tint, G.S., Mosbach, E.H.: A biochemical abnormality in cerebrotendinous xanthomatosis. Impairment of bile acid biosynthesis associated with incomplete degradation of the cholesterol side chain. J. clin. Invest. *53*, 1393–1401 (1974)

Primary Hemochromatosis

In 1865 Trousseau first described a patient with this disease [1].

Clinical Presentation. The features include cirrhosis of the liver, diabetes mellitus, and hypermelanotic pigmentation of the skin with a distribution similar to that of sunlight pigmentation. The signs and symptoms of the disease arise from organ damage occurring as a tissue reaction to hemosiderin deposits [2].

Plasma iron concentration is elevated. Plasma transferrin is decreased and completely saturated with iron.

Most patients with primary hemochromatosis become symptomatic between the ages of 40 and 60 years, since it takes years to accumulate the amount of iron that would produce the manifestations [2]. Ascites is a late complication of cirrhosis. Dyspnea and edema result from cardiac failure which develops rapidly and leads to death.

Hepatic impairment may result in loss of body hair; fine hair with female distribution; soft, atrophic, frequently dry, and finely desquamating skin; palmar erythema; and spider angiomas [2].

Pathology and Pathophysiology. There is excessive absorption of iron (2–3 mg per day). An accumulation of 20–60 g of iron is necessary to show clinical signs. The iron loss in females associated with menstruation, pregnancy, and lactation is partially protective, so that the clinical disease occurs 10 times more frequently in men than in women [2].

The pigmentation is due to increased melanin deposition in the skin and not to the deposition of iron. The latter imparts a metallic gray color [2].

Hemosiderin is deposited in the liver, pancreas, heart, pituitary, and adrenals.

Inheritance. It is generally thought that hemochromatosis is an autosomal recessive disease [3]. However, reports suggesting that the inheritance of adult-onset hemochromatosis may be dominant have been published [4, 5].

Treatment. Systematic venesection with loss of 500–1000 ml of whole blood per week usually arrests the development of the disease [2].

References

1. Trousseau, A.: Clinique médicale de l'Hôtel-Dieu de Paris, 2nd ed., p. 672. Paris: Baillière 1865
2. Pollycove, M.: Hemochromatosis. In: The metabolic basis of inherited disease. Stanbury, J.B., Wyngaarden, J.B., Fredrickson, D.S. (eds.), 4th ed., pp. 1127–1164. New York: McGraw-Hill Book Co. 1978
3. Saddi, R., Feingold, J.: Idiopathic hemochromatosis: an autosomal recessive disease. Clin. Genet. *5*, 234–241 (1974)
4. Williams, R., Scheuer, P.J., Sherlock, S.: The inheritance of idiopathic haemochromatosis: a clinical and liver biopsy study of 16 families. Quart. J. Med. *31*, 249–265 (1962)
5. Bothwell, T.H., Cohen, I., Abrahams, O.L., Perold, S.M.: A familial study in idiopathic hemochromatosis. Amer. J. Med. *27*, 730–738 (1959)

Other Metabolic Disorders

Acatalasemia

Takahara discovered this disorder in 1946 and first reported it in 1952 [1].

Clinical Presentation. The disease begins as a small painful ulcer in the crevices around the neck of a tooth or in tonsillar lacunae. The disease may appear in mild, moderate, and severe forms. In the mild type, ulcers appear in the dental alveoli. In the moderate form, alveolar gangrene and atrophy develop and the teeth fall out. In the severe cases, there may be widespread destruction with far-advanced gangrene of the maxilla and the soft oral tissues [2].

Pathology and Pathophysiology. The primary defect is a catalase deficiency in the blood and tissues. Bacteria proliferate in dental crevices and tonsillar lacunae and produce hydrogen peroxide which is not decomposed, because of the lack of catalase. Instead, the hydrogen peroxide oxidizes hemoglobin, thus depriving the infected area of oxygen and causing ulceration, necrosis, and decay [2].

Inheritance. Autosomal recessive [2].

Treatment. The treatment consists of surgical wound care of the affected areas in the mouth and administration of antibiotics [2].

References

1. Takahara, S.: Progressive oral gangrene probably due to lack of catalase in the blood (acatalasaemia). Report of nine cases. Lancet *1952 II*, 1101–1104
2. Aebi, H.E., Wyss, S.R.: Acatalasemia. In: The metabolic basis of inherited disease. Stanbury, J.B., Wyngaarden, J.B., Fredrickson, D.S. (eds.), 4th ed., pp. 1792–1807. New York: McGraw-Hill Book Co. 1978

Lesch-Nyhan Syndrome

In 1964 Lesch and Nyhan [1] described two brothers with mental retardation, choreoathetosis, a compulsive tendency to self-mutilation, hyperuricemia, and uricosuria. About 150 patients affected with this syndrome have been described [2]. Most patients are Caucasian, but the disease has also been found in Oriental and black families.

Clinical Presentation. Only males are affected. They generally have a normal motor development until the age of 6–8 months, at which time they start to develop progressive generalized spastic paresis, athetosis, chorea, tremor, and dysarthria. However, the most striking feature of the syndrome is a compulsion for self-mutilation. This is manifested by biting and mutilating the fingers and lips, resulting in extensive scarring (Figs. 15.27–15.29). Since pain perception is normal, there is extreme suffering and consequently these patients welcome any physical restraint that prevents self-mutilation. Most of them are mentally retarded [3]. The level of blood uric acid is usually (but not always) elevated (7–10 mg/100 ml). As a result of hyperuricemia and uricosuria, they develop tophi (Fig. 15.30), gouty arthritis, kidney stones, and gouty nephropathy. The increased ratio of urinary uric acid to creatinine is useful for screening [4]. Death usually occurs before puberty as a result of uremia or general debilitation.

Pathology and Pathophysiology. Complete deficiency of the X-linked enzyme hypoxanthine-guanine phosphoribosyltransferase (HGPRT) is associated with this syndrome [5]. This enzyme is essential in purine metabolism. The deficiency is found in the brain, liver, leukocytes, erythrocytes [6], cultured skin fibroblasts [4], and amniotic cells [2]. The excessive production of uric acid, characteristic of the Lesch-Nyhan syndrome, results from an accelerated rate of de novo purine biosynthesis. The pathogenesis of the central nervous system manifestations is not related to the presence of the hyperuricemia. Instead, it is probably due to the inadequate synthesis of inosinic acid (IMP) and guanylic acid (GMP) in the central nervous system, consequent to the severe deficiency in HGPRT.

Inheritance. X-linked recessive. The gene that codes for the enzyme HGPRT is also X-linked. Since this gene lyonizes (see p. 9), two different populations of somatic cells with respect to this enzyme are found in females heterozygous for the syndrome [7]. It has been found recently that heterozygotes may be detected by hair-root analysis. This method of heterozygote detection may help in proper genetic counseling [8].

Treatment. Symptomatic treatment consists of restraining the hands to prevent self-mutilation. Since prenatal diagnosis is achieved by amniocentesis and cell culture [9], one can resort to therapeutic abortion in the case of affected fetuses.

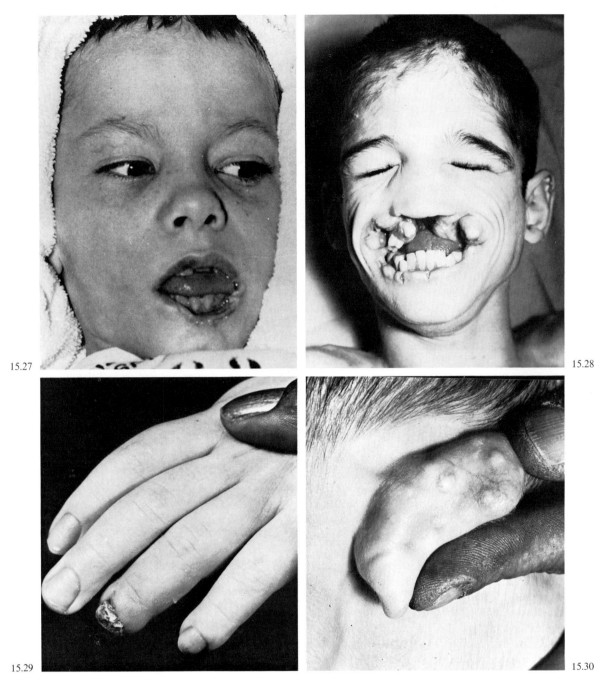

15.27

15.28

15.29

15.30

Figs. 15.27–15.30. Lesch-Nyhan syndrome

Figs. 15.27 and 15.28. Self-mutilation of the lips. (From Nyhan, W.L.: Fed. Proc. *27*, 1027–1033, 1968)

Fig. 15.29. Self-mutilation of the fingers. (From Nyhan, W.L.: Fed. Proc. *27*, 1027–1033, 1968)

Fig. 15.30. Tophi on pinna. (From Nyhan, W.L.: Fed. Proc. *27*, 1027–1033, 1968)

References

1. Lesch, M., Nyhan, W.L.: A familial disorder of uric acid metabolism and central nervous system function. Amer. J. Med. *36*, 561–570 (1964)
2. Boyle, J.A., Raivio, K.O., Astrin, K.H., Schulman, J.D., Graf, M.L., Seegmiller, J.E., Jacobsen, C.B.: Lesch-Nyhan syndrome: preventive control by prenatal diagnosis. Science *169*, 688–689 (1970)
3. Nyhan, W.L.: Clinical features of the Lesch-Nyhan syndrome. Introduction – clinical and genetic features. Fed. Proc. *27*, 1027–1033 (1968)
4. Kaufman, J.M., Greene, M.L., Seegmiller, J.E.: Urine uric acid to creatinine ratio – a screening test for inherited disorders of purine metabolism. J. Pediat. *73*, 583–592 (1968)
5. Seegmiller, J.E., Rosenbloom, F.M., Kelley, W.N.: Enzyme defect associated with a sex-linked human neurological disorder and excessive purine synthesis. Science *155*, 1682–1684 (1967)
6. Kelley, W.N.: Hypoxanthine-guanine phosphoribosyltransferase deficiency in the Lesch-Nyhan syndrome and gout. Fed. Proc. *27*, 1047–1052 (1968)
7. Migeon, B.R., Der Kaloustian, V.M., Nyhan, W.L., Young, W.J., Childs, B.: X-linked hypoxanthine-guanine phosphoribosyl transferase deficiency: heterozygote has two clonal populations. Science *160*, 425–427 (1968)
8. Silvers, D.N., Cox, R.P., Balis, M.E., Dancis, J.: Detection of the heterozygote in Lesch-Nyhan disease by hair-root analysis. New Engl. J. Med. *286*, 390–395 (1972)
9. DeMars, R., Sarto, G., Felix, J.S., Benke, P.: Lesch-Nyhan mutation: prenatal detection with amniotic fluid cells. Science *164*, 1303–1305 (1969)

Gout

Historically, gout was distinguished as an entity by Hippocrates and the treatment of the acute attack with colchicine was introduced in the fifth century A.D.

Clinical Presentation. Gout presents with acute, recurrent, characteristic attacks in different joints, eventually leading to the stage of chronic tophaceous gout. During the acute attack, the involved site shows the typical signs of an acute inflammatory process. As the attack subsides, the area becomes violaceous and the skin, scaly. In the chronic stage, the subcutaneous lesions are salmon pink and occur most commonly on the pinna of the ear, elbows, fingers, and toes. They may drain a chalky white material, identified as crystals of monosodium urate [1, 2].

Hyperuricemia is found in almost all gouty patients. Nephropathy and nephrolithiasis are frequent complications. Predisposing and provocative factors in gout include trauma, food, alcohol, medicinal preparations, and surgical operations. Slightly over 95% of all patients with gouty arthritis are males.

Pathology and Pathophysiology. Primary gout is biochemically and genetically heterogeneous. In

1973 two brothers were described [3] with marked purine overproduction and clinical gout. They showed phosphoribosylpyrophosphate (PRPP) synthetase activity in erythrocyte lysates 2.5–3 times greater than in normal persons. A daughter of one brother also showed increased enzymatic activity. Another variety of gout is characterized by the partial deficiency of hypoxanthine-guanine phosphoribosyltransferase (HGPRT). Accelerated purine biosynthesis also occurs due to a deficiency in glucose-6-phosphatase and the increased activity of glutathione reductase and a mutant glutamine phosphoribosylpyrophosphate amidotransferase [2].

Inheritance. Although there has been some debate as to whether the inheritance is polygenic or monogenic, classic familial gout is probably a monogenic dominantly inherited disorder [4].

Treatment. Colchicine and phenylbutazone are the most effective medications for the treatment of acute gouty arthritis. Between attacks, attempts are made to lower serum urate by using drugs that decrease either uric acid synthesis (allopurinol) or renal tubular reabsorption of urates (probenecid).

References

1. Seegmiller, J.E.: Skin lesions in gout. In: Dermatology in general medicine. Fitzpatrick, T.B., Arndt, K.A., Clark, W.H., Jr., Eisen, A.Z., Van Scott, E.J., Vaughan, J.H. (eds.), pp. 1167–1173. New York: McGraw-Hill Book Co. 1971
2. Wyngaarden, J.B., Kelley, W.N.: Gout. In: The metabolic basis of inherited disease. Stanbury, J.B., Wyngaarden, J.B., Fredrickson, D.S. (eds.), 4th ed., pp. 916–1010. New York: McGraw-Hill Book Co. 1978
3. Becker, M.A., Meyer, L.J., Seegmiller, J.E.: Gout with purine overproduction due to increased phosphoribosylpyrophosphate synthetase activity. Amer. J. Med. *55*, 232–242 (1973)
4. McKusick, V.A.: Mendelian inheritance in man, 5th ed., pp. 136–137. Baltimore: Johns Hopkins University Press 1978

Hereditary Angioedema

Osler [1], in 1888, documented the hereditary type of angioedema and distinguished it from the non-hereditary form of allergic or unknown etiology.

Clinical Presentation. The disease is characterized by recurrent acute attacks of localized edema of the skin, subcutaneous tissues, or mucous membranes, especially those of the pharynx, larynx, and gastrointestinal tract. The edema is remarkable in that it is nonpitting and for the total absence of symptoms of histamine release (pruritus, whealing, or erythema).

The sites commonly affected are the skin of the face and limbs. The attacks are usually precipitated by trauma. Involvement of the gastrointestinal mucosa leads to nausea, vomiting, and colic, but without fever or leukocytosis. Involvement of the mucosa of the larynx is associated with a high mortality rate. The onset of the disease is usually in infancy or childhood. The attacks may last one or several days; the interval between attacks varies from days to years.

Pathology and Pathophysiology. It is now accepted that the basic defect in individuals suffering from hereditary angioedema (HAE) is the absence in their sera of a functional inhibitor of the complement and kinin systems [2, 3]. Under the proper conditions, the first component of the complement is converted from an inactive form (C_1) to an active enzyme (C_1'). C_1' acts on synthetic amino acid ester substrates or natural substrates, the fourth and second components of complement (C_4 and C_2, respectively) [3]. These functions of C_1' are susceptible to inhibition by C_1' inhibitor (C_1' INH). In addition, C_1' INH, also described as $\alpha 2$-neuraminoglycoprotein, inhibits a number of serine histidine esterases found in plasma, like plasmin, kallikrein, activated Hageman factor, and activated plasma thromboplastin antecedent [4]. Affected individuals have low levels (but not complete absence) of C_1' INH. The attacks may be precipitated by exhaustion of the reduced inhibitor leading to the activation of C_4 and C_2 with the generation of kininlike substances [4]. Both the complement and the kinin systems participate in the pathogenesis of the disease [3], although the actual mediator remains unknown. Histologic examination of affected tissues reveals edema without any inflammatory reaction.

Laboratory diagnosis rests on the demonstration of low or absent functional C_1' INH by double immunodiffusion [5] or esterolytic techniques [4].

Studies of C_1' INH protein have demonstrated unique electrophoretic mobilities for some families, which are constant for all affected members of the kindred [3]. Thus, there seems to be a "genetic variant" form of HAE probably representing structural mutations.

The demonstration of reduced levels of C_2 and C_4, the natural substrates of C_1', is a useful indirect screening method.

Inheritance. Autosomal dominant with incomplete penetrance.

Treatment. Adrenalin, antihistamines, and corticosteroids are not helpful. During the attack, the administration of the inhibitor dramatically ends the attack. The readily available source of inhibitor is fresh-frozen plasma (400–1000 ml) [6]. Prophylactic treatment with ε-aminocaproic acid (30 g daily) or its analogue tranexamic acid (1–3 g daily) seems to reduce effectively the frequency of attacks [7].

References

1. Osler, W.: Hereditary angioneurotic edema. Amer. J. med. Sci. *95*, 362–367 (1888)
2. Donaldson, V.H., Evans, R.R.: A biochemical abnormality in hereditary angioneurotic edema: absence of serum inhibitor of C_1'-esterase. Amer. J. Med. *35*, 37–44 (1963)
3. Gigli, I.: Hereditary angioedema. J. invest. Derm. *60*, 516–521 (1973)
4. Lachmann, P.J.: Complement deficiencies. Brit. J. Derm. *92*, 593–594 (1975)
5. Ruddy, S., Gigli, I., Scheffer, A.L., Austen, K.F.: The laboratory diagnosis of hereditary angioedema. In: Excerpta medica international congress series, No. 162, pp. 351–359. Amsterdam: Excerpta Medica 1967
6. Pickering, R.J., Kelly, J.R., Good, R.A., Gewurz, H.: Replacement therapy in hereditary angioedema. Successful treatment of two patients with fresh frozen plasma. Lancet *1969 I*, 326–330
7. Champion, R.H., Lachmann, P.J.: Hereditary angio-oedema treated with ε-aminocaproic acid. Brit. J. Derm. *81*, 763–765 (1969)

Familial Carotenemia

Two pedigrees (four in three generations; and two sibs) have been described with high serum carotene levels and low vitamin A levels [1, 2]. The two sibs had keratodermia with a yellow discoloration [1]. A member of the other pedigree had generalized yellow-orange discoloration of her skin, varying from day to day and most marked over the palms, soles, and pressure areas but sparing the creases [2]. A defect in the conversion of carotene to vitamin A has been proposed [2]. Inheritance is probably autosomal dominant.

References

1. Frenk, E.: Etat kératodermique avec taux sérique abaissé de la vitamine A et hypercarotinémie. Dermatologica (Basel) *132*, 96–98 (1966)
2. Sharvill, D.E.: Familial hypercarotinaemia and hypovitaminosis A. Proc. roy. Soc. Med. *63*, 605–606 (1970)

Chapter 16   Chromosomal Anomalies

Contents

Chromosomal syndromes are not necessarily inherited, but they are obviously of genetic origin (see also p. 11). Many of them present with dermatologic, especially dermatoglyphic, abnormalities.

These syndromes may be due to anomalies of chromosomal number or structure; they may involve autosomes or sex chromosomes. Two of them (Down and Turner syndromes) are discussed here in greater detail. The others are presented in Table 16.1. Diseases in which there are nonspecific chromosomal anomalies confined to one tissue or system (Bloom syndrome, ataxia telangiectasia, Fanconi anemia, xeroderma pigmentosum, and Werner syndrome) are discussed separately. In scleroderma an increase in chromosomal breaks and other anomalies has been reported recently.

Down Syndrome (Mongolism)

In 1866 Down [1] described this syndrome which, in 1959, turned out to be the first recognized chromosomal anomaly [2]. It is the most common autosomal abnormality with a frequency of about 1 per 700 newborns [3].

Clinical Presentation. The most characteristic features of Down syndrome (Figs. 16.1–16.3) are brachycephaly; a characteristic facies with apparent hypertelorism, depressed bridge of the nose, epicanthic folds, and narrow and upward slanting palpebral fissures; hypoplasia of the iris stroma with Brushfield spots (white, elevated aggregates of stromal fibers in the pupillary margin of the iris) in 70% of cases; small ears with anomalies of the folds; protrusion of the tongue due to a relatively small mouth; scrotal tongue; protuberant abdomen, often with an umbilical hernia; small penis, scrotum,

and testes; broad and shortened hands, feet, and digits; hyperextensible joints; below normal height; and mental retardation ranging from mild to severe.

The following are the most common dermatologic features: a transverse palmar crease (simian crease), a single flexion crease of the fifth finger in association with clinodactyly, a distal axial triradius on the palms, ulnar loops on all fingers, and a tibial arch in the hallucal area of the soles [4, 5] (see also p. 302).

The skin is normal at birth. It is soft and velvety in early childhood but gradually becomes dry, inelastic, and, in early adulthood, shows mild ichthyosis. Patchy lichenification is present in 80% of adult patients. The patches occur mostly on the upper arm, the wrists, the front of the thighs, the back of the ankle, and the back of the neck. Cutis marmorata of the trunk and extremities is frequent. Acrocyanosis may also be present. The skin ages prematurely, showing lentigines and atrophy. Other associated dermatologic findings may be lichen simplex chronicus, keratosis follicularis, congenital erythrodermia, and elastosis perforans serpiginosa. Fissuring and thickening of the lips are frequent and increase in incidence and severity with age [6, 7].

The hair of the scalp is fine, silky, and straight. It becomes dry and sparse with age. The axillary hair is scanty and the pubic hair has a female distribution.

About 25–30% die during the first year of life. The most frequent causes of death are respiratory infections and congenital heart disease [8].

Pathology and Pathophysiology. No consistent brain abnormality has been observed. Acute leukemia is more common than in the normal population. The common internal anomalies are congenital heart disease, duodenal atresia, and Hirschsprung disease.

Ninety-five percent of patients with Down syndrome have 47 chromosomes with trisomy 21. Most of the remainder have 46 chromosomes with translocation of the long arm of an extra number 21 either to a D group or to another G group chromo-

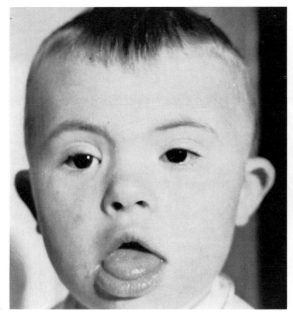

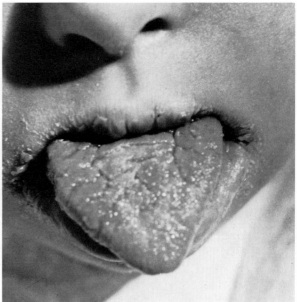

16.1   16.2

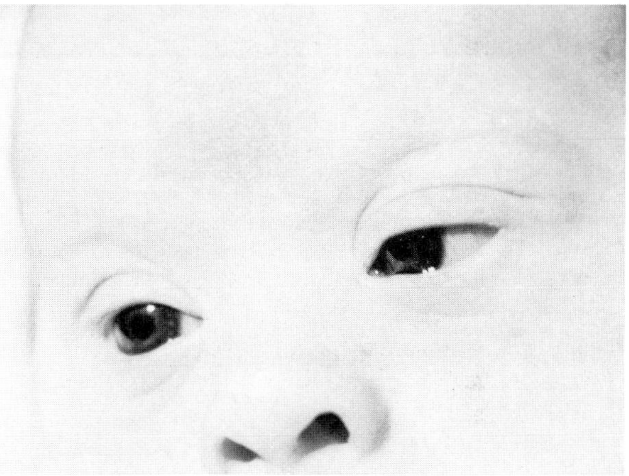

Fig. 16.1. Facies of patient with Down syndrome. Note protruding tongue. (Courtesy of Dr. F.C. Fraser)

Fig. 16.2. Scrotal tongue of patient with Down syndrome. (Courtesy of Dr. F.C. Fraser)

Fig. 16.3. Down syndrome. Note hypertelorism, narrow palpebral fissures, and epicanthic folds. (Courtesy of Dr. F.C. Fraser)

16.3

some [9]. However, it is also possible to have Down syndrome with 46 chromosomes and either 21/22 or 21/21 translocation. Mosaics with a normal cell line are usually milder.

In general, the incidence of trisomy 21 increases with maternal age. One study [10] states that a phenotypically normal female with 45 chromosomes and a D/21 translocation has a 9% risk of having a child with Down syndrome.

Inheritance. Males with Down syndrome are sterile. In the case of the few affected females who have had children, about half of the offspring have been affected.

Treatment. The treatment is directed generally to the cardiac and respiratory complications. Specialized institutions may help to teach simple trades to mildly retarded patients.

Turner Syndrome

In 1938 Turner [11] described this syndrome in seven young girls. Subsequently it was shown that patients with this syndrome are chromatin-negative and have a 45,X karyotype. The frequency of the 45,X Turner syndrome in newborns is 1 per 3300 [12].

Clinical Presentation. The characteristic physical findings (Figs. 16.4 and 16.5) in the Turner syndrome are as follows: small stature; broad chest with widely spread nipples which may be hypoplastic, inverted, or both; low posterior hairline with appearance of short neck; webbed posterior neck; and bone dysplasia with coarse trabecular pattern, most evident at the metaphyseal ends of the long bones.

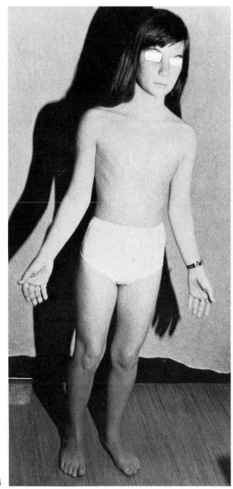

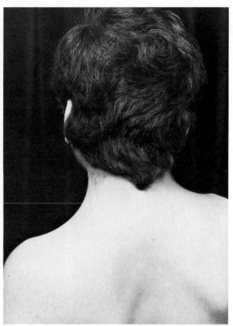

16.5

16.4

Fig. 16.4. Turner syndrome. Note webbed neck, shield chest, and increased carrying angles. (Courtesy of Dr. F.C. Fraser)

Fig. 16.5. Turner syndrome. Note low posterior hairline and webbed neck.

Lymphangiectatic edema of the hands and feet is present at birth and is due to dilatation of lymphatic capillaries. Resorption of this edema results in cutis laxa or hyperelastica. The nails are hypoplastic in the newborn and small and hyperconvex in the older patient.

The common dermatoglyphic findings are a distal axial triradius, associated with increased incidence of complex hypothenar patterns, high digital and *a–b* ridge counts [13], thenar exit to A-line, simian or variant palmar creases, large hallucal patterns, and absent *t* triradius (see p. 300).

Scattered small brown moles and pigmented nevi are common in older children and adults, but few are seen in young infants.

There may be very slight intellectual impairment.

Because of failure of gonad development, these patients are amenorrheic. Endocrinologic investigations reveal an increased output of pituitary gonadotropins accompanied by low estrogen levels.

Pathology and Pathophysiology. In place of normal gonads, ovarian streaks are present below the fallopian tubes. These are composed largely of collagenous tissue organized in whorls. Congenital heart disease and renal anomalies are found in one-third of the patients. The most common cardiovascular lesion is coarctation of the aorta [14].

The karyotype of these patients is mostly 45,X. Yet, many patients are mosaics (45,X/46,XX) or have 46 chromosomes with an isochromosome X [15]. Patients with 46,XXp– or 46,XXq– patterns may have features of the Turner syndrome [16].

Inheritance. Most of these patients are infertile. Mosaics with the 46,XX cell line may be fertile and have normal children.

Treatment. Estrogen therapy after the age of expected puberty is indicated to promote female secondary sex characteristics.

Table 16.1. Other syndromes with chromosomal anomalies[a]

Syndrome	Karyotype	Clinical presentation	Dermatologic findings	Dermatoglyphic anomalies	Ref.
Down	47,XY,+21	See p. 290	See p. 290	See p. 302	
Trisomy 13	47,XY,+13 or 46,XY, +(13/D)	Microcephaly, keel-shaped forehead; Cleft lip, hyper-telorism, shallow supraorbital ridges, small chin; Microphthalmus, iris colobomas, cataracts; sometimes unilateral anophthalmia; Small, low-set, malformed ears; Inguinal and umbilical hernias; Polydactyly (post-axial) and flexion deformity of fingers; Fibular polydactyly; Clubfoot deformity	Capillary hemangioma, especially over the forehead; Localized scalp defects in the parieto-occipital area; Loose skin over posterior neck; Hyperconvex narrow fingernails; Cleft between 1st and 2nd toes; Hypoplastic toenails; Cleft lip and palate	Distal palmar axial tri-radii; Increased number of arches; Simian crease; Hypoplastic dermal ridges; Single 5th finger crease; Hypoplastic dermal ridges; Radial loop on other than 2nd digit; Thenar exit to A-line	[17–20]
Trisomy 18	47,XY,+18	Prominent occiput; Hypoplastic supra-orbital ridges, ptosis, small chin; Corneal opacities, cataracts, microphthalmus; Small, low-set, malformed ears; Inguinal and abdominal hernias; Undescended testes in males; hypoplastic labia in females; Rocker-bottom feet; Index finger over-lying middle finger	Hypoplasia of nails, especially of 5th finger and toes; Small nipples; Mild hirsutism of forehead and back; Cutis marmorata; Epicanthic folds; Excess or paucity of eyebrows and eyelashes; Webbing of neck in 1/3 cases; Capillary hemangiomas	Absence of distal crease in 5th finger, occasionally of 3rd and 4th; Low-arch dermal ridge pattern on 6 or more fingertips; Transverse palmar crease (simian) in 50%; Increased incidence of radial loops on thumbtips; Paucity of whorls on fingertips; Very low TRC; Distal axial triradius; Hypoplasia of dermal ridge; Increased incidence of hallucal arches on open field	[21, 22]
Group G monosomy	45,XX,−G	Syndactyly between 2nd and 3rd toes; Large, low-set, mis-shapen ears; Hypospadias, crypt-orchidism; Mental retardation	Epicanthic folds; Dystrophic nails		[23, 24]
Chromosome 4 short arm deletion syndrome	46,XY,4p−	Microcephaly and severe mental retardation; Prominent glabella, hypertelorism, blepharoptosis; Hypospadias in all males, cryptor-chidism in some; Occasional short metacarpals, meta-tarsals	Epicanthic folds; Carp-shaped mouth; Ptosis of eyelids; Preauricular sinuses; Preauricular tags; Cleft lip and/or palate in 50%; Capillary hemangiomas; Oblique ridges on nails	Hypoplastic dermal ridges; Increased incidence of digital arches with low dermal ridge count; Simian crease	[25, 26]

[a] See p. 290 for general principles on chromosomes and p. 299 for dermatoglyphics.

Table 16.1. (continued)

Syndrome	Karyotype	Clinical presentation	Dermatologic findings	Dermatoglyphic anomalies	Ref.
Cri-du-Chat syndrome	46,XY,5p−	Catlike cry Microcephaly and severe mental retardation Hypertelorism and downward eye slant Beaklike profile in infants Scoliosis in adults Occasional short metacarpals and metatarsals Clinodactyly, partial syndactyly of hands and feet	Cleft lip and palate Epicanthic folds Preauricular skin tags Premature graying of hair Modification of cutaneous elastic fibers	Simian crease in 81% Distal axial triradius in 40% Increased incidence of arches and whorls on digits Low TRC Fusion of b and c triradii with or without syndactyly	[27, 28]
Chromosome 18 long arm deletion syndrome	46,XY,18q−	Microcephaly and severe mental retardation Underdeveloped midportion of face Prominent antihelix and antitragus; poorly developed helix Cleft palate Females: small labia and clitoris; males: small penis and scrotum, undescended testes Low levels of IgA in serum and saliva	Carp-shaped mouth Eczema (25%) Skin dimples over acromion and knuckles Widely separated nipples Lipomas at lateral border of feet	High incidence of whorl digital pattern Distal axial triradius, deviated to radial margin of palm Increased incidence of simian crease Increased incidence of missing or misplaced triradii at base of digits Increased frequency of exit to A-line	[29–33]
Chromosome 21 long arm deletion syndrome (antimongolism)	46,XY,21q−		Blepharochalasis Dysplastic nails Preauricular tags	Distal axial triradii	
Cat eye syndrome	47,XY,+?G	Retarded psychomotor development Hypertelorism, downward palpebral fissure, strabismus Unilateral or bilateral iris and choroid colobomas Imperforate anus	Preauricular fistula and skin tags		[34]
Chromosome 13 long arm deletion and ring D	46,XX,13q− and 46,XY,r13	Microcephaly and severe mental retardation Hypertelorism, narrow palpebral fissures, prominent nasal bridge Ophthalmic pathology: microphthalmus, iris colobomas, cataract, retinoblastoma	Epicanthic folds		[35, 36]

Table 16.1. (continued)

Syndrome	Karyotype	Clinical presentation	Dermatologic findings	Dermatoglyphic anomalies	Ref.
Chromosome 18 short arm deletion	46,XY,18p−	Microcephaly, brachycephaly, mental retardation (IQ 35–75) Hypertelorism, flat nasal bridge Strabismus Large, floppy or small, low-set ears Short, broad fingers; syndactyly; cubitus valgus; congenital dislocation of the hips; talipes equinovarus; pes planus Absence of serum and salivary IgA	Epicanthic folds Blepharoptosis Webbing of neck with low posterior hairline	Distal axial triradius Simian crease Absent c triradius	[37–40]
Turner	45,X0	See p. 291	See p. 291	See p. 291	
XXX syndrome	47,XXX	Some may be mentally retarded or have psychiatric disorders		Reduced total finger ridge count	
XXXX syndrome	48,XXXX	Absence or hypoplasia of thumb IQ ranging from 30–80 Normal or irregular menses Dislocated hips, short middle and distal phalanges		Reduced total finger ridge count	[41, 42]
XXXXX syndrome	49,XXXXX	Mental retardation and microcephaly Clinodactyly of 5th finger	Epicanthic folds Scanty pubic hair	Unilateral or bilateral transverse palmar creases 10 digital arches	
Klinefelter syndrome	47,XXY	Bilateral or unilateral breast enlargement Small testes Eunuchoid proportions Psychiatric disorders	Hair growth on trunk, limbs, and beard tends to be below average Feminine distribution of pubic hair in 40%	Increased number of arches with low total digital count	[43, 44]
XXXY syndrome	48,XXXY	Flat nasal bridge Gynecomastia Small testes	Epicanthic folds Facial and body hair less than normal	Increased arches with decreased total digital ridge count	[45, 46]
XXXXY syndrome	49,XXXXY	Mental retardation Upward eye slant, strabismus Abnormalities of ears Abnormalities of teeth and mandible Kyphosis, scoliosis Limitation of movement of elbow and clinodactyly	No consistent dermatologic defects; some patients hypotrichotic Epicanthic folds Mild degree of webbing	High frequency of low-arch pattern on fingertips Mean total ridge count of only 50 vs. normal average of 144	[47, 48]

Table 16.1. (continued)

Syndrome	Karyotype	Clinical presentation	Dermatologic findings	Dermatoglyphic anomalies	Ref.
XYY syndrome	47,XYY	Tall stature Mental retardation Aggressive behavior Gonadal defects Bony abnormalities	Nodulocystic acne (Figs. 16.6–16.8)	Normal	[49]
XXYY syndrome	48,XXYY	Unilateral or bilateral gynecomastia Small testes Eunuchoid proportions Mild to severe mental retardation	Sparse body hair Multiple cutaneous angiomas Acrocyanosis Webbing of neck	Predominance of arches and very small loops on fingers Low total ridge count Increased incidence of certain hypothenar patterns (ulnar triradius, loop carpal, loop radial, arch radial)	[50, 51]

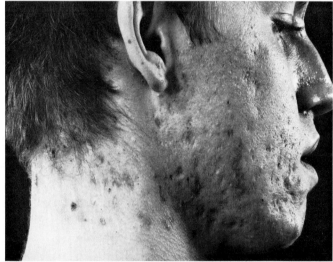

16.6

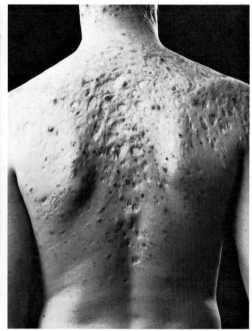

16.8

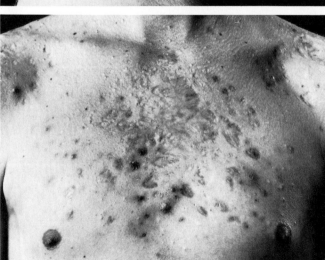

16.7

Figs. 16.6–16.8. Nodulocystic acne on face, chest, and back of a patient with XYY syndrome. (From Voorhees, J.J., et al.: In: The clinical delineation of birth defects. Bergsma, D. (ed.), Vol. VII, No. 8, pt. XII, pp. 186–192. Baltimore: Williams & Wilkins Co. 1971)

References

1. Down, J.L.H.: Observations on an ethnic classification of idiots. Clin. Lect. Rep. Lond. Hosp. *3*, 259–262 (1866)
2. Lejeune, J., Gautier, M., Turpin, R.: Les chromosomes somatiques des enfants mongoliens. C. R. Acad. Sci. [D] (Paris) *248*, 1721–1722 (1959)
3. Fabia, J.: Illegitimacy and Down's syndrome. Nature (Lond.) *221*, 1157–1158 (1969)
4. Beckman, L., Gustavson, K.H., Norring, A.: Dermal configurations in the diagnosis of the Down syndrome: an attempt at a simplified scoring method. Acta Genet. Statist. med. *15*, 3–12 (1965)
5. Smith, G.F., Bat-Miriam, M., Ridler, M.A.: Dermal patterns on the fingers and toes in mongolism. J. ment. Defic. Res. *10*, 105–115 (1966)
6. Butterworth, T., Leoni, E.P., Beerman, H., Wood, M.G., Strean, L.P.: Cheilitis of mongolism. J. invest. Derm. *35*, 347–352 (1960)
7. Zeligman, I., Scalia, S.P.: Dermatologic manifestations of mongolism. Arch. Derm. Syph. *69*, 342–344 (1954)
8. Lilienfeld, A.J.: Epidemiology of mongolism. pp. 104–105. Baltimore: Johns Hopkins University Press 1969
9. Hamerton, J.L.: Human cytogenetics, Vol. II, pp. 196–275. New York: Academic Press 1971
10. Hamerton, J.L.: Fetal sex. Lancet *1970I*, 516–517
11. Turner, H.H., A syndrome of infantilism, congenital webbed neck, and cubitus valgus. Endocrinology *23*, 566–574 (1938)
12. Court Brown, W.M.: Sex chromosome aneuploidy in man and its frequency with special reference to mental subnormality and criminal behavior. In: International review of experimental pathology. Richter, G.W., Epstein, M.A. (eds.), Vol. 7, pp. 31–97. New York: Academic Press 1969
13. Forbes, A.P.: Fingerprints and palm prints (dermatoglyphics) and palmar-flexion creases in gonadal dysgenesis, pseudohypoparathyroidism and Klinefelter's syndrome. New Engl. J. Med. *270*, 1268–1277 (1964)
14. Goldberg, M.B., Scully, A.L., Solomon, I.L., Steinbach, H.L.: Gonadal dysgenesis in phenotypic female subjects. A review of eighty-seven cases, with cytogenetic studies in fifty-three. Amer. J. Med. *45*, 529–543 (1968)
15. Hecht, F., MacFarlane, J.P.: Mosaicism in Turner's syndrome reflects the lethality of X0. Lancet *1969II*, 1197–1198
16. Hecht, F., Jones, D.L., Delay, M., Klevit, H.: Xq-Turner's syndrome: reconsideration of hypothesis that Xp− causes somatic features in Turner's syndrome. J. med. Genet. *7*, 1–4 (1970)
17. Patau, K., Smith, D.W., Therman, E., Inhorn, S.L., Wagner, H.P.: Multiple congenital anomaly caused by an extra autosome. Lancet *1960I*, 790–793
18. Taylor, A.I.: Autosomal trisomy syndromes: a detailed study of 27 cases of Edward's syndrome and 27 cases of Patau's syndrome. J. med. Genet. *5*, 227–252 (1968)
19. Magenis, R.E., Hecht, F., Milham, S., Jr.: Trisomy 13 (D_1) syndrome: studies on parental age, sex ratio, and survival. J. Pediat. *73*, 222–228 (1968)
20. Miller, D.A., Allderdice, P.W., Miller, O.J., Breg, W.R.: Quinacrine fluorescence patterns of human *D* group chromosomes. Nature (Lond.) *232*, 24–27 (1971)
21. Passarge, E., True, C.W., Sueoka, W.T., Baumgartner, N.R., Keer, K.R.: Malformation of the central nervous system in trisomy 18 syndrome. J. Pediat. *69*, 771–778 (1966)
22. Ross, L.J.: Dermatoglyphic observations in a patient with trisomy 18. J. Pediat *72*, 862–863 (1968)
23. Thorburn, M.J., Johnson, B.E.: Apparent monosomy of a G autosome in a Jamaican infant. J. med. Genet. *3*, 290–292 (1966)
24. Hall, B., Fredga, K., Svenningen, N.: A case of monosomy G? Hereditas *57*, 356–364 (1967)

25. Miller, O.J., Breg, W.R., Warburton, D., Miller, D.A., deCapoa, A., Allderdice, P.W., Davis, J., Klinger, H.P., McGilvray, E., Allen, F.H., Jr.: Partial deletion of the short arm of chromosome No. 4 (4p−): clinical studies in five unrelated patients. J. Pediat. *77*, 792–801 (1970)
26. Guthrie, R.D., Aase, J.M., Asper, A.C., Smith, D.W.: The 4p− syndrome. A clinically recognizable chromosomal deletion syndrome. Amer. J. Dis. Child. *122*, 421–425 (1971)
27. Lejeune, J., Lafourcade, J., Berger, R., Vialatte, J., Boeswillwald, M., Seringe, P., Turpin, R.: Trois cas de délétion partielle du bras court d'un chromosome 5. C. R. Acad. Sci [D] (Paris) *257*, 3098–3102 (1963)
28. Vissian, L., Manassero, J., Kermarec, J., Duplay, H., Vaillaud, J.-C.: Modifications des fibres élastiques cutanées dans la maladie du "cri du chat" (à propos d'un nouveau cas). Ann. Derm. Syph. (Paris) *98*, 53–56 (1971)
29. de Grouchy, J., Royer, P., Salmon, C., Lamy, M.: Délétion partielle des bras longs du chromosome 18. Path. Biol. (Paris) *12*, 579–582 (1964)
30. de Grouchy, J.: The 18p−, 18q− and 18r syndromes. In: The clinical delineation of birth defects. Bergsma, D. (ed.), Vol. V, No. 5, pt. V, pp. 74–87. Baltimore: Williams & Wilkins Co. 1969
31. Mavalwala, J., Wilson, M.G., Parker, C.E.: The dermatoglyphics of the 18q− syndrome. Amer. J. phys. Anthropol. *32*, 443–449 (1970)
32. Wertelecki, W., Gerald, P.S.: Clinical and chromosomal studies of the 18q− syndrome. J. Pediat. *78*, 44–52 (1971)
33. Feingold, M., Schwartz, R.S., Atkins, L., Anderson, R., Bartsocas, C.S., Page, D.L., Littlefield, J.W.: IgA deficiency associated with partial deletion of chromosome 18. Amer. J. Dis. Child. *117*, 129–136 (1969)
34. Gerald, P.S., Davis, C., Say, B.M., Wilkins, J.L.: A novel chromosomal basis for imperforate anus (the "cat's eye" syndrome). Pediat. Res. *2*, 297 (1968)
35. Allderdice, P.W., Davis, J.G., Miller, O.J., Klinger, H.P., Warburton, D., Miller, D.A., Allen, F.H., Jr., Abrams, C.A.L., McGilvray, E.: The 13q− deletion syndrome. Amer. J. hum. Genet. *21*, 499–512 (1969)
36. Grace, E., Drennan, J., Colver, D., Gordon, R.R.: The 13q− deletion syndrome. J. med. Genet. *8*, 351–357 (1971)
37. de Grouchy, J., Lamy, M., Thieffry, S., Arthuis, M., Salmon, C.: Dysmorphie complexe avec oligophrénie: délétion des bras courts d'un chromosome 17–18. C. R. Acad. Sci. [D] (Paris) *256*, 1028–1029 (1963)
38. Ruvalcaba, R.H.A., Thuline, H.C.: IgA absence associated with short arm deletion of chromosome No. 18. J. Pediat. *74*, 964–965 (1969)
39. Uchida, I.A., McRae, K.N., Wang, H.C., Ray, M.: Familial short arm deficiency of chromosome 18 concomitant with arhinencephaly and alopecia congenita. Amer. J. hum. Genet. *17*, 410–419 (1965)
40. Migeon, B.R.: Short arm deletions in group E and chromosomal "deletion" syndromes. J. Pediat. *69*, 432–438 (1966)
41. Carr, D.H., Barr, M.L., Plunkett, E.R.: An XXXX sex chromosome complex in two mentally defective females. Canad. med. Ass. J. *84*, 131–137 (1961)
42. Telfer, M.A., Richardson, C.E., Helmken, J., Smith, G.F.: Divergent phenotypes among 48,XXXX and 47,XXX females. Amer. J. hum. Genet. *22*, 326–335 (1970)
43. Becker, K.L., Hoffman, D.L., Albert, A., Underdahl, L.O., Mason, H.L.: Klinefelter's syndrome. Clinical and laboratory findings in 50 patients. Arch. intern. Med. *118*, 314–321 (1966)
44. Cushman, C.J., Soltan, H.C.: Dermatoglyphics in Klinefelter's syndrome (47,XXY). Hum. Heredity *19*, 641–653 (1969)

45. Ferguson-Smith, M.A., Johnston, A.W., Handmaker, S.D.: Primary amentia and micro-orchidism associated with an XXXY sex-chromosome constitution. Lancet *1960II*, 184–187

46. Carr, D.H., Barr, M.L., Plunkett, E.R., Grumbach, M.M., Morishima, A., Chu, E.H.Y.: An XXXY sex chromosome complex in Klinefelter subjects with duplicated sex chromatin. J. clin. Endocr. Metab. *21*, 491–505 (1961)

47. Barr, M.L., Carr, D.H., Pozsonyi, J., Wilson, R.A., Dunn, H.G., Jacobson, T.S., Miller, J.R. (with Appendix by Lewis, M., Chow, B.): The XXXXY sex chromosome abnormality. Can. med. Ass. J. *87*, 891–901 (1962)

48. Scherz, R.G., Roeckel, I.E.: The XXXXY syndrome. A report of a case and review of the literature. J. Pediat. *63*, 1093–1098 (1963)

49. Voorhees, J.J., Wilkins, J.W., Jr., Hayes, E., Harrel, E.R.: Nodulocystic acne as a phenotypic feature of the XYY genotype. Report of five cases, review of all known XYY subjects with severe acne, and discussion of XYY cytodiagnosis. Arch. Derm. *105*, 913–919 (1972)

50. Peterson, W.C., Jr., Gorlin, R.J., Peagler, F., Bruhl, H.: Cutaneous aspects of the XXYY genotype. A variant of Klinefelter's syndrome. Arch. Derm. *94*, 695–698 (1966)

51. Parker, C.E., Mavalwala, J., Melnyk, J., Fish, C.H.: The 48, XXYY syndrome. Amer. J. Med. *48*, 777–781 (1970)

Chapter 17   Dermatoglyphics

Contents

Dermatoglyphics is the study of epidermal ridges and the patterns formed by them. The lifelong permanence of the pattern features was first scientifically demonstrated by Sir Francis Galton in 1892 in his book *Finger Prints* [1]. Although Galton was the first to suggest a hereditary basis for pattern types, it was Wilder [2] who, at the turn of this century, attempted, by pedigree studies, to demonstrate the role of hereditary factors in ridge arrangements. The term "dermatoglyphics," meaning "skin carving," was coined by the anatomist Harold Cummins. The book *Finger Prints, Palms and Soles* by Cummins and Midlo [3], published in 1943, has been for many years the source of all relevant information in the field. Holt and Penrose subsequently made important contributions to the genetics of dermatoglyphics in normal populations [4, 5]. Recently, there has been a tremendous upswing in the number of reports on dermatoglyphics, stressing in particular their value in diagnosing various diseases [6, 7].

Dermatoglyphics is significant in the fields of multigenic inheritance, identification of individuals, zygosity determination, population studies, chromosomal anomalies, and certain nonchromosomal disorders.

Embryology

The differentiation of the dermal ridges begins in the third fetal month and is complete by the end of the fourth month. The alignment of ridges is strongly influenced by the relative growth rates of the skeletal and muscular elements of the hand and foot. Developmental disturbances of genetic or environmental etiology occurring during ridge differentiation can produce abnormalities of dermal patterns [8, 9].

Ridge Patterns

If a finger, palm, or sole is inked and then pressed on to paper, the resulting reproduction of the ridge pattern is the print. Several methods for making a permanent record of dermatoglyphic patterns have been outlined [10–12].

The simplest procedure for obtaining permanent prints quickly and efficiently has been the Faurot or inkless method (sensitized paper and resensitizing fluid supplied by Faurot Inc., 299 Broadway, New York, N.Y. 10007). It is of particular value in large-scale studies. The Hollister method (Hollister Inc., 211 E. Chicago, Chicago, Ill. 60611) gives clearer prints and is particularly useful in printing small areas with indistinct patterns [11].

Ridge patterns can be classified into three main types: *arches*, *loops*, and *whorls* (Fig. 17.1). Arches may be simple or tented; loops may be ulnar or radial according to the direction they open. The whorls are of three main kinds: symmetric, spiral, and double loop. The classification of the patterns is according to the number of *triradii*. (A triradius is a point formed by the meeting of three different ridge fields at angles greater than 90°. Thus, a simple arch has no triradius, a loop has one, and a whorl has two or more triradii.)

The commonest pattern type is the loop. Certain patterns occur more frequently on some fingers than on others. Thus, whorls are most frequent on thumbs and ring fingers, while radial loops and arches are most common on the index fingers. The little fingers have the highest frequency of ulnar loops and the lowest frequency of other patterns.

The size of a finger pattern may be expressed as the *ridge count*. To make a ridge count one draws a straight line from the core or center of a fingerprint pattern to the triradius and then counts the number of ridges transected or touched by this line. In this

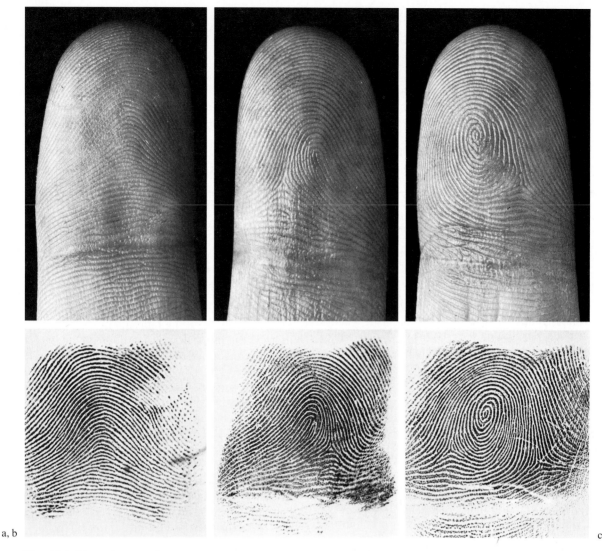

a, b   c

Fig. 17.1. Fingertips and fingerprints demonstrating the three basic digital pattern types: *a*, arch; *b*, loop; *c*, whorl. Note the two triradial points in the whorl pattern and the single triradius in the loop pattern. (From Miller, J.R., Giroux, J.: J. Pediat. *69*, 302–312, 1966)

count, the triradius and the core are not included. The finger ridge count is considered a classic example of polygenic inheritance [4], although a single major autosomal locus with two additive alleles may account for over half the variation in absolute ridge count [13]. The total ridge count (TRC) (including all 10 fingers) is about 145 in males and 127 in females. The TRC depends mainly on a number of additive genes, while the environment plays a relatively small part. This proposition is backed, in family studies, by correlation coefficients that measure hereditary likeness. In parents and their children and in sib pairs this coefficient is expected to be 0.5. This relationship is very closely approached when total ridge counts are compared.

Similarly, the correlation between monozygotic twins is very high and the correlation between dizygotic twins is of the same order as that between ordinary sibs. Using this information, statistical tables were developed for the use of fingerprints in zygosity determination [1, 14].

The palmprint (Fig. 17.2) usually reveals a triradius at the base of each digit except the thumb. These are called the "digital triradii" and are designated as *a*, *b*, *c*, and *d* for the index, middle, ring, and small fingers, respectively. Another triradius is usually found at the base of the palm and is called the "axial triradius" (*t* or *p*). If more than one axial triradius is present, the most distal one is used in the dermatoglyphic analysis. The position of the triradius

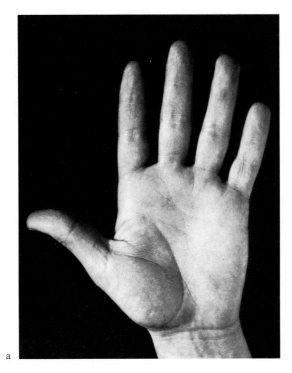

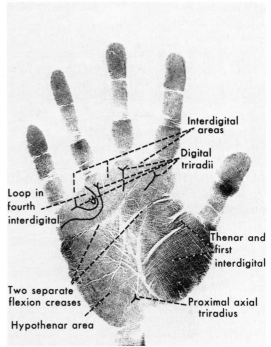

a

b

Fig. 17.2. a Normal palm. (From Miller, J.R., Giroux, J.: J. Pediat. *69*, 302–312, 1966). **b** Print of normal palm showing the main topographic areas. (From Miller, J.R., Giroux, J.: J. Pediat. *69*, 302–312, 1966)

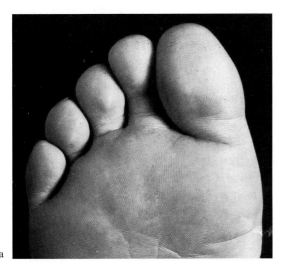

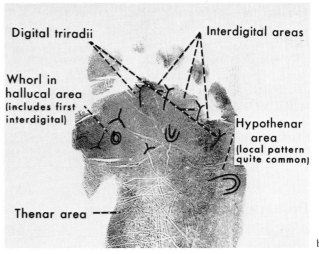

a

b

Fig. 17.3. a Normal sole. (From Miller, J.R., Giroux, J.: J. Pediat. *69*, 302–312, 1966.) **b** Print of normal sole showing the main topographic areas. (From Miller, J.R., Giroux, J.: J. Pediat. *69*, 302–312, 1966)

can be described in one of two ways, both of which have their merits [11]:

1. A measurement can be made of the distance from the distal wrist crease to the axial triradius as the percentage of the total vertical distance from the distal wrist crease to the base of the middle finger. A lower limit of 40% is set for a "high" axial triradius.

2. A measurement can be made of the atd angle formed between lines drawn from triradii a and d to the axial triradius t [15]. The more distal the axial triradius, the larger the angle. Positions of the axial triradii which form an angle greater than 56° are designated "distal" [11]. The atd angle is age-dependent, getting smaller with time [15].

Plantar patterns (Fig. 17.3), although potentially as informative as palmar patterns, have been less extensively studied chiefly because they are less readily obtained. The topographic areas and the triradii of the soles are similar to those of the palms. The hallucal area is the area of the sole shown to be of greatest importance at present.

Technically, flexion creases on the palms and soles are not part of dermatoglyphics. However, the two are generally considered together. The flexion creases represent the point where the skin is attached to the underlying structures. A recent study [16] has revealed that creases are related to the flexion movements of the hands of the late embryo and early fetus.

Different races have differences in the frequency of various dermatoglyphic patterns. However, it is not possible to determine to which race a particular individual belongs from a study of the fingerprints alone, since no one ridge pattern is exclusively characteristic of any particular racial group [17, 18].

Dermatoglyphics in Chromosomal Aberration Syndromes[1]

In 1939 it was pointed out [3] for the first time that certain dermatoglyphic features in Down syndrome differed from those in controls (Figs. 17.4 and 17.5). Although no single feature of the dermal patterns of Down syndrome is unique, the frequency with which it appears in controls is quite different from its frequency in patients. Thus, a radial loop is found on the second digit in 2% of Down syndrome patients, whereas it is found in 20% of controls. A radial loop on the fifth finger occurs in 4% of patients with Down syndrome but in only

3 per 1000 controls. The most common digital pattern combination in Down syndrome is that of 10 ulnar loops. The palm bears more frequently an axial triradius which is displaced distally, lies near the middle of the palm, and thus gives an atd angle of more than 45°. Fifty percent of patients with Down syndrome have an "arch tibial" (A^t) pattern (Fig. 17.5b). This is the single most useful dermal pattern in this syndrome since it is very rare (0.3%) in controls [19–21]. In 1970 a discriminate analysis was used [22] to develop a "dermatoglyphic nomogram" for the diagnosis of the syndrome. This nomogram is based on four areas: the right hallucal, the right atd angle, and the right and left index fingers. In 1971 a mathematical method of discrimination was developed which separated Down syndrome patients from controls, with less overlap [23].

Dermatoglyphic Anomalies in Nonchromosomal Disorders

Dermatoglyphic abnormalities have been reported in the Rubinstein-Taybi syndrome [6, 24], anonychia, nail-patelly syndrome, Coffin-Lowry syndrome, Holt-Oram syndrome [25], Cornelia de Lange syndrome [6], Smith-Lemli-Opitz syndrome [6], cerebrohepatorenal syndrome [6], and arthrogryposis multiplex congenita (AMC) [6]. Although not confirmed or well-established, dermatoglyphic abnormalities have also been reported in the following disorders: sickle cell amunia [26], hypohidrotic or anhidrotic ectodermal dysplasia, schizophrenia, carcinoma of the breast, leukemia [27], congenital heart disease [28], alopecia areata, psoriasis [20], camptodactyly [29], cerebral gigantism [30], systemic lupus erythematosus [31], Wilson disease, phenylketonuria, Ehlers-Danlos syndrome, celiac disease, Waardenburg syndrome, neurofibromatosis, and Huntington chorea [32].

In the syndrome called dermal "ridges-off-the-end," the fingertip ridges, instead of running transversely, run vertically to the ends of the fingertips. Bilateral radial loops on the ring and little fingers, although very rare in controls, are common in this syndrome. The condition is thought to follow the autosomal dominant pattern of inheritance [33].

Injuries to the skin such as cuts and burns and conditions such as leprosy, Darier disease, and adult acanthosis nigricans may alter epidermal ridges. Pedigrees may show absent dermal ridges [34]; ectodermal dysplasia, absent dermatoglyphic pattern, changes in the nails, and a simian crease (the Basan syndrome) [35]; and patternless dermal

---

1 See also tables on pp. 293–296.

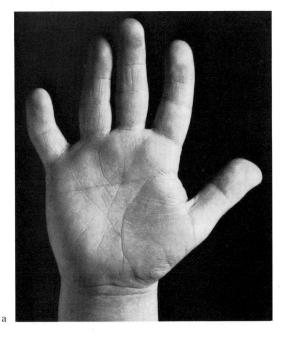

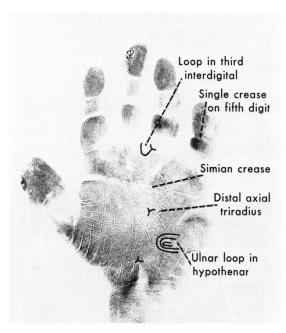

Fig. 17.4. a Palm of a child with Down syndrome. Note simian crease on the palm and single interphalangeal crease of the little finger. (From Miller, J.R., Giroux, J.: J. Pediat. *69*, 302–312, 1966.) b Palm print of a child with Down syndrome showing the typical dermatoglyphic features. (From Miller, J.R., Giroux, J.: J. Pediat. *69*, 302–312, 1966)

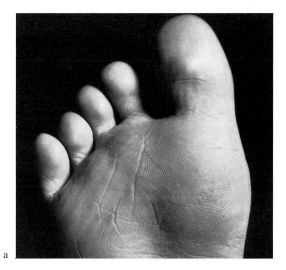

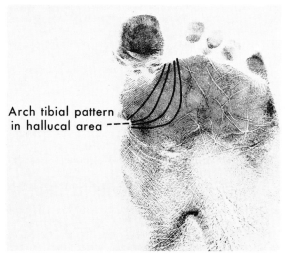

Fig. 17.5. a Sole of a child with Down syndrome. (From Miller, J.R., Giroux, J.: J. Pediat. *69*, 302–312, 1966.) b Sole print of the hallucal area of a child with Down syndrome, demonstrating the typical arch tibial pattern. (From Miller, J.R., Giroux, J.: J. Pediat. *69*, 302–312, 1966)

ridges consisting of scattered short ridges or ridges consisting only of irregular dots [4, 36]. However, patternless ridge formation and the congenital absence of ridged skin are extremely rare [20]

The importance of dermatoglyphics to genetics and medicine should not be overemphasized, since many pathogenetic factors still remain unknown. Yet, if used correctly, it remains a significant tool in research and diagnosis.

References

1. Galton, F.: Finger prints. London: Macmillan Co. 1892
2. Wilder, H.H.: Physical correspondence in two sets of duplicate twins. J. Hered. *10*, 410–420 (1919)
3. Cummins, H., Midlo, C.: Finger prints, palms and soles. New York: Blakiston 1943; republished New York: Dover Publications Inc. 1961
4. Holt, S.B.: The genetics of dermal ridges. Springfield: Charles C Thomas 1968
5. Penrose, L.S., Loesch, D.: Classification of normal and abnormal dermatoglyphics. In: Proceedings of the second congress of the international association for the scientific study of mental deficiency. Primrose, D.A.A. (ed.), pp. 355–360. Warsaw: Polish Medical Publishers 1972
6. Preus, M., Fraser, F.C.: Dermatoglyphics and syndromes. Amer. J. Dis. Child. *124*, 933–943 (1972)
7. Holt, S.B.: The significance of dermatoglyphics in medicine. A short survey and summary. Clin. Pediat. (Philadelphia) *12*, 471–484 (1973)
8. Mulvihill, J.J., Smith, D.W.: The genesis of dermatoglyphics. J. Pediat. *75*, 579–589 (1969)
9. Hirsch, W., Schweichel, J.U.: Morphological evidence concerning the problem of skin ridge formation. J. ment. Defic. Res. *17*, 58–72 (1973)
10. Walker, N.F.: Inkless methods of finger, palm and sole printing. J. Pediat. *50*, 27–29 (1957)
11. Uchida, I.A., Soltan, H.C.: Dermatoglyphics in medical genetics. In: Endocrine and genetic diseases of childhood. Gardner, L.I. (ed.), pp. 579–592. Philadelphia: Saunders, W.B. Co. 1969
12. Miller, J.R., Giroux, J.: Dermatoglyphics in pediatric practice. J. Pediat. *69*, 302–312 (1966)
13. Spence, M.A., Elston, R.C., Namboodiri, K.K., Pollitzer, W.S.: Evidence for a possible major gene effect in absolute finger ridge count. Hum. Heredity *23*, 414–421 (1972)
14. Smith, M., Penrose, L.S.: Monozygotic and dizygotic twin diagnosis. Ann. hum. Genet. *19*, 273–289 (1955)
15. Penrose, L.S.: Familial studies on palmar patterns in relation to mongolism. Proc. 8th Int. Congr. Genetics, Hereditas (Suppl.), 412, 1949
16. Popich, G.A., Smith, D.W.: The genesis and significance of digital and palmar hand creases: preliminary report. J. Pediat. *77*, 1017–1023 (1970)
17. Holt, S.B.: Palm-prints and their uses in medical biology. Cereb. Palsy Bull. *3*, 333–347 (1961)
18. Naffah, J.: Dermatoglyphics and flexion creases in the Lebanese population. Amer. J. phys. Anthropol. *41*, 391–409 (1974)
19. Miller, J.R.: Dermatoglyphics. J. invest. Derm. *60*, 435–442 (1973)
20. Verbov, J.: Clinical significance and genetics of epidermal ridges – a review of dermatoglyphics. J. invest. Derm. *54*, 261–271 (1970)
21. Thompson, J.S., Thompson, M.W.: Genetics in medicine, 2nd ed., pp. 320–332. Philadelphia: Saunders, W.B. Co. 1973
22. Reed, T.E., Borgaonkar, D.S., Conneally, P.M., Yu, P.-L., Nance, W.E., Christian, J.C.: Dermatoglyphic nomogram for the diagnosis of Down's syndrome. J. Pediat. *77*, 1024–1032 (1970)
23. Borgaonkar, D.S., Davis, M., Bolling, D.R., Herr, H.M.: Evaluation of dermal patterns in Down's syndrome by predictive discrimination. I. Preliminary analysis based on frequencies of patterns. Johns Hopk. med. J. *128*, 141–152 (1971)
24. Giroux, J., Miller, J.R.: Dermatoglyphics of the broad thumb and great toe syndrome. Amer. J. Dis. Child. *113*, 207–208 (1967)
25. Gall, J.C., Jr., Stern, A.M., Cohen, M.M., Adams, M.S., Davidson, R.T.: Holt-Oram syndrome: clinical and genetic study of a large family. Amer. J. hum. Genet. *18*, 187–200 (1966)
26. Zizmor, J.: The extra transverse digital crease: a skin sign found in sickle cell disease. Cutis *11*, 447–449 (1973)
27. Wertelecki, W., Plato, C.C., Fraumeni, J.F., Niswander, J.D.: Dermatoglyphics in leukemia. Pediat. Res. *7*, 620–626 (1973)
28. Preus, M., Fraser, F.C., Levy, E.P.: Dermatoglyphics in congenital heart malformations. Hum. Heredity *20*, 388–402 (1970)
29. Goodman, R.M., Katznelson, M.B.-M., Manor, E.: Camptodactyly: occurrence in two new genetic syndromes and its relationship to other syndromes. J. med. Genet. *9*, 203–212 (1972)
30. Bejar, R.L., Smith, G.F., Park, S., Spellacy, W.N., Wolfson, S.L., Nyhan, W.L.: Cerebral gigantism: concentrations of amino acids in plasma and muscle. J. Pediat. *76*, 105–111 (1970)
31. Dubois, R.W., Weiner, J.M., Dubois, E.L.: Dermatoglyphic study of systemic lupus erythematosus. Arthr. and Rheum. *19*, 83–87 (1976)
32. Shiono, H., Kadowaki, J.-I.: Dermatologic uses of dermatologlyphics. Int. J. Derm. *17*, 134–136 (1978)
33. David, T.J.: "Ridges-off-the-end" – a dermatoglyphic syndrome. Hum. Heredity *21*, 39–53 (1971)
34. Baird, H.W., III: Kindred showing congenital absence of the dermal ridges (fingerprints) and associated anomalies. J. Pediat. *64*, 621–631 (1964)
35. Jorgenson, R.J.: Ectodermal dysplasia with hypotrichosis, hypohydrosis, defective teeth, and unusual dermatoglyphics (Basan syndrome?). In: The clinical delineation of birth defects. Bergsma, D. (ed.), Vol. X, No. 4, pt. XVI, pp. 323–325. Baltimore: Williams & Wilkins Co. 1974
36. Dodinval, P., Leblanc, P., Delree, C., Deslypere, P.: Dysplasie des crêtes épidermiques, à l'hérédité dominante autosomique. Etude des dermatoglyphes d'une famille. Humangenetik *11*, 230–236 (1971)

Chapter 18   Cancer, Genetics, and the Skin

Contents

Hereditary Skin Diseases Associated with Cancer

Since the skin is an easily accessible organ and its lesions are usually apparent to the naked eye, a thorough knowledge of the different types of skin cancer and their distinctive identifying characteristics helps in their early detection, timely diagnosis, and prompt therapy. Certain syndromes have specific dermatologic signs and a predisposition to the development of cancer in other organs. Awareness of these syndromes helps in cancer detection. In all such cases, judicious medical action may be lifesaving. When these diseases are inherited, proper genetic counseling and screening of relatives may again prove to be very rewarding.

Although the details are discussed separately elsewhere, a list of the hereditary skin diseases associated with cancer may be helpful for quick reference (modified from Lynch and Szentivanyi [1]).

Table 18.1. Disorders with autosomal dominant inheritance

Disorder	Predominant cancers
Cutaneous malignant melanoma	Cutaneous malignant melanomas
Epidermolysis bullosa dystrophica	Carcinomas of mucous membranes, multiple basal and squamous cell carcinomas of skin
Gardner syndrome	Adenocarcinomas of colon
Generalized keratoacanthoma	Rare occurrences of squamous cell carcinomas
von Hippel-Lindau syndrome	Hemangioblastomas of cerebellum, hypernephromas, and pheochromocytomas
Kaposi sarcoma (multiple idiopathic hemorrhagic sarcoma of Kaposi)	Sarcomas
Multiple nevoid basal cell carcinoma syndrome	Multiple basal cell carcinomas
Neurofibromatosis	Sarcomas, acoustic neuromas, pheochromocytomas
Peutz-Jeghers syndrome	Adenocarcinomas of duodenum and colon
Porphyria cutanea tarda	Basal cell carcinomas of skin, hepatomas
Tuberous sclerosis (Bourneville disease)	Intracranial neoplasms (astrocytomas, glioblastomas)
Tylosis and esophageal carcinoma (keratosis palmaris et plantaris)	Esophageal cancer

Table 18.2. Disorders with autosomal recessive inheritance

Disorder	Predominant cancers
Albinism	Basal and squamous cell carcinomas of skin
Ataxia telangiectasia (Louis-Bar syndrome)	Acute leukemias and lymphomas
Bloom syndrome (congenital telangiectatic erythema and stunted growth)	Acute leukemias
Chédiak-Higashi syndrome	Lymphomas
Fanconi aplastic anemia	Leukemias
Werner syndrome (progeria of the adult)	Sarcomas, meningiomas
Xeroderma pigmentosum	Basal and squamous cell carcinomas of skin and malignant melanomas

Table 18.3. Disorders with X-linked recessive inheritance

Disorder	Predominant cancers
Aldrich syndrome (Wiskott-Aldrich syndrome)	Leukemias, lymphomas
Bruton agammaglobulinemia	Acute leukemias

Table 18.4. Disorders with possible genetic etiology — mode of inheritance unknown

Disorder	Predominant cancers
Dermatomyositis	Adenocarcinomas of viscera and sarcomas of soft tissues in adult onset dermatomyositis
Giant pigmented nevi (bathing trunk nevi)	Melanomas in children
Scleroderma	Bronchiolar carcinomas, malignant carcinoids
Sjögren syndrome (keratoconjunctivitis sicca)	Lymphomas
Systemic lupus erythematosus	Thymic tumors, leukemias, and lymphomas

The last decade has witnessed genetic studies related to carcinogenesis in two special directions: enzymatic and chromosomal.

The discovery of defective DNA repair in patients with xeroderma pigmentosum (XP) has brought forward the attractive hypothesis of a relationship between actinic carcinogenesis and defective DNA repair [2]. (See also p. 1 and p. 151.)

The following observations support this hypothesis.

1. At least six different mutations resulting in defective DNA repair are associated with a high risk for skin cancer [2].

2. Dutch investigators have found that the lower the residual levels of DNA repair in the cells from patients with XP, the severer their clinical symptoms [3, 4]. The severity of the cancerous lesions is evaluated on the basis of the age of onset of malignancies, the rate of tumor production, and the age at death. However, investigators in the United States [5] did not find this inverse correlation. The discrepancy between the results of these two groups may be due to differences in environmental factors influencing the phenotypic expression of the XP genotype [2].

3. Exposure of human cells in vitro to various carcinogenic agents generates an excision repair process [6, 7] and, possibly, a mechanism that resembles postreplication repair [8, 9]. Studies in bacteria have shown that DNA repair mechanisms are not free from errors. The more the damage, the more the risk of erroneous repair. The extrapolation of these facts to man may explain the high incidence of skin cancer in sailors and fishermen who are continuously exposed to the sun.

Thus, both a defective repair of sunlight-induced DNA lesions and an excess of these lesions with a normal repair mechanism result in carcinogenesis. Yet, the direct pathogenetic mechanism of malignant cellular transformation remains to be discovered [1]. XP data can be further extrapolated in two directions: (a) genetic changes may arise through mutations or chromosomal changes resulting from unrepaired damage in DNA; (b) unrepaired damage to DNA may potentiate the transformation of cells by oncogenic viruses [10]. This latter postulate has been tested but no such potentiation found [11].

Many diseases displaying chromosomal instability, whether induced genetically or environmentally (irradiation, certain viruses, oncogenic chemicals), are associated with cancer and may have an etiologic significance [12]. Certain inherited skin diseases fit this observation. Among them the most striking and interesting are the Bloom syndrome, Fanconi anemia, ataxia telangiectasia (Louis-Bar syndrome), and xeroderma pigmentosum [13]. Different types of chromosomal anomalies (quadriradial configurations, chromatid gaps and breaks) are found in lymphocyte and fibroblast cultures from patients with these diseases (see also p. 11). The emergence in these disorders of new *marker* chromosomes not represented in the normal complement may be significant in the pathogenesis of cancer [13]. UV light induces both chromatid breaks and exchanges in XP cells, but precise quantitative data from normal and XP cells are not yet available [10].

Although Bloom syndrome, Fanconi anemia, and ataxia telangiectasia are individually rare conditions, collectively, the homozygous patients and the heterozygous carriers of the mutant genes may represent a significant group. In some obligate heterozygotes for the gene for Bloom syndrome, i.e., parents of affected persons, more chromosomal rearrangements were observed than exist in ordinary individuals [13]. If the heterozygotes of these diseases show an increased predisposition to cancer, the detection of chromosomal instability in the general population may be undertaken for a more effective and efficient control of cancer.

From the observations mentioned above, a two or more step model has been proposed for the pathogenesis of cancer [14, 15]. It may explain the existence of both hereditary and nonhereditary forms of every cancer. The first step is called "mutational" and may represent a point mutation, frameshift mutation, deletion, duplication, rearrangement, or addition of a viral genome (see p. 3). The other steps might be "mutational" also, but there is no conclusive evidence for this. They represent the effects of a chemical carcinogen, a tumor virus, or radiation. The first step mutation is supposed to occur in germinal cells in the hereditary forms and somatic cells in the nonhereditary forms. The second step occurs in somatic cells in both forms.

References

1. Lynch, H.T., Szentivanyi, J.: Genetics as guide to early diagnosis and cancer control – cutaneous syndromes. Cutis *6*, 179–185 (1970)

2. De Weerd-Kastelein, E.A.: Genetic heterogeneity in the human skin disease xeroderma pigmentosum. Doctoral thesis, pp. 14–15. Rotterdam: Bronder-Offset B. V. 1974

3. Bootsma, D., Mulder, M.P., Pot, F., Cohen, J.A.: Different inherited levels of DNA repair replication in xeroderma pigmentosum cell strains after exposure to ultraviolet irradiation. Mutat. Res. *9*, 507–516 (1970)

4. Kleijer, W.J., Hoeksema, J.L., Sluyter, M.L., Bootsma, D.: Effects of inhibitors on repair of DNA in normal human and xeroderma pigmentosum cells after exposure to x-rays and ultraviolet irradiation. Mutat. Res. *17*, 385–394 (1973)

5. Robbins, J.H., Kraemer, K.H., Lutzner, M.A., Festoff, B.W., Coon, H.G.: Xeroderma pigmentosum. An inherited disease with sun sensitivity, multiple cutaneous neoplasms, and abnormal DNA repair. Ann. intern. Med. *80*, 221–248 (1974)

6. Setlow, R.B., Regan, J.D.: Defective repair of *N*-acetoxy-2-acetylaminofluorene-induced lesions in the DNA of xeroderma pigmentosum cells. Biochem. biophys. Res. Commun. *46*, 1019–1024 (1972)

7. Stich, H.F., San, R.H.C., Kawazoe, Y.: Increased sensitivity of xeroderma pigmentosum cells to some chemical carcinogens and mutagens. Mutat. Res. *17*, 127–137 (1973)

8. Buhl, S.N., Regan, J.D.: DNA replication in human cells treated with methyl methanesulfonate. Mutat. Res. *18*, 191–197 (1973)

9. Van den Berg, H.W.: Alkaline sucrose gradient sedimentation studies of DNA from Hela S$_3$ cells exposed to methyl methanesulphonate or methylazoxymethanol acetate. Biochim. biophys. Acta (Amst.) *353*, 215–226 (1974)

10. Cleaver, J.E.: Xeroderma pigmentosum – progress and regress. J. invest. Derm. *60*, 374–380 (1973)

11. Key, D.J., Todaro, G.J.: Xeroderma pigmentosum cell susceptibility to SV40 virus transformation: lack of effect of low dosage ultraviolet radiation in enhancing viral-induced transformation. J. invest. Derm. *62*, 7–10 (1974)

12. German, J.: Genes which increase chromosomal instability in somatic cells and predispose to cancer. In: Progress in medical genetics. Steinberg, A.G., Bearn, A.G. (eds.), Vol. VIII, pp. 61–101. New York: Grune & Stratton 1972

13. German, J.: Genetic disorders associated with chromosomal instability and cancer. J. invest. Derm. *60*, 427–434 (1973)

14. Knudson, A.G., Jr., Strong, L.C., Anderson, D.E.: Heredity and cancer in man. In: Progress in medical genetics. Steinberg, A.G., Bearn, A.G. (eds.), Vol. IX, pp. 113–158. New York: Grune & Stratton 1973

15. Knudson, A.G., Jr.: Genetics and the etiology of childhood cancer. Pediat. Res. *10*, 513–517 (1976)

Chapter 19   Miscellaneous

Contents

Leiner Disease (Erythrodermia Desquamativa)

Clinical Presentation. This disorder appears during the first 3 months of life. The lesions may be limited to the scalp and face or the diaper area, but most patients have a diffuse erythrodermia with desquamation of fine scales. Thick greasy scales accumulate on the scalp. Affected infants usually have a protracted severe diarrhea.

The familial form emphasizes the generalized skin involvement (seborrheic dermatitis), intractable diarrhea, marked wasting, and increased susceptibility to infection [1, 2].

Pathology and Pathophysiology. The skin shows a picture of chronic or subacute dermatitis: hyper- and parakeratosis, acanthosis with mild spongiosis, and a mild perivascular inflammatory infiltrate.

In the familial cases, there is a deficiency of the phagocytosis-enhancing activity of serum related to dysfunction of the fifth component of complement (C_5) [1, 2]. The serum opsonic function is markedly deficient with yeast particles, and this is corrected by the addition of C_5 [2]. This defect is present in other members of the affected family.

Inheritance. Inheritance is probably autosomal recessive.

Treatment. Treatment consists of topical corticosteroids, appropriate antibiotics to combat infections, and, in cases of C_5 deficiency, frequent transfusions with fresh plasma [2].

References

1. Miller, M.E., Koblenzer, P.J.: Leiner's disease and deficiency of C_5. J. Pediat. *80*, 879–880 (1972)
2. Jacobs, J.C., Miller, M.E.: Fatal familial Leiner's disease: a deficiency of the opsonic activity of serum complement. Pediatrics *49*, 225–232 (1972)

Deafness and Dermatitis

In three of four sibs, familial nonprogressive neural hearing loss has been described in association with "atypical atopic dermatitis" [1]. The dermatitis, which had its onset between 9 and 11 years of age, affected the waist, antecubital fossae, forearms, dorsa of wrists, hands, and fingers, and was clinically and histologically a chronic lichenified dermatitis [1]. The diagnosis of "atypical" atopic dermatitis was made because of the late onset and peculiar distribution of the dermatitis. Inheritance in this syndrome is probably autosomal recessive.

Reference

1. Konigsmark, B.W., Hollander, M.B., Berlin, C.I.: Familial neural hearing loss and atopic dermatitis. J. Amer. med. Ass. *204*, 953–957 (1968)

Granulosis Rubra Nasi

Clinical Presentation. This uncommon disorder usually begins in childhood as small, discrete, reddish macules or papules. Pustules and vesicles may also appear. The nose is usually involved and is characteristically hyperhidrotic. Other sites, such as the cheeks, upper lip, and chin, may also be affected.

The disease usually clears after puberty and rarely persists into late adult life. Familial occurrence has been reported [1, 2].

Pathology and Pathophysiology. The main feature is dilatation of the blood vessels and sweat ducts. Mild inflammatory changes may be present.

Inheritance. Probably autosomal dominant [2].

Treatment. There is no effective treatment.

References

1. Lebet, A.: Contribution à l'étude de l'hidrocystome (avec une note sur la granulosis rubra nasi). Ann. Derm. Syph. (Paris) *4*, 273–282 (1903)
2. Hellier, F.F.: Granulosis rubra nasi in a mother and daughter. Brit. med. J. *1937 II*, 1068

Wrinkly Skin Syndrome

This recently described syndrome is characterized by wrinkled skin present at birth. The skin of the hands and feet is first affected, but the skin over most of the body is easily wrinkled [1]. The affected skin is dry and shows decreased extensibility. Palmar creases also increase in number. Other features of the syndrome include poor muscle development and short stature. Light microscopy of the skin shows no characteristic abnormalities [1]. Inheritance is autosomal recessive.

Reference

1. Gazit, E., Goodman, R.M., Katznelson, M.B.-M., Rotem, Y.: The wrinkly skin syndrome: a new heritable disorder of connective tissue. Clin. Genet. *4*, 186–192 (1973)

Geroderma Osteodysplastica

In 1950 Bamatter et al. [1] described a Swiss family with lax, wrinkled skin, osteoporosis, and a marked susceptibility to fractures and coined the name "gérodermie ostéodysplastique héréditaire." Later, in 1978, two more affected families were described by Hunter et al. [2].

Clinical Presentation. The major features of the syndrome include thin, creased skin with decreased turgor and elasticity, most marked over the hands and feet; a sad face with droopy eyelids and jowly appearance; malocclusion, delayed dental eruption, and a high palate; a span greater than height; dislocated hips; and joint laxity, especially of the hands and feet but also of the knees and sternoclavicular joint. Intelligence is normal. Radiologic findings include generalized osteoporosis, frequent compression fractures, occasional biconcavity of the vertebrae, and minor variations of the ossification centers at the wrist.

Inheritance. Although, after the report of the first family [1], the inheritance of this condition was thought to follow the X-linked recessive pattern, the more recent report of two additional families favors very strongly the autosomal recessive mode.

Treatment. No specific treatment is available.

References

1. Bamatter, F., Franceschetti, A., Klein, D., Sierro, A.: Gérodermie ostéodysplastique héréditaire. Ann. Paediat. *174*, 126–127 (1950)
2. Hunter, G.W., Martsoff, J.T., Baker, C.G., Reed, M.H.: Geroderma osteodysplastica. Hum. Genet. *40*, 311–324 (1978)

Stiff Skin Syndrome

In 1971 Esterly and McKusick [1] described four patients with localized areas of stony-hard skin, mild hirsutism, and limitation of joint mobility.

Clinical Presentation. Rock-hard skin is observed at birth. The buttocks and upper thighs are the most severely involved areas, but the posterior neck, upper arms, trunk, and lower legs may also be involved. The skin of the hands and feet is normal. There is some increased hair growth on the thighs [1].

A variable number of joints are involved, in particular the elbows, knees, and hips (Figs. 19.1 and 19.2). Neck and lumbar spine movements are also limited. A lordotic stance is characteristic of affected individuals.

The patients are neurologically normal and have a normal intelligence. The skin and joint findings are not progressive.

All radiologic examinations are normal. There is no abnormal mucopolysacchariduria.

Pathology and Pathophysiology. Histologic examination of the skin reveals a normal stratum corneum and epidermis. The interstitial ground substance of the upper dermis is slightly granular and eosinophilic, with deposition of hyaluronic acid.

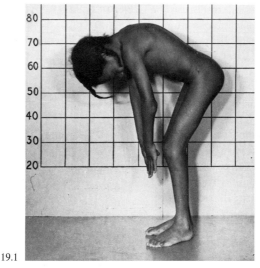
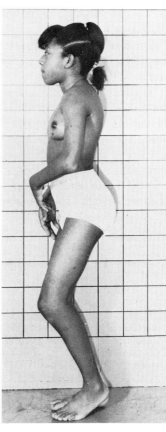

Figs. 19.1 and 19.2. Stiff skin syndrome. Note limited joint movements and inability of normal extension of the knees and elbows. (Courtesy of Dr. V.A. McKusick, from Esterly, N.B.: In: The clinical delineation of birth defects. Bergsma, D. (ed.), Vol. VII, No. 8, pt. XII, pp. 306–307. Baltimore: Williams & Wilkins Co. 1971)

Defective synthesis of acid mucopolysaccharides by fibroblasts is suggested by the presence of large numbers of metachromatic granules in cultured fibroblasts.

Inheritance. Most probably autosomal dominant. But the autosomal recessive mode cannot presently be ruled out [1].

Treatment. The treatment is symptomatic.

Reference

1. Esterly, N.B., McKusick, V.A.: Stiff skin syndrome. Pediatrics *47*, 360–369 (1971)

Winchester Disease

In 1969 Winchester et al. [1] described this syndrome characterized by short stature, joint stiffness with contractures, corneal opacities, coarsened facial features, dissolution of the carpal and tarsal bones, and generalized osteoporosis. Less than ten cases have been described to date.

Clinical Presentation. The onset is in infancy with arthralgias, joint stiffness, dwarfism, peripheral corneal opacities, symmetric flexion contractures of major and minor joints, generalized osteoporosis, carpal-tarsal osteolysis, marked intra- and periarticular small joint destruction, and skin lesions. The intelligence is normal [2].

The characteristic skin lesions are plaques of thickened skin with a leathery feeling. These plaques are usually hyperpigmented, hypertrichotic, and involve the face, trunk, and extremities. Such lesions are extensive and symmetrically distributed. They usually appear with the arthralgias and are chronic, but do not increase with time [2]. Other skin lesions are firm nodules.

Angiographic studies demonstrate hypervascularity apparently associated with osteolysis at large joints.

Pathology and Pathophysiology. The leathery skin lesions show focal areas of fibroblastic proliferation deep in the dermis by morphologically normal fibroblasts which replace the normal heavy collagen bundles. No epidermal atrophy is observed. A mild perivascular chronic infiltrate is seen in many areas [2]. Ultrastructural peculiarities of fibroblasts include dilated and vacuolated mitochondria, the presence of varying amounts of myofilaments in the cytoplasm, and a prominent fibrous nuclear lamina. Cells other than fibroblasts display no abnormalities [3].

The basic defect in this disorder is unknown. It may be related to abnormal function of fibroblasts. On the basis of cellular metachromasia and a twofold increase in cellular uronic acid in cultured fibroblasts, the syndrome was postulated to represent a new acid mucopolysaccharidosis. However, further data suggest that it does not appear to be a lysosomal storage disease and should be removed from the current list of mucopolysaccharidoses [2].

Inheritance. Autosomal recessive.

Treatment. Treatment is symptomatic.

References

1. Winchester, P., Grossman, H., Lim, W.N., Danes, B.S.: A new acid mucopolysaccharidosis with skeletal deformities simulating rheumatoid arthritis. Amer. J. Roentgenol. *106*, 121–128 (1969)
2. Hollister, D.W., Rimoin, D.L., Lachman, R.S., Cohen, A.H., Reed, W.B., Westin, G.W.: The Winchester syndrome: a nonlysosomal connective tissue disease. J. Pediat. *84*, 701–709 (1974)
3. Cohen, A.H., Hollister, D.W., Reed, W.B.: The skin in the Winchester syndrome. Histologic and ultrastructural studies. Arch. Derm. *111*, 230–236 (1975)

Parana Hard-Skin Syndrome

This condition has been described in seven families in Paranà, Brazil [1]. Onset is around the second or third month with the infant's skin becoming firm, thick, and gradually very hard and immovable. All of the skin is involved except that of the eyelids, neck, and ears. The affected patients cannot walk and their posture is fixed in flexion at the hips, knees, ankles, and elbows. There is restriction in the movement of the chest (with sternal protrusion) that may lead to pulmonary insufficiency, osteoarthropathy, and death [1]. Other features are round facies; hirsutism of thorax, limbs, face, and forehead; straight wide eyebrows; malar flush; corners of the mouth turned down; widely spaced nipples; generalized hyperpigmentation, especially over the abdomen and lumbar area; mild scaliness of the legs; and lichenification in flexural areas [1]. There are no signs of visceral or nervous system involvement. Ultrastructurally, the skin collagen fibrils appear normal. Inheritance is probably autosomal recessive. (See also Stiff Skin Syndrome.)

Reference

1. Cat, I., Rodrigues Magdalena, N.I., Parolin Marinoni, L., Wong, M.P., Freitas, O.T., Malfi, A., Costa, O., Esteves, L., Giraldi, D.J., Opitz, J.M: Parana hard-skin syndrome: study of seven families. Lancet *1974I*, 215–216

Dermochondrocorneal Dystrophy of François

François [1] described this syndrome in 1949. The clinical features are (a) skeletal deformity of the hands and feet; (b) xanthomatous nodules on the pinnae, dorsal surface of the metacarpophalangeal and interphalangeal joints, posterior surface of the elbows, etc.; and (c) corneal dystrophy. The condition follows the autosomal recessive pattern of inheritance.

Reference

1. François, J.: Dystrophie dermo-chondro-cornéenne familiale. Ann. Oculist. *182*, 409–442 (1949)

Rubinstein-Taybi Syndrome

In 1963 Rubinstein and Taybi [1] reported this syndrome in seven children. By 1968 more than 100 cases had been reported [2]. Although the syndrome is sometimes called "the broad thumbs and toes syndrome," the eponym is favored.

Clinical Presentation. The characteristic features of the syndrome are microcephaly and mental retardation; typical facies with hypertelorism, downward palpebral slant, heavy eyebrows, beaked nose, and retrognathia (Figs. 19.3 and 19.4); certain eye abnormalities such as strabismus, refractive errors, and cataracts; and broad terminal phalanges of the thumbs and great toes (Figs. 19.5 and 19.6). The nails of the enlarged digits are usually short, flat, and wide. The thumb and great toe are radially deviated in many patients [2, 3].

Cutaneous findings noted in these patients are a flat capillary hemangioma over the forehead, nape of neck, or back (in 36 out of 79 cases) and hirsutism of the trunk (Fig. 19.7) and limbs at all ages, and of the face in infants (in 46 out of 72 cases) [4]. Less frequently, the following skin findings are noted: eczema, warts, freckles, increased pigmentation of the abdomen and lumbar area, vitiligo, anal tags, keloids, hairy nevus of the cheek, recurrent paronychia, lymphedema of the legs, cavernous angio-

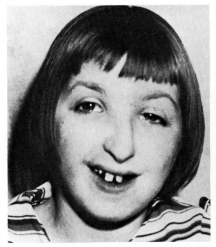
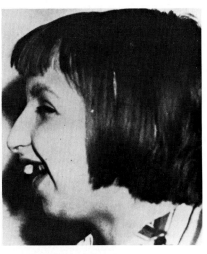

19.3   19.4

Figs. 19.3 and 19.4. Rubinstein-Taybi syndrome. Note typical facies with antimongoloid slant of the eyes, beaked nose, and micrognathia. (From Rubinstein, J.H.: In: The clinical delineation of birth defects. Bergsma, D. (ed.), Vol. V, No. 2, pt. II, pp. 25–41. Baltimore: Williams & Wilkins Co. 1969)

ma, café-au-lait spots, striae, stasis ulcer, and cutis verticis gyrata [4].

In relation to hair [5], there is a medial eyebrow flare in 60% of patients studied, anterior scalp upsweep in 45%, low anterior hairline in 20%, widow's peak in 15%, anterior scalp whorl in 15% (Fig. 19.8), and lateral frontal backsweep in 15%. Keratosis pilaris has also been reported [6].

The most important dermatoglyphic feature is a high frequency of pattern formations in the thenar and first interdigital areas. Double patterns may be present on the tips of the thumbs or the fifth fingers [7].

X-rays show enlargement of the phalangeal bones and skeletal anomalies like an enlarged foramen magnum, flat acetabular angles, flared ilia, and vertebral rib anomalies [2].

Pathology and Pathophysioloid. No consistent pathologic changes have been observed. Congenital heart disease and the absence of the corpus callosum were noted in several patients [2].

Inheritance. Polygenic [8] and monogenic autosomal recessive [3] patterns of inheritance have been suggested. The syndrome is probably heterogeneous [3].

Treatment. There is no available treatment.

References

1. Rubinstein, J.H., Taybi, H.: Broad thumbs and toes and facial abnormalities. A possible mental retardation syndrome. Amer. J. Dis. Child. *105*, 588–608 (1963)
2. Rubinstein, J.H.: The broad thumbs syndrome – progress report 1968. In: The clinical delineation of birth defects. Bergsma, D. (ed.), Vol. V, No. 2, pt. II, pp. 25–41. Baltimore: Williams & Wilkins Co. 1969
3. Der Kaloustian, V.M., Afifi, A.K., Sinno, A.A., Mire, J.: The Rubinstein-Taybi syndrome. A clinical and muscle electron microscopic study. Amer. J. Dis. Child. *124*, 897–902 (1972)
4. Rubinstein, J.H.: Personal communication (1976)
5. Smith, D.W., Gong, B.T.: Scalp-hair patterning: its origin and significance relative to early brain and upper facial development. Teratology *9*, 17–34 (1974)
6. Naveh, Y., Friedman, A.: A case of Rubinstein-Taybi syndrome. Clin. Pediat. (Philad.) *15*, 779–783 (1976)
7. Padfield, C.J., Partington, M.W., Simpson, N.E.: The Rubinstein-Taybi syndrome. Arch. Dis. Child. *43*, 94–101 (1968)
8. Roy, F.H., Summitt, R.L., Hiatt, R.L., Hughes, J.G.: Ocular manifestations of the Rubinstein-Taybi syndrome. Case report and review of the literature. Arch. Ophthal. *79*, 272–278 (1968)

Noonan Syndrome

In 1963 Noonan and Ehmke [1] reported nine patients of both sexes affected with valvular pulmonic stenosis, short stature, hypertelorism, ptosis, skeletal anomalies, and mental retardation. Although phenotypically these patients resemble individuals with the Turner syndrome, they have normal karyotypes (46,XY or 46,XX).

Clinical Presentation. The face is quite characteristic with hypertelorism, a downward palpebral slant,

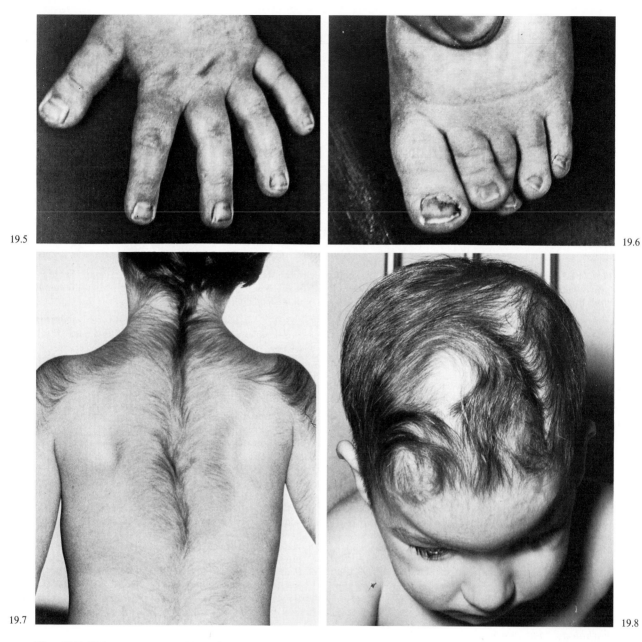

19.5

19.6

19.7

19.8

Figs. 19.5–19.8. Rubinstein-Taybi syndrome

Figs. 19.5 and 19.6. Broad thumb and large toe. (Courtesy of Dr. J.H. Rubinstein)

Fig. 19.7. Hirsutism. (Courtesy of Dr. F.C. Fraser)

Fig. 19.8. Peculiar hair whorls – see text. (Courtesy of Dr. J.H. Rubinstein)

blepharoptosis, epicanthic folds, and a small chin. A narrow palate and a cleft uvula are common findings [2].

Webbing of the neck is present in some patients, whereas others have a short, broad neck with excessive skin folds. Most patients have a pectus carinatum deformity of the upper sternum and excavatum of the lower sternum. Valvular pulmonic stenosis is common. Some patients have scoliosis, kyphosis, and vertebral anomalies [2].

Cryptorchidism is common in males, whereas some females have a delayed onset of menarche [2].

Clinodactyly and cubitus valgus are frequently found. Several patients are reported to have had congenital lymphedema of the hands and feet. The nails are short and poorly developed. The hair is often coarse.

Dermatoglyphic examination reveals a distally placed axial triradius, a high incidence of arches, and a low ridge count [3].

Although most patients are mentally retarded, the intelligence ranges from normal to severe mental retardation.

Pathology and Pathophysiology. The most common cardiac abnormality found at cardiac catheterization or surgery is valvular pulmonary stenosis [4].

Inheritance. Autosomal dominant [5].

Treatment. The treatment is symptomatic, aimed mainly at cardiac and respiratory problems.

References

1. Noonan, J.A., Ehmke, D.A.: Associated noncardiac malformations in children with congenital heart disease. J. Pediat. *63* (Abstr.), 468–470 (1963)
2. Abdel-Salam, E., Temtamy, S.A.: Familial Turner phenotype. J. Pediat. *74*, 67–72 (1969)
3. Nora, J.J., Sinha, A.K.: Direct familial transmission of the Turner phenotype. Amer. J. Dis. Child. *116*, 343–350 (1968)
4. Noonan, J.A.: Hypertelorism with Turner phenotype. A new syndrome with associated congenital heart disease. Amer. J. Dis. Child. *116*, 373–380 (1968)
5. Baird, P.A., De Jong, B.P.: Noonan's syndrome (XX and XY Turner phenotype) in three generations of a family. J. Pediat. *80*, 110–114 (1972)

Leprechaunism (Donohue Syndrome)

In 1948 Donohue [1] first described this condition. Since then, 15 similar cases have been reported [2]. The clinically descriptive term of "leprechaunism" is generally accepted.

Clinical Presentation. This syndrome is characterized by grotesque elfin facies, a flat nasal bridge, flaring nostrils, thick lips, hirsutism, large low-set ears, scanty subcutaneous tissue with loose and wrinkled skin (Figs. 19.9 and 19.10), hypoplastic nails, enlarged external genitalia, and psychomotor retardation. One child presented with camptodactyly of the third, fourth, and fifth fingers of both hands, short distal phalanges of the fifth fingers, and absent nails on the fifth fingers and toes [3]. All reported cases had a delayed bone age.

Pathology and Pathophysiology. The most consistently reported pathologic finding in autopsied female patients is the large and cystic ovaries. The pancreas was normal in three reported cases and showed hyperplasia of the islets of Langerhans in six. Excessive hepatic glycogen was found in four patients. In both newborn and older infants, the mammary tissue and the nipples were abnormally prominent. The autopsy findings in the adrenals, pituitary, and kidneys revealed inconsistent abnormalities in different reports.

The finding of an abnormally large metacentric chromosome in a male infant with leprechaunism [4] is considered coincidental and of no significance in the causation of the disease.

Considering the variety and inconsistency of the findings, leprechaunism is probably a heterogeneous condition.

Inheritance. Not definite. The involvement of several siblings and the consanguinity of the parents are suggestive of an autosomal recessive pattern of inheritance.

Treatment. Treatment is symptomatic. Most patients die in the first 6 months of life.

References

1. Donohue, W.L.: Clinicopathologic conference at the Hospital for Sick Children. Dysendocrinism. J. Pediat. *32*, 739–748 (1948)
2. Der Kaloustian, V.M., Kronfol, N.M., Takla, R., Habash, A., Khazin, A., Najjar, S.S.: Leprechaunism. Amer. J. Dis. Child. *122*, 442–445 (1971)
3. Summit, R.L., Favara, B.E.: Leprechaunism (Donohue's syndrome): a case report. J. Pediat. *74*, 601–610 (1969)
4. Ferguson-Smith, M.A., Hamilton, W., Ferguson, I.C., Ellis, P.M.: An abnormal metacentric chromosome in an infant with leprechaunism. Ann. Génét. (Paris) *11*, 195–200 (1968)

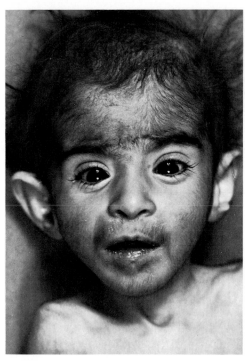 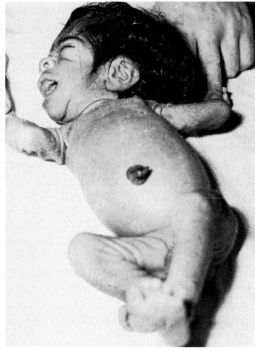

19.9

19.10

Figs. 19.9 and 19.10. Leprechaunism. Note elfin facies, hirsutism, large low-set ears, and scanty subcutaneous tissue with loose and wrinkled skin. (From Der Kaloustian, V.M., et al.: Amer. J. Dis. Child. *122*, 442–445, 1971)

Coffin-Lowry Syndrome

This syndrome was described in 1966 by Coffin et al. [1] and in 1971 by Lowry et al. [2]; these reports were thought to represent two entities. In 1975 Temtamy et al. [3] suggested that they represented one and the same entity which they called the Coffin-Lowry syndrome.

Clinical Presentation. The main features of the syndrome, which are more marked in males and progressive with age, involve the face, hands, nervous system, skeleton, orodental area, and skin [3]. The facial features display progressive coarsening, with thick lips and pouting lower lip. The hands are broad and thick, with distally tapered and hyperextensible fingers. The chest may reveal pectus excavatum or carinatum. Mental retardation is severe in all affected males and variable in affected females. There may be an internal communicating hydrocephalus with progressive motor deterioration. Partial cleft tongue, bilateral winging of the upper central incisors, and poor alignment of the upper anterior teeth may be present.

A frequent dermatoglyphic change is a transverse hypothenar crease. The *atd* angle is increased. Increased interdigital patterns, an increase of the

a–b ridge count, and a low total ridge count are also significant changes [3].

In males, the skin is loose and easily stretched. The veins may be dilated and readily seen, with capillary telangiectasia and extensive varicose veins of the legs. Cutis marmorata and discoloration of the hands and feet, when held dependent, are present in both sexes. The hair is straight and coarse in all affected males [3].

Other associated findings may be congenital heart disease, inguinal hernias, or prolapse of the uterus. Roentgenologic examinations reveal the following: hypertelorism, thickened facial bones, hyperostosis frontalis interna, kyphoscoliosis, narrowed intervertebral spaces, short distal phalanges with prominent tufting, retarded bone age, sternal abnormalities, narrow iliac wings, short wide femoral necks, coxa valga, and short great toe [3].

Pathology and Pathophysiology. By light microscopy, conjunctival and skin biopsy specimens demonstrate hypercellularity of the subepithelial connective tissue. Many of the cells are filled with small intracytoplasmic inclusions. By electron microscopy, the intracytoplasmic inclusions appear as single membrane-limited bodies (0.3–0.5 μ in diameter) with pleomorphic contents, predominantly fine fibrillogranular material, and intensely electron-dense bodies. These histopathologic changes suggest that this is a lysosomal storage disorder.

Inheritance. X-linked or sex-influenced autosomal dominant inheritance is suggested by severe expression in males and transmission through mildly affected females [3].

Treatment. No specific treatment is available.

References

1. Coffin, G.S., Siris, E., Wegienka, L.C.: Mental retardation with osteocartilaginous anomalies. Amer. J. Dis. Child. *112*, 205–213 (1966)
2. Lowry, B., Miller, J.R., Fraser, F.C.: A new dominant gene mental retardation syndrome. Association with small stature, tapering fingers, characteristic facies, and possible hydrocephalus. Amer. J. Dis. Child. *121*, 496–500 (1971)
3. Temtamy, S.A., Miller, J.D., Hussels-Maumenee, I.: The Coffin-Lowry syndrome: an inherited faciodigital mental retardation syndrome. J. Pediat. *86*, 724–731 (1975)

Familial Mediterranean Fever (Familial Paroxysmal Polyserositis)

Familial Mediterranean fever (FMF) or familial paroxysmal polyserositis (FPP) was first described as a separate syndrome in 1945 by Siegal [1].

Clinical Presentation. This is a familial disease manifested by recurrent episodes of fever accompanied by signs of peritonitis, pleuritis, and synovitis and sometimes complicated by amyloidosis. The symptoms usually appear in the first two decades and are of lifelong duration [2–5].

The attacks last not less than 24 h and usually not more than 72 h. The usual picture is that of abdominal pain with or without pleuritic and arthritic manifestations, diffuse in nature, with rigidity, direct and rebound tenderness, a mild paralytic ileus, and fever. Pleuritis or arthritis of the large joints may occur independently from the abdominal manifestations [2–5].

The laboratory picture during the attacks is characterized by nonspecific elevation of febrile reactants: erythrocyte sedimentation rate, white blood cell count, fibrinogen, and C-reactive protein.

Other rarer manifestations include hematuria during the attacks, pericarditis, lymphadenitis, and febrile attack with no serous inflammation.

Cutaneous manifestations include erythematous and purpuric skin rashes [5], an erysipelaslike erythema [6] during the attacks, urticaria [7], angio-neurotic edema [8], Henoch-Schönlein purpura [3], nonspecific purpura [9], subcutaneous nodules [3], and herpes simplex labialis [7].

The disease has been reported in almost all Middle Eastern ethnic groups, but especially Armenians and Jews. In addition, sporadic cases have been reported among the Dutch, Swedes, and others of non-Middle Eastern or non-Mediterranean extraction [4].

Pathology and Pathophysiology. The pathogenetic and pathophysiologic mechanisms are unknown. The incidence of amyloidosis varies: 26% [3] among Jewish patients to 8% [4] among Armenian patients.

Inheritance. The mode is not definitely established. Most reports favor the autosomal recessive pattern [3, 4]. Some suggest that it may be autosomal dominant [2, 10]. The disease may be genetically heterogeneous.

Treatment. The treatment should consist mainly of providing understanding and psychological support to the patient to prevent depressive episodes. Drugs known to suppress the attacks include clofibrate (Atromid S), hormones [cyclic therapy (in women)], and colchicine [5].

References

1. Siegal, S.: Benign paroxysmal peritonitis. Ann. intern. Med. *23*, 1–21 (1945)
2. Reimann, H.A., Moadié, J., Semerdjian, S., Sahyoun, P.F.: Periodic peritonitis – heredity and pathology. Report of seventy-two cases. J. Amer. med. Ass. *154*, 1254–1259 (1954)
3. Sohar, E., Gafni, J., Pras, M., Heller, H.: Familial Mediterranean fever. A survey of 470 cases and review of the literature. Amer. J. Med. *43*, 227–253 (1967)
4. Khachadurian, A.K., Armenian, H.K.: Familial paroxysmal polyserositis (familial Mediterranean fever) incidence of amyloidosis and mode of inheritance. In: The clinical delineation of birth defects. Vol. X, No. 4, pt. XVI, pp. 62–66. Baltimore: Williams & Wilkins Co. 1974
5. Armenian, H.K., Uthman, S.M.: Familial paroxysmal polyserositis (FPP). Leb. med. J. *28*, 439–442 (1975)
6. Azizi, E., Fisher, B.K.: Cutaneous manifestations of familial Mediterranean fever. Arch. Derm. *112*, 364–366 (1976)
7. Siegal, S.: Familial paroxysmal polyserositis. Analysis of fifty cases. Amer. J. Med. *36*, 893–918 (1964)
8. Reimann, H.A.: Periodic disease. Med. (Baltimore) *30*, 219–245 (1951)
9. Mamou, H., Maret, R.: Étude anatomo-clinique d'une épanalepsie méconnue chez un Arménien. Sem. Hôp. Paris *32*, 3197–3204 (1956)
10. Naffah, J.: Personal communication (1977)

Atopic Dermatitis

This is a common disorder that is adequately covered in textbooks of dermatology. Thus, only a very brief clinical discussion will be given here.

Clinical Presentation. The manifestations of atopic dermatitis are rather characteristic. In infants (2 months to 2 years), there is an exudative oozing dermatitis mainly over the face and neck. In children (3–10 years), the eruption is papular with lichenified plaques especially over the extremities. As the patients grow older (12 years and on), the involved sites are usually the flexural areas of the arms and legs, as well as the neck. The eruption is in the form of thick lichenified plaques. In general, the skin is dry, and itching is a prominent sign. Patients with atopic dermatitis have a number of associated stigmas: ocular (cataract, keratoconus); vascular (white dermographism, delayed blanch to acetylcholine, etc.); and others (flat oral glucose tolerance, hypotension). Patients with atopic dermatitis have increased susceptibility to herpes simplex and vaccinia viruses.

Pathology and Pathophysiology. Atopic dermatitis is closely associated with atopy. Atopy signifies an increased liability to form IgE antibodies and an increased susceptibility to bronchial asthma, hay fever, and atopic dermatitis. It is not clear as yet whether atopic dermatitis is due to an immunologic mechanism or whether the latter plays only a minor role. Even though the serum level of IgE is elevated in patients with atopic dermatitis, there is no correlation between IgE levels and severity of the disease [1]. Cell-mediated immunity is depressed in these patients [2, 3].
The histopathologic skin changes are not characteristic but are those of acute dermatitis in the infantile form and of chronic dermatitis in the childhood and adult forms.

Inheritance. The genetics of atopic dermatitis is not simple. It was thought [4] that each of the three forms of atopy is determined by homozygosity at a single and separate locus. However, others [5] suggest a more general increased risk of allergic manifestations.
Dominant inheritance has also been proposed [6]. Demonstration of immune response genes [7] supports the heritability of atopy and its autosomal dominant inheritance.

Treatment. The main aims in the treatment of atopic dermatitis are to eliminate aggravating factors, decrease pruritus, and control the inflammation. The proper use of topical steroids and lubrication of the skin are effective in controlling the dermatitis provided that the patient's emotional and physical environment are kept as near optimum as possible.

There are several syndromes and diseases in which atopic dermatitis is a feature. These have been discussed in their respective places (see also Appendix, p. 319). One other syndrome, Dubowitz syndrome, has not been mentioned. In this syndrome [8] there is an atopic dermatitislike eruption on the face and flexural areas of the extremities, sparsity of hair especially over the lateral parts of the eyebrows, peculiar facies (small facies, shallow supraorbital ridge, short palpebral fissures, variable ptosis, blepharophimosis, and micrognathia), mild microcephaly, prenatal growth deficiency, mental deficiency, lag in eruption of teeth, and other variable features. The inheritance follows the autosomal recessive pattern.

References

1. Stone, S.P., Gleich, G.J., Muller, S.A.: Atopic dermatitis and IgE: relationship between changes in IgE levels and severity of disease. Arch. Derm. *112*, 1254–1255 (1976)
2. McGeady, S.J., Buckley, R.H.: Depression of cell-mediated immunity in atopic eczema. J. Allergy clin. Immunol. *56*, 393–406 (1975)
3. Rogge, J.L., Hanifin, J.M.: Immunodeficiencies in severe atopic dermatitis: depressed chemotaxis and lymphocyte transformation. Arch. Derm. *112*, 1391–1396 (1976)
4. Tips, R.L.: A study of the inheritance of atopic hypersensitivity in man. Amer. J. hum. Genet. *6*, 328–343 (1954)
5. Lubs, M.-L.E.: Empiric risks for genetic counseling in families with allergy. J. Pediat. *80*, 26–31 (1972)
6. Schwartz, M.: Heredity in bronchial asthma. Copenhagen: Munksgaard 1952
7. McDevitt, H.O., Bodmer, W.F.: HL-A, immune-response genes, and disease. Lancet *19741*, 1269–1275
8. Dubowitz, V.: Familial low birth weight with an unusual facies and a skin eruption. J. med. Genet. *2*, 12–17 (1965)

Appendix

Differential Diagnoses of Disorders Based on Dermatologic Signs

Glossary

Acantholysis: Dissolution of the intercellular cement or bridges leading to loss of cohesion between epithelial (or epidermal) cells. This process results in the formation of vesicles and lacunae within the epidermis as in keratosis follicularis and benign familial chronic pemphigus.

Acanthosis: Increase in the thickness of the basal, squamous, and granular cell layers of the epidermis.

Alcian blue stain: A histochemical stain used to demonstrate the presence of acid mucopolysaccharides.

Alleles: Alternative forms of genes which occur at the same locus.

Anisocoria: Unequal pupils.

Anomalad: A condition formed of a malformation together with different structural changes that are secondary to it.

Bulla: A fluid-filled cavity within or beneath the epidermis. The fluid may be serum, plasma, or blood. Often inflammatory cells are also present. If smaller than 5 mm it is called "vesicle"; if narrow and slitlike (as in keratosis follicularis) it is called "lacuna."

Camptodactyly: Permanent flexion of finger(s).

Clinodactyly: Permanent deviation or deflection (medial or lateral) of finger(s).

Corps ronds: A peculiar type of dyskeratosis (see dyskeratosis).

Dopa (dihydroxyphenylalanine) reaction: A histochemical reaction to demonstrate the presence of tyrosinase by the oxidation of dopa to dopa-melanin.

Dyskeratosis: Abnormal keratinization of individual keratinocytes. In keratosis follicularis and benign familial chronic pemphigus, the dyskeratosis is in the form of *corps ronds*: a central, homogeneous basophilic mass surrounded by a clear halo.

Dystopia canthorum: Faulty position of canthi.

Ectrodactyly: Congenital absence of digit(s).

Endoreduplication: Multiplication of chromosomes without cell division. Thus, the cell ends up by having a multiple of the normal number of chromosomes.

Founder effect: With isolation and inbreeding of certain populations, any variants present in the original group remain in the growing population in a high proportion. The Ellis-van Creveld syndrome, Mal de Meleda, and cartilage-hair hypoplasia are examples

Granular cell layer: The outermost layer of the viable part of the epidermis. The cells are flattened and contain keratohyaline granules that are deeply basophilic.

Hemizygote: The state of the male with regard to the X chromosome.

Hypertelorism, ocular: Abnormal wide spacing of the eyes.

Karyorrhexis: Fragmentation of nuclei resulting in nuclear dust.

Lacuna: A narrow slitlike bulla (as in keratosis follicularis and Hailey-Hailey disease).

Langerhans cells: Dendritic cells in the upper stratum Malpighii. In routine stains, these appear as clear cells.

Lysosomes: Membrane-bound intracytoplasmic structures containing hydrolytic enzymes that can digest endogenous or exogenous material.

Ophiasis: Baldness in winding streaks.

Papillae, dermal: Dermal protrusions into the epidermis surrounded by rete ridges.

Papillary bodies: See papillae.

Papillomatosis: Irregularly undulated epidermis due to proliferation of dermal papillae.

Parakeratosis: Incomplete or faulty keratinization characterized by retention of nuclei in the stratum corneum (horny layer).

Periodic acid-Schiff (PAS) stain or Schiff reaction: A histochemical stain to demonstrate the presence of polysaccharides, especially glycogen and neutral mucopolysaccharides.

Phagosome: Detached surface membrane engulfing intracellular material to be digested. The fusion of lysosome with phagosome (phagolysosome) allows the hydrolytic enzymes of the lysosome to digest the contents of the phagosome.

Phrynoderma (toad skin): Papular dry skin with follicular hyperkeratosis, due to vitamin A deficiency.

Prickle cell layer: The major part of the viable epidermis. It is 5–10 layers thick and the cells are polygonal and flatten toward the surface. Intercellular bridges are demonstrable by light microscopy in this layer.

Pyknosis: Nucleus shrinks in size and the chromatin condenses. A sign of degeneration of a cell.

Rete pegs: See rete ridges.

Rete ridges: Pits on the under surface of the epidermis that surround the dermal papillas.

Squamous cell layer: See prickle cell layer.

Stratum Malpighii: The nucleated or viable part of the epidermis comprising the basal, prickle, and granular cell layers.

Syndactyly: Two or more digits grown together or adherent.

Synophrys: Eyebrows joining together at midline.

Ultraviolet light (UV): Radiation in the electromagnetic spectrum with wavelengths ranging from 100–400 nm. Conventionally, UV is divided into
UVA: long wave, black light 320–400 nm
UVB: middle wave, sunburn 290–320 nm
UVC: short wave 100–290 nm

Vesicle: A fluid-filled cavity within or beneath the epidermis, up to 5 mm in diameter.

Wood's light: Ultraviolet light through Wood's filter (black light) with wavelength peak around 360 nm.

Subject Index

Boldface type indicates the principal discussion of each subject. *Italic* type indicates illustrative material.

F. Vogel, A. G. Motulsky

Human Genetics

Problems and Approaches

1979. 451 figures., 213 tables. Approx. 800 pages
ISBN 3-540-09459-8

Biologic, medical and behavioral aspects of the principles of human genetics are treated comprehensively in this book. Various developments are discussed in a historical and social context. An overview of the different fields comprising human genetics is offered.

Unsolved problems and concepts, feasible solutions, and the influences of human genetics on medicine and society are discussed in detail. Research approaches and methodology are presented critically. A comprehensive bibliography enhances the value of this standard work on human genetics.

The book is intended for those students of medicine, biology, psychology, anthropology, and biostatistics who want a critical assessment of the principles of modern human genetics, for university instructors in biology and genetics, for researchers in human and medical genetics, and for phsyicians who are interested in the many ways in which human genetics influences all areas of medicine.

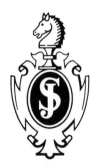

Springer-Verlag
Berlin
Heidelberg
New York

Physical Modalities in Dermatologic Therapy

Radiotherapy – Electrosurgery – Phototherapy – Cryosurgery
Editor: H. Goldschmidt
1978. 317 figures, 16 in color, 62 tables.
XV, 290 pages
ISBN 3-540-90267-8

Effects of Ionizing Radiation on DNA

Physical, Chemical and Biological Aspects
Editors: A. J. Bertinchamps, J. Hüttermann,
W. Köhnlein, R. Téoule
With contributions by numerous experts
1978. 74 figures, 48 tables. XXII, 383 pages
(Molecular Biology, Biochemistry and Biophysics,
Vol. 27)
ISBN 3-540-08542-4

Tumors of the Male Genital Systems

(7th International Symposium of the Gesellschaft
zur Bekämpfung der Krebskrankheiten Nord-
rhein-Westfalen e.V., Düsseldorf, October
24/25, 1975)
Editors: E. Grundmann, W. Vahlensieck
1977. 123 figures, 63 tables. XII, 268 pages
(Recent Results in Cancer Research, Vol. 60)
ISBN 3-540-08029-5

B. Schaumann, M. Alter
Dermatoglyphics in Medical Disorders

1976. 74 figures, 51 tables. XI, 258 pages
ISBN 3-540-07555-0

R. G. Freemann, J. M. Knox
Treatment of Skin Cancer

1967. 32 figures. VIII, 50 pages
(Recent Results in Cancer Research, Vol. 11)
ISBN 3-540-03959-7

J. Petres, M. Hundeiker
Dermatosurgery

With a foreword by K. W. Kalkoff
Translation from the German
1978. 112 figures. XVII, 152 pages
ISBN 3-540-90296-1

G. Plewig, A. M. Kligman
Acne

Morphogenesis and Treatment
1975. 110 plates, mostly in color. XII, 333 pages
ISBN 3-540-07212-8

Methods in Human Cytogenetics

Editors: H. G. Schwarzacher, U. Wolf
Coeditor of the English Version: E. Passarge
With contributions by numerous experts
1974. 59 figures. XV, 295 pages
ISBN 3-540-06610-1

R. Rieger, A. Michaelis, M. M. Green
Glossary of Genetics and Cytogenetics

Classical and Molecular
4th completely revised edition. 1976. 100 figures,
8 tables. 647 pages
ISBN 3-540-07668-9
Distribution rights for India, Sri Lanka, Pakistan,
Bangladesh and Nepal:
Narosa Publishing House, New Delhi
Distribution rights for the socialist countries:
VEB Georg Fischer Verlag, Jena

W. Fuhrmann, F. Vogel
Genetic Counseling

A Guide for the Practicing Physician. Translation
from the German by S. Kurth
2nd edition
1976. 34 figures, 20 tables. XIII, 138 pages
(Heidelberg Science Library, Vol. 10)
ISBN 3-540-90151-5

H. G. Schwarzacher
Chromosomes

in Mitosis and Interphase
1976. 116 figures, 3 tables. VIII, 182 pages
(Handbuch der mikroskopischen Anatomie des
Menschen, Band 1, Teil 3)
ISBN 3-540-07456-2

Prices are subject to change without notice

Springer-Verlag
Berlin Heidelberg New York